Eating Disorders

Core interventions in the treatment and management of anorexia nervosa, bulimia nervosa, and related eating disorders

National Clinical Practice Guideline Number CG9

developed by

National Collaborating Centre for Mental Health

commissioned by the

National Institute for Clinical Excellence

published by

The British Psychological Society and Gaskell

British Library Cataloguing-in-Publication Data

A catalogue record for this book is available from the British Library.

ISBN 1 85433 398 4

Distributed in North America by Balogh International Inc.

Printed in Great Britain by Stanley L. Hunt (Printers) Ltd, Rushden, Northamptonshire.

developed by   National Collaborating Centre for Mental Health
Royal College of Psychiatrists' Research Unit
6th Floor
83 Victoria Street
London
SW1H 0HW

commissioned by   National Insitute for Clinical Excellence
11 Strand
London
WC2N 5HR
www.nice.org.uk

published by   The British Psychological Society
St Andrews House
48 Princess Road East
Leicester
LE1 7DR
www.bps.org.uk

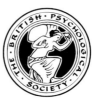

and

The Royal College of Psychiatrists
17 Belgrave Square
London
SW1X 8PG
www.rcpych.ac.uk

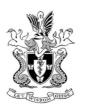

Contents

Eating Disorders Guideline Development Group Members

Professor Simon Gowers (Guideline Development Chair)

Professor of Adolescent Psychiatry, University of Liverpool.
Cheshire and Merseyside Eating Disorders Service for Adolescents.
Cheshire and Wirral Partnership Trust.

Mr Stephen Pilling (Guideline Facilitator)

Co-Director, National Collaborating Centre for Mental Health, University College London.
Camden and Islington Mental Health and Social Care Trust.

Professor Janet Treasure (Lead, Topic Group on Physical Management)

Professor of Psychiatry, Eating Disorders Unit, Guys' King's and St. Thomas School of Medicine, Kings College London, South London and Maudsley NHS Trust.

Professor Christopher Fairburn (Lead, Topic Group on Psychological Interventions)

Wellcome Principal Research Fellow and Professor of Psychiatry,
Department of Psychiatry, Oxford University.

Dr Bob Palmer (Lead, Topic Group on Service-level Interventions)

Senior Lecturer in Psychiatry, University of Leicester.

Dr Lorraine Bell

Consultant Clinical Psychologist, Eating Disorders Team,
Portsmouth Health Care NHS Trust.

Ms Nicky Bryant

Chief Executive, Eating Disorders Association (March 2002–2003).

Dr Rachel Bryant-Waugh

Consultant Clinical Psychologist, West Hampshire NHS Trust, Honorary Senior Lecturer, University of Southampton.

Mr Peter Honig

Family Therapist, Phoenix Centre Eating Disorders Service,
Cambridgeshire and Peterborough Mental Health Partnership NHS Trust

Dr Pippa Hugo

Child and Adolescent Psychiatrist, St. George's Eating Disorder Service,
South West London and St. George's Mental Health NHS Trust.

Dr Robert Mayer

General Practitioner, Highgate Group Practice, London.

Mr Ciaran Newell

Consultant Nurse, Eating Disorder Service, Dorset Healthcare NHS Trust.

Ms Jane Nodder

Patient representative, London.

Dr Deborah Waller

General Practitioner, 19 Beaumont Street, Oxford.

Ms Susan Ringwood

Chief Executive, Eating Disorders Association (December 2002–January 2004).

Dr Ulrike Schmidt

Senior Lecturer in Eating Disorders, Eating Disorders Unit, Institute of Psychiatry.

National Collaborating Centre for Mental Health staff

Dr Catherine Pettinari **Senior Project Manager**

Dr Craig Whittington **Senior Systematic Reviewer**

Dr Judit Simon **Health Economist**

Ms Heather Wilder **Information Scientist**

Ms Ellen Boddington **Research Assistant**

Mr Lawrence Howells **Research Assistant**

1 Introduction

This guideline has been developed to advise on the identification, treatment and management of the eating disorders anorexia nervosa, bulimia nervosa and related conditions. The guideline recommendations have been developed by a multidisciplinary group of health care professionals, patients and their representatives, and guideline methodologists after careful consideration of the best available evidence. It is intended that the guideline will be useful to clinicians and service commissioners in providing and planning high quality care for those with eating disorders while also emphasising the importance of the experience of care for patients and carers.

Eating disorders comprise a range of syndromes encompassing physical, psychological and social features. Whilst the acute physical complications of these disorders may provoke great concern in family members and health service staff, anorexia nervosa and bulimia nervosa are frequently chronic conditions with substantial long-term physical and social sequelae, from which recovery is difficult. Long-term disabilities include negative effects on employment, fertility, relationships and parenting. The impact of a person's eating disorder on home and family life is often considerable and family members may carry a heavy burden over a long period of time. Family members are often at a loss to know how to help and offer support to an affected relative.

About 1 in 250 females and 1 in 2000 males will experience anorexia nervosa, generally in adolescence or young adulthood. About five times that number will suffer from bulimia nervosa. Other atypical eating disorders are more common still, though many will not receive treatment. As eating disorders commonly develop during adolescence, they can blight physical and social development and many sufferers fail to reach their academic potential. Depressed mood is a common feature, partly because of these adverse consequences and also because of the distressing nature of the central symptoms of these disorders. The adverse physical consequences of dieting, weight loss and purging behaviours are notable and sometimes prove fatal. Indeed, anorexia nervosa has the highest mortality rate of any psychiatric disorder of adolescence.

The treatment experience of those with eating disorders is extremely variable. In part, this relates to the inherent ambivalence to treatment commonly experienced by those with these conditions. It is also due to the uneven provision of effective psychiatric treatments that range from high quality age-appropriate specialist eating disorder services, to basic generic provision in areas of the country where skills and experience are scarce. Sadly, a number of those with eating disorders will receive negative attitudes from inexperienced clinical staff and they may on occasion fear being trapped in treatment rather than helped by it.

This guideline addresses aspects of service provision, physical management and therapeutic approaches for those with eating disorders from the age of 8 upwards. Although the evidence base is rapidly expanding, there are a number of major gaps and future revisions of this guideline will incorporate new scientific evidence as it develops. The guideline makes a number of research recommendations specifically to address these gaps in the evidence base. In the meantime, we hope that the guideline will assist clinicians, patients and carers by identifying the merits of particular treatment approaches where the evidence from research and clinical experience exists.

1.1 National guidelines

1.1.1 What are clinical practice guidelines?

Clinical practice guidelines are 'systematically developed statements that assist clinicians and patients in making decisions about appropriate treatment for specific conditions' (NHS Executive, 1996). They are derived from the best available research evidence, using predetermined and systematic methods to identify and evaluate the evidence relating to the specific condition in question. Where evidence is lacking, the guidelines will incorporate statements and recommendations based upon the consensus statements developed by the guideline development group.

Clinical guidelines are intended to improve the process and outcomes of health care in a number of different ways. Clinical guidelines can:

- Provide up-to-date evidence-based recommendations for the management of conditions and disorders by health care professionals

- Be used as the basis to set standards to assess the practice of health care professionals

- Form the basis for education and training of health care professionals

- Assist patients and carers in making informed decisions about their treatment and care

- Improve communication between health care professionals, patients and carers

- Help identify priority areas for further research.

1.1.2 Uses and limitations of clinical guidelines

Guidelines are not a substitute for professional knowledge and clinical judgment. Guidelines can be limited in their usefulness and applicability by a number of different factors: the availability of high quality research evidence, the quality of the methodology used in the development of the guideline, the generalisability of research findings and the uniqueness of individual patients.

Although the quality of research in eating disorders is variable, the methodology used here reflects current international understanding on the appropriate practice for guideline development (AGREE: Appraisal of Guidelines for Research and Evaluation Instrument; www.agreecollaboration.org), ensuring the collection and selection of the best research evidence available, and the systematic generation of treatment recommendations applicable to the majority of patients and situations. However, there will always be some people and situations for which clinical guideline recommendations are not readily applicable. This guideline does not, therefore, override the individual responsibility of health care professionals to make appropriate decisions in the circumstances of the individual patient, in consultation with the patient and/or carer.

In addition to the clinical evidence, cost-effectiveness information, where available, is taken into account in the generation of statements and recommendations of the clinical guidelines. While national guidelines are concerned with clinical and cost-effectiveness, issues of affordability and implementation costs are to be determined by the NHS.

In using guidelines, it is important to remember that the absence of empirical evidence for the effectiveness of a particular intervention is not the same as evidence for ineffectiveness. In addition, of particular relevance in mental health, evidence-based treatments are often delivered within the context of an overall treatment programme including a range of activities, the purpose of which may be to help engage the patient, and provide an appropriate context for the delivery of specific interventions. It is important to maintain and enhance the service context in which these interventions are delivered; otherwise the specific benefits of effective interventions will be lost. Indeed, the importance of organising care, so as to support and encourage a good therapeutic relationship, is at times as important as the specific treatments offered.

1.1.3 Why develop national guidelines?

The National Institute for Clinical Excellence (NICE) was established as a Special Health Authority for England and Wales in 1999, with a remit to provide a single source of authoritative and reliable guidance for patients, professionals and the public. NICE guidance aims to improve standards of care, to diminish unacceptable variations in the provision and quality of care across the NHS and to ensure that the health service is patient centred. All guidance is developed in a transparent and collaborative manner using the best available evidence and involving all relevant stakeholders.

NICE generates guidance in a number of different ways, two of which are relevant here. First, national guidance is produced by the Technology Appraisal Committee to give robust advice about a particular treatment, intervention, procedure or other health technology. Second, NICE commissions the production of national clinical practice guidelines focused upon the overall treatment and management of a specific condition. To enable this latter development, NICE has established seven National Collaborating Centres in conjunction with a range of professional organisations involved in health care.

1.1.4 The National Collaborating Centre for Mental Health

This guideline has been commissioned by NICE and developed within the National Collaborating Centre for Mental Health (NCCMH). The NCCMH is a collaboration of the professional organisations involved in the field of mental health, national patient and carer organisations, a number of academic institutions and NICE. The NCCMH is funded by NICE and is led by a partnership between the Royal College of Psychiatrists' research unit (College Research Unit – CRU) and the British Psychological Society's equivalent unit (Centre for Outcomes Research and Effectiveness – CORE). Members of the NCCMH reference group come from the following organisations:

- Royal College of Psychiatrists (RCPsych)

- British Psychological Society (BPS)

- Royal College of Nursing (RCN)

- Social Care Institute of Excellence (SCIE)

- College of Occupational Therapists (COT), now replaced by the Clinical Effectiveness Forum for the Allied Health Professions (CEFAHP)

- Royal College of General Practitioners (RCGP)

- Royal Pharmaceutical Society (RPS)

- Rethink Severe Mental Illness

- Manic Depression Fellowship (MDF)

- MIND

- Centre for Evidence Based Mental Health (CEBMH)

- Centre for the Economics of Mental Health (CEMH)

- Institute of Psychiatry (IoP).

The NCCMH reference group provide advice on a full range of issues relating to the development of guidelines, including the membership of experts, professionals, patients and carers within guideline development groups.

1.1.5 From national guidelines to local protocols

Once a national guideline has been published and disseminated, local health care groups will be expected to produce a plan and identify resources for implementation, along with appropriate timetables. Subsequently, a multidisciplinary group involving commissioners of health care, primary care and specialist mental health care professionals, patients and carers should undertake the translation of the implementation plan into local protocols taking into account both the recommendations set out in this guideline and the priorities set in the National Service Framework for Mental Health and related documentation. The nature and pace of the local plan will reflect local health care needs and the nature of existing services; full implementation may take a considerable time, especially where substantial training needs are identified.

1.1.6 Auditing the implementation of guidelines

This guideline identifies key areas of clinical practice and service delivery for local and national audit. Although the generation of audit standards is an important and necessary step in the implementation of this guidance, a more broadly-based implementation strategy will be developed. Nevertheless, it should be noted that the Commission for Healthcare Audit and Inspection (CHAI) will monitor the extent to which these guidelines have been implemented by NHS Trusts and Local Health Boards and specialist secondary care trusts responsible for mental health and social care.

1.2 The national eating disorders guideline

1.2.1 Who has developed this guideline?

The Guideline Development Group (GDG) was convened by the NCCMH based upon advice from the Centre's reference group representatives, and supported by funding from NICE. The GDG included members from the following professional groups: psychiatry, clinical psychology, nursing, family therapy, social work and general practice. In addition, the GDG included a patient[1] and a representative of the Eating Disorders Association.

Staff from the NCCMH provided leadership and support throughout the process of guideline development, undertaking systematic searches, information retrieval, appraisal and systematic review of the evidence. Members of the GDG received training in the process of guideline development from the Centre for Evidence-Based Mental Health (CEBMH), and support from the NICE Patient Involvement Unit. The NICE Guidelines Technical Advisor provided advice and assistance regarding aspects of the guideline development process.

All GDG members made formal declarations of interest at the outset, which were updated at every GDG meeting. The GDG met a total of 23 times throughout the process of guideline development. The GDG formed sub-groups, or 'Topic Groups' for ease of evidence identification and analysis and to address identifiable treatment approaches. Each Topic Group was led by a national expert in the relevant topic and the groups supported by the NCCMH technical team, with additional expert advice from special advisors where necessary. Topic Groups oversaw the production and synthesis of research evidence before presentation to the wider GDG. All statements and recommendations in this guideline have been generated and agreed by the whole GDG.

1.2.2 For whom is this guideline intended?

This guideline will be of relevance to all people with a diagnosis of anorexia nervosa, bulimia nervosa or related eating disorders aged eight years of age and over. The guideline will not explicitly provide guidance on the diagnosis or treatment of people with eating disorders if there is a separate physical or other primary mental disorder of which a disorder of eating is a symptom. This may be dealt with in a future guideline.

---

1 The term 'patient' was the preferred term for use in the guideline based on a survey of Eating Disorders Association members.

The guideline will review the issue of diagnosis and assessment, as many people suffer with eating disorders that fall outside established diagnostic criteria.

In sum, this guideline is intended for use by:

●   Individuals with a diagnosis of anorexia nervosa, bulimia nervosa or related conditions aged eight years and over and their families/carers.

●   Professional groups who share in the treatment and care for people with a diagnosis of an eating disorder, including psychiatrists, clinical psychologists, mental health nurses, community psychiatric nurses, social workers, practice nurses, dietitians, secondary care medical, dental, nursing and paramedical staff, occupational therapists, pharmacists, paediatricians, other physicians, general medical and dental practitioners, physiotherapists and family/other therapists.

●   Professionals in other health and non-health sectors who may have direct contact with or are involved in the provision of health and other public services for those diagnosed with eating disorders. These may prison doctors, the police and professionals who work in the criminal justice and education sectors.

●   Those with responsibility for planning services for people with a diagnosis of an eating disorder and their carers, including directors of public health, NHS trust managers and managers in PCTs.

The 'Information for the Public' version of this guideline, published by NICE, is a good starting point in providing patients with written information about the sort of care they can expect.

1.2.3 Specific aims of this guideline

The guideline makes recommendations for the identification, treatment and management of eating disorders. Specifically, it aims to:

●   Evaluate the role of specific psychological interventions in the treatment and management of eating disorders.

●   Evaluate the physical management and role of specific pharmacological agents in the treatment of eating disorders.

●   Evaluate the role of specific service delivery systems and service-level interventions in the management of eating disorders.

●   Integrate the above to provide best practice advice on the care of individuals with a diagnosis of an eating disorder throughout the course of the disorder.

●   Promote the implementation of best clinical practice through the development of recommendations tailored to the requirements of the NHS in England and Wales.

2 Eating disorders

This guideline is concerned with the identification, treatment and management of anorexia nervosa and bulimia nervosa as defined in the 10th edition of the *International Classification of Diseases* (ICD 10) (WHO, 1992). The guideline does not address the management of loss of appetite, psychogenic disturbance of appetite or other conditions that involve significant weight loss but which are due to known physical illness. The guideline is also concerned with other related disorders that do not fulfil diagnostic criteria for anorexia nervosa or bulimia nervosa. These are generally called 'atypical eating disorders' (Fairburn & Harrison, 2003) or 'eating disorder not otherwise specified' (EDNOS) (APA, 1994). The American Psychiatric Association's *Diagnostic and Statistical Manual 4th Revision* (DSM-IV; APA, 1994) further describes the diagnostic category 'binge eating disorder' as a research diagnosis within EDNOS. (See Appendix 17 for further details on these diagnostic systems.)

2.1 Anorexia nervosa

2.1.1 Symptoms, presentation and patterns of illness

Anorexia nervosa is a syndrome in which the individual maintains a low weight as *a result of a pre-occupation with body weight*, construed either as a fear of fatness or pursuit of thinness. In anorexia nervosa, weight is maintained at least 15 per cent below that expected, or in adults body mass index (BMI) – calculated as weight in kilograms divided by height in metres squared – is below 17.5 kg/m^2. In younger people, the diagnosis may be made in those who fail to gain weight during the expected growth spurt of puberty, as they can become underweight without weight loss.

Weight loss in anorexia nervosa is induced by avoiding 'fattening foods', sometimes supported by excessive exercising or self-induced purging (by vomiting or misuse of laxatives). As a consequence of poor nutrition, a widespread endocrine disorder involving the hypothalamic-pituitary-gonadal axis develops, manifest in women by amenorrhoea and in men by a lack of sexual interest or potency. In prepubertal children, puberty is delayed and growth and physical development are usually stunted.

The subjective experience of anorexia nervosa is often at odds with the assessment of others. The conviction that weight control is desirable is usually strongly held, particularly when challenged and others are seen as mistaken in believing the person should gain weight, particularly where there is a marked disturbance of body image. Weight loss is experienced as a positive achievement and, therefore, may be strongly reinforcing to someone with low confidence and poor self-esteem. As a result, they will often deny the seriousness of the condition. The essential role of 'weight phobia' is increasingly being questioned however, and is believed by some to be culture specific.

The condition generally starts with dieting behaviour that may evoke no concern. Indeed, some will experience reinforcing compliments. After a while, however, the commitment to dieting increases, often with a number of secondary features such as social withdrawal, rigidity and obsessionality, particularly where these traits have previously been features of the person's personality. A number of secondary difficulties may develop including physical adverse effects, social isolation, compromise of educational and employment plans and occupation in the areas of leisure, self-care, daily living and productivity of employment and/or education. A smaller number will enter anorexia nervosa through a pattern of purging behaviour without dieting, following a viral illness, which resulted in weight loss that then became positively valued, or in the context of a chronic illness such as diabetes or Crohn's disease.

Typically individuals are persuaded to seek help by concerned family members, teaching staff or general practitioners with whom they consult about physical consequences. Sometimes, however, the person begins to appreciate the damaging effects of the disorder and may seek help in their own right. Children and adolescents are almost always brought to treatment, very rarely actively seeking help initially and can present more complex diagnostic challenges (Bryant-Waugh *et al.*, 1992).

2.1.2 Diagnosis

The diagnosis of anorexia nervosa in its typical form is a relatively straightforward one in older adolescents and adults. The diagnosis has good validity and reliability, the main obstacle to diagnosis being the person's own willingness or otherwise to disclose his or her motives, symptoms and behaviours. Thus, engagement in a supportive, empathic assessment interview is crucial in enabling the person to reveal fears around weight, dieting behaviour and any purging or other maladaptive behaviour such as excessive exercising. In the absence of this engagement, the individual may fail to reveal weight-controlling behaviours and collude with the doctor in pursuing physical investigations to explain the weight loss. In women, the presence of secondary amenorrhoea (i.e. cessation of menstruation after it has been established) or other physical features of starvation should always alert the physician to the possibility of this diagnosis. Diagnosis may be more problematic in children and younger adolescents, as the existing diagnostic criteria are insufficiently developmentally sensitive (Lask & Bryant-Waugh, 2000).

The diagnosis is made on the basis of the history, supported where possible by a corroborative account from a relative or friend. Physical examination, with measurement of weight and height and calculation of body mass index (BMI), can reveal the extent of emaciation. On occasion, clinical observation during a hospital assessment can enable characteristic behaviours to be observed. Physical investigations are less useful in making the diagnosis but are crucial in assessing the physical impact of the disorder and its complications. Depending on the results of the physical examination, these may include haematological tests, electrocardiography, radiological assessment and ultrasound (Royal College of Psychiatrists, 2002).

A diagnostic challenge occurs in those with comorbid physical disorders, such as diabetes, chronic bowel or thyroid disorder. In diabetes, the patient may be tempted to restrict insulin intake in order to lose calories, whilst on occasions the symptoms of organic intestinal disorder may mask the psychological condition.

The weight loss that occurs with the anorexia of depression can usually be distinguished from that resulting from the dietary control of anorexia nervosa, but the condition can sometimes be difficult to distinguish from post-viral and other chronic fatigue syndromes where food intake is poor. Weight loss and limited food intake secondary to a brain tumour are also known to have been mistaken for anorexia nervosa.

2.1.3 Physical and social consequences

Although in the acute stages of anorexia nervosa subjective distress may be limited, emotional disturbance is common, chiefly comprising anxiety and mood symptoms. With time, emotional difficulties usually increase along with a range of physical and social difficulties, including becoming unable to care for oneself adequately, reducing or stopping leisure activities, interrupting educational goals and losing personal autonomy. These affect the person's quality of life and increase the reliance on and the importance of the eating disorder.

Depression is a common comorbid diagnosis, with rates of up to 63 per cent in some studies (Herzog *et al.*, 1992), while obsessive-compulsive disorder (OCD) has been found to be present in 35 per cent of patients with anorexia nervosa (Rastam, 1992).

Physical problems can be classified as those due to the effects of starvation and the consequences of purging behaviour. Starvation affects every system in the body. In the musculo-skeletal system, this will be evident as weakness, loss of muscle strength (which also affects heart muscle), loss of bone density and impairment of linear growth. Young women with anorexia nervosa are at increased risk of bone fractures later in life (Lucas *et al.*, 1999). The effects on the endocrine system have their impact on target organs, causing infertility, a risk of polycystic ovaries and loss of bone mineralisation. Where pubertal development has not been completed, incomplete development of secondary sexual characteristics may occur (Goldbloom & Kennedy, 1995) and permanent stunting of growth is common. Patients with anorexia nervosa have disorders in the reproductive hormones (low LH and FSH), suppressed TSH, growth hormone resistance and raised corticol levels. The effects of purging are described in Section 7.5.2, including long-term disabilities such as erosion of tooth enamel sometimes amounting to destruction of the whole dentition. Worn painful teeth can be a considerable concern to the patient in terms of comfort, appearance and, therefore, self-esteem.

Brain volume is reduced in anorexia nervosa (Dolan, Mitchell & Wakeling, 1988; Kohn *et al.*, 1997; Kingston, Szmukler, Andrewes, Tress & Desmond, 1996; Krieg, Pirke, Lauer & Backmund, 1988; Swayze *et al.*, 1996). There are two small longitudinal studies, which have examined the structural changes in the brain of adolescents after full weight gain (Golden *et al.*, 1996; Katzman *et al.*, 1996). Both found persistent deficits in grey matter (cell bodies of neurons and glial cells) although there was recovery of white matter (mainly myelinated axons). This supports the finding of grey matter deficits in people who have made a full recovery from their eating disorder (Lambe, Katzman, Mikulis, Kennedy & Zipursky, 1997). One post-mortem study reported that there was a reduction in basal dendritic fields and dendritic spine density (Neumarker *et al.*, 1997).

Many of the cognitive deficits in anorexia nervosa are restored after weight recovery. However, some abnormalities in executive function remain after weight restoration. For example, people with eating disorders have scores greater than one standard deviation from the norms on tests of perceptual rigidity, perseveration and set shifting and the neurological sign dysdiadokinesis (Tchanturia, Morris, Surguladze & Treasure, 2002).

Although little is known of the effects short or long term of extreme weight loss on brain development and function in children, it is possible that such weight loss may have both short and long-term effects on cognitive functioning.

Social difficulties may result in continued dependence on family of origin into adult life and often include difficulties engaging in intimate relationships. Employment prospects may be adversely affected either because of the limitations of the disorder or the disruption caused by lengthy hospitalisations.

2.1.4 Course and prognosis

The course of anorexia nervosa is very variable. There is no good evidence on the prognosis for people with anorexia nervosa who do not access formal medical care (Treasure & Schmidt, 2002). A summary of 68 treatment studies published before 1989 with a length of follow-up of one to 33 years, found that 43 per cent of people recover completely, 36 per cent improve, 20 per cent develop a chronic eating disorder and five per cent die from anorexia nervosa (Steinhausen, 1995). The overall mortality in these long-term studies ranged from 0 21 per cent from a combination of physical complications and suicide. The all-cause standardised mortality ratio anorexia nervosa has been estimated at 9.6 (95 per cent Confidence Interval 7.8 to 11.5) Nielsen (2001), about three times higher than other psychiatric illnesses. The average annual risk of mortality has been calculated at 0.59 per cent per year in females averaged from 10 samples, with a minimum follow-up of six years (Neilsen et al., 1998). The mortality rate appears to be higher for people with lower weight during their illness and those presenting between 20 and 29 years of age.

A number of those with anorexia nervosa progresses to other eating disorders, particularly bulimia nervosa, but also binge eating disorder, highlighting the relationship between the disorders. Movement in the other direction is less common, but a number of those with anorexia nervosa gives a premorbid history of obesity in childhood or adolescence.

2.1.5 Anorexia nervosa in children and adolescents

Although the essential psychological features are similar, children and younger adolescents may present with delayed puberty or stunted growth as well as weight loss. Parents or teachers are generally the ones who raise concern and the young person may resist medical attention. Some young people will voice anxieties around unwanted aspects of development, particularly if they have experienced early puberty or feel unable to engage with their peers' increasing adolescent independence and social experimentation. In some, bullying or teasing about weight may have provoked this concern.

Although the principles of making the diagnosis are the same as in adults and are often straightforward, the greatest diagnostic difficulty occurs in the youngest cases. In children between the ages of around eight and 12, the condition is less common than in older individuals and should be distinguished from other types of eating disturbance seen in middle childhood, such as selective eating and food avoidance emotional disorder. By definition feeding disorder of infancy and childhood has onset below age six. In pubescent cases with primary amenorrhoea, it can sometimes be difficult to judge whether puberty has been delayed from the normal variation in timing of puberty.

Reference to height and weight centile charts is useful in evaluating weight in comparison to height. It is particularly helpful to compare presenting centiles for weight and height with historical values, as these may identify stunting of height (where the young person has crossed height centile lines). The result of such stunting is that the person may not appear unduly thin, though his or her weight may be considerably below the projected level as indicated by premorbid height and weight. It is also helpful to plot body mass index on BMI centile charts, as BMI norms are not stable over age. Average BMI increases with age during childhood and adolescence, a BMI of 17.5 kg/m^2 being close to the mean for a child at the age of 12 (Cole *et al.*, 1995).

In children and adolescents with atypical presentations of an eating disorder, consideration should be given to the possibility of separate underlying physical pathology. In these circumstances the involvement of a paediatrician should be considered.

The prognosis for children and adolescents with anorexia nervosa is variable. Some (particularly those with a rapid and early onset) will make a full recovery from a first episode. This is most likely where early physical and psychosocial development has been healthy and where there is an identified precipitating negative life event such as bereavement (North *et al.*, 1997). In such cases and where onset is pre-pubertal, physical consequences such as stunted growth and pubertal delay are usually fully reversible. Others with a more insidious onset, with earlier social difficulties or abnormal personality development, may go on to have a more chronic course into middle age (Gowers *et al.*, 1991).

2.2 Bulimia nervosa

2.2.1 Symptoms, presentation and pattern of illness

Bulimia nervosa is characterised by recurrent episodes of binge eating and secondly by compensatory behaviour (vomiting, purging, fasting or exercising or a combination of these) in order to prevent weight gain. Binge eating is accompanied by a subjective feeling of loss of control over eating. Self-induced vomiting and excessive exercise, as well as the misuse of laxatives, diuretics, thyroxine, amphetamine or other medication, may occur. As in anorexia nervosa, self-evaluation is unduly influenced by body shape and weight, and there may indeed have been an earlier episode of anorexia nervosa. The diagnosis of anorexia nervosa is given precedence over bulimia nervosa; hence in bulimia nervosa BMI is maintained above 17.5 kg/m^2 in adults and the equivalent in children and adolescents (see Section 2.1.5). There is some controversy concerning whether those who binge eat but do not purge should be included within this diagnostic category. The ICD10 criteria (WHO, 1992) stress the importance of purging behaviour on the grounds that vomiting and laxative misuse are considered pathological behaviours in our society in comparison to dieting and exercise. The DSM-IV criteria (APA, 1994) agree about the importance of compensatory behaviour but distinguish between the purging type of bulimia nervosa in which the person regularly engages in self-induced vomiting or the misuse of laxatives, diuretics or enemas, from the non-purging type in which other inappropriate compensatory behaviours such as fasting or excessive exercise occur but not vomiting or laxative misuse.

People with bulimia nervosa tend to not disclose their behaviour nor to seek out treatment readily although may be more likely to do so than those with anorexia nervosa. The condition appears to be subjectively less 'valued' than anorexia nervosa; indeed binge eating and purging are commonly associated with extreme subjective guilt and shame. These emotions are sometimes reinforced by the pejorative language used by relatives and others including some clinicians, who may refer to 'confessing' or 'admitting' to purging behaviour. A person's ambivalence towards treatment often arises from the fear that they will be stopped from vomiting and purging and then left to face the consequences of their binge eating, i.e. excessive weight gain.

The condition usually develops at a slightly older age than anorexia nervosa (the mean age of onset is 18 to 19, compared to 16 to 17 for anorexia nervosa). Bulimia nervosa sometimes arises from a pre-existing anorexic illness. Where this is not the case the development of the disturbance is often essentially similar to that of anorexia nervosa, arising from a background of attempts to restrain eating. In bulimia nervosa however, dietary restriction cannot be maintained and is broken by episodes of reactive binge eating, which result from a combination of physiological and psychological factors. Compensatory behaviours follow in order to counteract the effect of binge eating on weight. The person, therefore, maintains a weight, usually within the normal range despite overeating but commonly progresses into a vicious cycle of attempted dieting, binge eating and compensatory purging, frequently on a daily basis. As these behaviours dominate daily life, the person becomes preoccupied with thoughts of food and life may be re-organised around shopping, eating and purging behaviour. Initially, those with bulimia nervosa are generally secretive about their bulimic episodes, though some may leave obvious signs of their disorder such as empty food packaging and occasionally bags of vomit for other family members to discover.

Bulimic episodes are frequently planned, with food purchased or prepared in order to be consumed without interruption. The individual may also avoid situations in which they are likely to be exposed to food or will find it difficult to control their eating, such as when eating out with others. This avoidance behaviour tends to add to any social and relationship difficulties that may be present.

Mood disturbance is extremely common in bulimia nervosa and symptoms of anxiety and tension are frequently experienced. Self-denigratory thoughts may develop out of disgust at overeating or purging whilst low self-esteem and physical self-loathing may in some be rooted in the past experience of physical or sexual abuse. Self-harm, commonly by scratching or cutting, is common. A significant proportion of those with bulimia nervosa have a history of disturbed interpersonal relationships with poor impulse control. Some will abuse alcohol and drugs.

2.2.2 Diagnosis

As in anorexia nervosa, the diagnosis depends on obtaining a history supported, as appropriate, by the corroborative account of a parent or relative. This will require an empathic, supportive, non-judgemental interview style in which the person is enabled to reveal the extent of his or her symptoms and behaviours. Although those with bulimia nervosa generally have fewer serious physical complications than those with anorexia nervosa, they commonly report more physical complaints when first seen. They may complain of fatigue, lethargy, or feeling bloated, and they may suffer constipation, abdominal pain and on occasions swelling of the hands and feet or irregular menstruation. There may also be erosion of dental enamel in which the lingual surface of the upper teeth is mainly affected, and it has been argued that this is virtually pathognomonic of vomiting (Mitchell, 1995).

Physical examination is often normal, though the salivary glands (particularly the parotid glands) may be enlarged. Calluses on the back of the hand may be found; these result from the use of the hand to stimulate the gag reflex and induce vomiting. Oedema is common in those who have used laxatives or diuretics whilst these behaviours also lead to fluid loss and subsequent dehydration, which in turn may result in a metabolic alkalosis. This is generally accompanied by hypochloraemia and hypokalaemia. Overall, about 10 per cent of those with bulimia nervosa have electrolyte abnormalities detected on routine screening (Mitchell, 1995). Metabolic acidosis can also occur in patients who are abusing laxatives as a result of the loss of bicarbonate from the bowel. Less commonly hyponatraemia, hypocalcaemia, hypophosphataemia and hypomagnesaemia may develop.

In the gastrointestinal system, oesophagitis may occur. Gastric dilatation that poses the risk of gastric rupture and death occurs rarely but may be the most common cause of fatality (Mitchell, 1997). Constipation is extremely common, mainly due to dehydration; steatorrhoea and protein losing gastroenteropathy have also been reported secondary to laxative abuse. Severe use of laxatives has been reported to cause cardiomyopathy and other types of myopathic disorder as a result of storage of Ipecac in muscle tissue (Mitchell, 1995). Electrocardiography may indicate heart conduction abnormalities and possibly an increase in the risk of mitral valve prolapse.

Abnormal electroencephalographic (EEG) findings have been reported probably secondary to fluid and electrolyte abnormalities; there does not seem to be an association between bulimia nervosa and epilepsy.

Endocrine abnormalities are variable. These include abnormalities in the menstrual cycle and blunting of the thyroid stimulating hormone and growth hormone response to thyroid releasing hormone.

2.2.3 Impairment and disability

There is considerable overlap between the long-term disabling consequences of bulimia nervosa and those of anorexia nervosa. Mood and anxiety symptoms are very common. These symptoms, low self-esteem and body image disturbance can all have a negative effect on social relationships, which in turn may be damaged by a lifestyle that may be chaotic and characterised by impulsivity.

The adverse physical consequences of purging behaviour have been identified in Section 7.5.2. In addition, those with bulimia nervosa may be at risk from the effects of alternating weight loss and weight gain.

Lissner et al. (1991) in a series of 3130 participants found that both all-cause and coronary heart disease mortality were increased significantly in both men and women with high levels of weight variability. Morbidity from coronary heart disease was also increased.

Estimates of the prevalence of the diagnoses of personality disorder in people with bulimia nervosa have ranged from 21 per cent to 77 per cent. Obsessive-compulsive and avoidant personality disorders (Cluster C) have been described frequently (Braun *et al.*, 1994). The relationship of borderline personality disorder to bulimia nervosa has been a source of considerable debate (Wonderlich, 1995) with reported rates ranging from two per cent to 47 per cent, these rates apparently influenced by subject and measurement variability across studies, thus BPD probably occurs no more frequently than other PDs in bulimia nervosa.

2.2.4 Course and prognosis

There have been few studies with a lengthy follow-up period of the course and outcome of bulimia nervosa in the community. Many people with bulimia nervosa are not receiving any form of help (Hsu, 1995). Of these, the majority will suffer chronicity or a relapsing course, maintained by over-valued belief in the importance of appearance and thinness in particular (Fairburn *et al*, 2000). With the most effective treatments about 50 per cent of people with bulimia nervosa can be expected to be asymptomatic two to 10 years after assessment. Twenty per cent are likely to continue with the full form of bulimia nervosa whilst the remainder (30 per cent) have a course of illness characterised either by remissions or relapses or persistent but subdiagnostic bulimia (Hsu, 1995). One 10-year follow-up study of 50 people with bulimia nervosa found that 52 per cent had fully recovered and only nine per cent continued to experience symptoms of bulimia nervosa (Collings & King, 1994). A larger study of 222 followed-up for a mean of 11 years revealed that 11 per cent still met criteria for bulimia nervosa whereas 70 per cent were in full or partial remission (Keel *et al.*, 1999).

There are few consistent predictors of longer-term outcome, though a number of studies have shown strong associations between weight fluctuation (which commonly occurs in bulimia nervosa) and negative health outcomes. Patients with the uni-impulsive form of the illness without additional control difficulties are also thought to do better. The mortality rate associated with bulimia is uncertain but may be higher than in the matched general population (Hsu, 1995).

2.2.5 Bulimia nervosa in children and adolescents

The full syndrome of bulimia nervosa is rarely seen in young people under the age of 14 (Bryant-Waugh & Lask, 1995). Indeed in these authors' uniquely specialised clinic fewer than five per cent of children under the age of 14 presenting with eating disorders were diagnosed with bulimia nervosa. Where these presentations occurred the clinical features were the same as found in the older age group. Young people with this disorder were also, in common with adults with the same diagnosis, depressed and suffered poor self image (Bryant-Waugh & Lask, 1995). There is no substantial literature on treatment or outcome in this age group. Adolescents with bulimia nervosa may sometimes be considered to be suffering incipient personality disorder, though caution should be exercised in diagnosing personality disorder before development is completed. In these cases it can be difficult to judge whether the eating disorder is contributing to abnormal personality development or conversely, if the personality difficulties have acted as a risk factor for the development of bulimia nervosa.

Since bulimia nervosa is very rarely seen in children and uncommonly in younger adolescents, and there has been no research on the treatment of adolescents with bulimia nervosa, in line with much current clinical practice and taking into account the above issues, the GDG took the view that, subject to adaptation to their age, circumstances and level of development, adolescent patients with bulimia nervosa should receive the same type of treatment as adults with the disorder along with appropriate family involvement.

2.3 Atypical eating disorders (eating disorders not otherwise specified; EDNOS) including binge eating disorder

2.3.1 Symptoms, presentation and pattern of illness

A number of people suffer from eating disorders that closely resemble anorexia nervosa and bulimia nervosa, but which are considered atypical, as they do not meet the precise diagnostic criteria for these conditions (Fairburn & Harrison, 2003; Turner & Bryant-Waugh, 2003; Ricca et al., 2001). In Europe, these are often termed 'atypical eating disorders' (Fairburn & Harrison, 2003), the equivalent American term being 'eating disorders not otherwise specified' (American Psychiatric Association, 1994). For example, the patient's weight might be just above the diagnostic threshold for anorexia nervosa or she might still be menstruating. Binge eating and purging may occur less frequently than specified for a diagnosis of bulimia nervosa. Over concern with weight and shape is generally present in these disorders, although in some the primary focus is on maintaining strict control over eating. Although the diagnostic criteria may not be met, many atypical eating disorders are as severe and long lasting as anorexia nervosa and bulimia nervosa. Patients' treatment needs and prognosis may be virtually identical.

Binge eating disorder (BED) is a recently described condition, first defined as a research category in DSM-IV (APA, 1994), though there is some overlap with the ICD 10 category 'Overeating associated with other psychiatric disturbance' (F50.4) (WHO, 1992). In BED, individuals engage in uncontrollable episodes of binge eating but do not use compensatory purging behaviours. These binge eating episodes are associated with three or more of the following:

● Eating much more rapidly than normal

● Eating until feeling uncomfortably full

● Eating large amounts of food when not physically hungry

● Eating alone through embarrassment at the amount one is eating

● Feeling disgust or extreme guilt after overeating.

Marked distress regarding binge eating is present and social avoidance is common.

2.3.2 Diagnosis

Atypical eating disorders are conditions of clinical severity that do not conform to the diagnostic criteria for anorexia nervosa or bulimia nervosa. An example would be someone with extreme dietary restraint, who exercised excessively to control weight, which was maintained in the low normal range. This condition would also include those with the features of anorexia nervosa at low weight who are still menstruating. Many people with atypical eating disorders have suffered with anorexia nervosa or bulimia nervosa in the past.

In comparison with anorexia nervosa and bulimia nervosa, far less is known about binge eating disorder (Fairburn & Harrison, 2003). Apart from binge eating, its systematic profile overlaps little with the other eating disorders. Defining binge eating can be problematic and there may be a discrepancy between the subjective experience and clinical assessment of a binge. The onset of binge eating disorder is usually in the teenage years or early 20s, but people tend to present later, typically in their 30s or 40s, when they have become overweight or obese. The sex ratio is more even and binge eating generally occurs against a background of a tendency to overeat rather than of dietary restraint. Many people with binge eating disorder are obese. By definition self induced vomiting and laxative misuse are not present or only occasionally present. Depressive features and dissatisfaction with shape is common, though over-evaluation of the importance of weight and shape is less marked than in bulimia nervosa.

As with the other eating disorders, the diagnosis of binge eating disorder is made on the basis of the history, with physical investigations being used to assess any physical consequences. Observation and assessment in hospital is rarely indicated, though where available as part of a day programme, assessment of meal preparation and eating may be a useful adjunct to treatment planning.

2.3.3 Impairment and disability

Where atypical eating disorders are similar to the full syndromes of anorexia and bulimia nervosa, the physical dangers and psychosocial impairments closely resemble those of the diagnostic conditions. Many of those with BED will suffer similar physical complications of binge eating to those with bulimia nervosa, though purging carries greater physical risk than binge eating. Those who are obese are at risk of the psychological and physical disabilities associated with this condition, namely low self-esteem, diabetes, heart disease, hypertension and stroke.

2.3.4 Course and prognosis

The prognosis for those disorders that resemble anorexia nervosa and bulimia nervosa depends on the severity of the associated physical and psychological features. Those with binge eating disorder typically give long histories of proneness to binge eating but these may alternate with extended periods free from binge eating. The spontaneous remission rate may be high (Fairburn et al., 2000). Short-term response to treatment appears better than for anorexia nervosa and bulimia nervosa but there are as yet no studies of long-term course or outcome. There is a certain amount of movement from one diagnosis to another, thus those with atypical eating disorders may go on to develop bulimia nervosa, or more rarely anorexia nervosa.

2.3.5 Atypical eating disorders in children and adolescents

Atypical eating disorders are relatively commonly diagnosed in childhood, in part because of the difficulty in strictly applying existing diagnostic criteria for anorexia nervosa and bulimia nervosa, and in part because of an ongoing lack of clarity about the classification of eating disturbances in this age group. Children and younger adolescents may present with a range of other types of clinical eating disturbance, which may be different in terms of psychopathology to anorexia nervosa/bulimia nervosa presentations (Cooper *et al.*, 2002). They frequently develop in those who have suffered feeding disorders of childhood and sometimes the distinction (particularly in middle childhood) can be a difficult one. Some have suggested that atypical eating disorders probably occur more commonly (Bryant-Waugh, 2000) and some have suggested modification to the ICD10 criteria for the diagnosis of eating disorders in children is required. Binge eating disorder has not been systematically investigated in this age group.

2.4 Incidence and prevalence of eating disorders

The incidence of anorexia nervosa in the general population has been calculated from 12 cumulative studies at 19 per 100,000 per year in females and two per 100,000 per year in males (Pawluck & Gorey, 1998). The highest rates in this study were in female teenagers aged 13 to 19 years where there were 50.8 cases per 100,000 per year. A large Swedish cohort of 16-year-old schoolchildren who were assessed in a two stage screening process gave a prevalence for anorexia nervosa of seven per 1000 girls and one per 1000 boys (Rastam *et al.*, 1989). Anorexia nervosa has long been considered a culture bound syndrome; until recently the condition was thought to be extremely rare in developing countries and black populations. Although there is growing evidence of the existence of eating disorders in a range of cultures, little is known of the incidence or prevalence in Asia, South America or Africa (Treasure & Schmidt, 2002), owing in part to differential rates of awareness and detection.

In community-based studies, the prevalence of bulimia nervosa has been estimated between 0.5 per cent and 1.0 per cent in young women with an even social class distribution (Hay & Bacaltchuk, 2001). About 90 per cent of people diagnosed with bulimia nervosa are female. The numbers of presentations of people with bulimia nervosa in developed countries increased steadily during the 1980s and 1990s; in addition, community surveys suggest a true increase in incidence during this period (Hall & Hay, 1991). The prevalence of eating disorders appears to be lower in developing countries and in rural areas. In Britain, young Muslim Asian women may be at particularly high-risk of developing bulimia nervosa (Mumford & Whitehouse, 1988).

Less is known about the prevalence of binge eating than of bulimia nervosa (Fairburn, Hay & Welch, 1993). This is because two stage surveys designed to detect cases of bulimia nervosa have not generated figures for the prevalence of binge eating and secondly because of variability in interpretation of the term 'binge eating'. Often self-report questionnaires are employed to elicit this behaviour with the possibility of discrepancy between lay and clinical uses of the term. Beglin and Fairburn (1992) have shown that there is relatively poor agreement between self-reported binge eating and the eliciting of this behaviour by the Eating Disorder Examination administered by interview. Probably because of these problems of definition and assessment Fairburn and

Beglin (1990) found great variability in the figures available on the prevalence of binge eating. A review of 16 studies reported a range of seven per cent to 79 per cent for current 'binge eating' and 11 studies revealed a range of five per cent to 39 per cent reporting at least weekly binge eating. Within the normal weight sub group (i.e. those with a BMI below 25 kg/m^2) only 1.7 per cent of a subsequent study (Fairburn, Beglin & Davies, 1992) reported weekly binge eating. Thus, binge eating does not appear to be a common behaviour even among young women, though further research is necessary to estimate its prevalence with confidence.

Despite some shortcomings in epidemiological measurement in the area of binge eating, two large population-based studies have estimated the prevalence of binge eating disorder using semi-structured interviews. Hay (1998) gives a prevalence of one per cent for women, while Kinzl et al. (1999) estimate this at 3.3 per cent for women and 8.5 per cent for those with obesity. A further epidemiological study by Fairburn et al. (1992) sampled 285 women aged 16 to 35 years at random from general practice case registers. In total, 243 agreed to be interviewed using the EDE. Twenty-one (8.6 per cent) reported at least one binge over the previous month whilst 10 reported at least an average of one weekly binge and four (1.7 per cent) at least eight episodes in four weeks, a rate sufficient to make a diagnosis of bulimia nervosa or binge eating disorder.

2.5 The aetiology of eating disorders

The aetiology of eating disorders in common with most other psychiatric disorders is generally considered to be multifactorial; no single aetiological factor in isolation can account for the development of the disorder in an individual, nor can it be seen to account for the variation among individuals (Cooper, 1995). Whether or not a person develops an eating disorder will depend on their individual vulnerability, consequent on the presence of biological or other predisposing factors, their exposure to particular provoking risk factors and 'on the operation of protective factors. Following the establishment of the disorder a further combination of risk and protective factors may act to maintain the condition or determine whether an individual recovers.

Much of the research in this area suffers from methodological weakness. Firstly much of it has been based on clinical samples often attending specialist eating disorder clinics, which may result in selection biases. Few studies have included the appropriate control groups required to judge whether any putative aetiological factor is specific to eating disorders or might play a role in the development of psychiatric disorder in general. Secondly, a great deal of the published literature concerns cross-sectional or retrospective research. Where the onset of disorder is insidious, it is not always clear whether such factors are causes or consequences of the disorder. This is particularly true of family or life event research where the independence of any event may not be clear. Finally, few studies have included the person's own perspective about his or her eating disorder. One recent study (Tozzi et al., 2003), suggested that those with anorexia nervosa perceived dysfunctional families, dieting behaviour and stressful life events as the main causes of their condition.

A recent meta-analysis of prospective and experimental studies has systematically reviewed the evidence for aetiological and maintaining factors (Stice, 2002).

2.5.1 Genetic factors

The majority of family studies have shown that eating disorders run in families. In a large case-control family study (Strober *et al.*, 2000), female relatives of those with anorexia nervosa were 11.4 times as likely to suffer the disorder than relatives of control subjects, while female relatives of those with bulimia nervosa were 3.7 times as likely to suffer with bulimia. Some family studies have also reported familial aggregation of milder sub-diagnostic eating disorders or related concerns (Strober, 2000). The prevalence of full and partial bulimia nervosa has been shown to be more common in female relatives of those with anorexia nervosa than in relatives of control subjects and vice versa. These findings suggest that eating disorders form a spectrum of clinical severity in which there is a continuum of familial liability. The aggregation of full and subclinical eating disorders suggests that genetic factors are likely to be involved in causation. A twin study of anorexia nervosa has estimated the heritability to be 58 per cent (95 per cent Confidence Interval 33 per cent to 77 per cent) with the remaining variance explained by non-shared environment (Wade *et al.*, 2000). Genetic factors are also purported to play a role in the aetiology of bulimia nervosa (Kendler *et al.*, 1991). Fifty-four per cent to 83 per cent of the variance in liability has been thought to be due to common genetic factors (Bulik *et al.*, 2000), but again the confidence intervals around the estimation of heritability are broad, thus the relative contribution of genetic to other factors is unclear. The contribution of twin studies to the estimates of heritability of eating disorders has been criticised (e.g. Fairburn *et al.*, 1999) on the grounds of ascertainment bias, small sample sizes or violation of the equal environment assumption, which assumes that both identical and non-identical twins are equally exposed to aetiological environmental factors.

2.5.2 Physical risk factors

A history of premorbid obesity has been documented in series of those with both anorexia nervosa (seven to 20 per cent) and bulimia nervosa (18 to 40 per cent) (Cooper, 1995) as has constitutional leanness/thinness. There is prospective evidence that this experience leads to a propensity to an increase in body dissatisfaction and likelihood of dieting behaviour (Stice, 2002) as well as greater self-evaluation in terms of weight. However, there is little prospective evidence that high body mass leads to an increase in eating pathology.

Early feeding difficulties in infancy or early childhood are often documented but it is unclear whether this constitutes a physical risk factor or is related to the mother child relationship.

Although a range of neuro-endocrine and metabolic disturbances occurs in those with eating disorders, the evidence suggests that these disturbances are secondary rather than primary to the disorder.

Early menarche has long been considered a risk factor for eating disorder through a putative relationship with adiposity and body dissatisfaction.

The dietary restraint model suggests that calorie restriction increases the risk for binge eating and bulimia nervosa. Although dieting appears to increase negative affect and may contribute to eating difficulties, dieting has a small effect size in the contribution to the development of eating pathology (Stice, 2002).

2.5.3 Adverse life events and difficulties

Severe life stresses have been implicated in the aetiology of both anorexia nervosa and bulimia nervosa, with approximately 70 per cent of cases being triggered by severe life events or difficulties. These stresses most commonly occur in the area of close relationships with family or friends (Schmidt *et al.*, 1997, Welch *et al.*, 1997). One controlled study of anorexia nervosa in adolescents (North *et al.*, 1997) suggested that a severe independent negative life event had occurred in the year before onset of approximately one quarter of an adolescent series and this was associated with a good prognosis. Particular attention has focused on the experience of childhood sexual abuse as a potential predisposing factor. There is little persuasive evidence that either sexual abuse or other stressful life events are specific predisposing factors for eating disorders rather than psychiatric disorder *per se*. Childhood sexual abuse did not emerge as a significant predictor of the onset of binge eating in the only prospective study to date (Vogelantz-Holm *et al.*, 2000)

2.5.4 Family factors

Mounting evidence from family studies suggests increased rates of affective disorder among first and second degree relatives of people with both anorexia nervosa and bulimia nervosa. This is three times greater than for relatives of normal control participants (Cooper, 1995). Several family studies have revealed higher rates of alcohol abuse among first degree relatives of those with bulimia nervosa but again, the specificity to eating disorder as opposed to psychiatric disorder in general is unclear. A family history of substance abuse may however be a specific risk factor for bulimia nervosa (Cooper, 1995).

A number of studies have looked at family environment and functioning. There are difficulties extrapolating from disturbance within the family after the disorder has developed and assuming that it predated the onset of disorder. Prospective studies have to date failed to provide support for the causative role of dysfunctional family systems (Stice, 2002). Familial faddy eating and undue concern about the importance of weight and shape have been described in family members of those with eating disorders and may contribute to weight and shape concern in vulnerable adolescents (Gowers & Shore, 2001). There is also growing evidence of disturbance of eating in the children of mothers with eating disorders (Stein, 1995) but it is as yet unclear whether these children will be at risk of anorexia and bulimia nervosa in their own adolescence. One controlled study demonstrated a style of 'high concern' parenting in a number of adolescent cases of anorexia nervosa, which arose in infancy and long predated the onset of eating difficulties. In a quarter of cases, this followed an earlier severe obstetric tragedy prior to the subject's birth. These rates were significantly higher than in a matched control group (Shoebridge & Gowers, 2000) and challenge the notion that observed parenting styles are solely a response to the development of an eating disorder in adolescents.

2.5.5 Socio-cultural factors

A number of socio-cultural theories have been put forward to explain the aetiology of eating disorders. Such theories include the meaning of weight and shape for women in different cultures and the impact of advertising and other media. It is argued that societal pressure to be thin fosters an internalisation of a thin ideal and body dissatisfaction, which in turn leads to dieting behaviour and places the person at risk for eating pathology (Striegel-Moore *et al.*, 1986). This perceived pressure does appear to predict dieting and eating pathology (Stice, 2002). Furthermore, in prospective studies perceived pressure to be thin predicted the onset of binge eating, bulimic symptoms and increases in eating pathology (Stice, 2002).

2.5.6 Perfectionism

This personality trait has long been considered a risk factor for eating pathology as it may promote the relentless pursuit of the 'thin ideal'. Fairburn (1997) has implicated perfectionism as a maintenance factor for bulimic pathology as it encourages rigid dieting thought to underlie the binge-purge cycle. Meta-analysis of prospective studies provides support for the notion of perfectionism as a risk factor for bulimic pathology and a maintenance factor for more general eating pathology (Stice, 2002).

2.5.7 Impulsivity

General problems in the area of impulse control have been proposed as risk factors for eating pathology as they may render the individual vulnerable to episodes of uncontrollable binge eating (Hawkins & Clement, 1984). The empirical support for this association is weak (Stice, 2002), however some indirect support is offered by the finding of an association between substance use and bulimic pathology (Stice & Agras, 1998)

2.6 Use of health service resources

Eating disorders can be chronic, recurrent mental disorders with important psychiatric co-morbidities (depression, generalised anxiety disorder, alcoholism, phobias, panic disorder and post-traumatic stress disorder) and physical complications such as cardio-vascular and renal problems, gastrointestinal disturbance, fluid and electrolyte abnormalities, menstrual and fertility problems, osteoporosis and osteopenia, dental and dermatological abnormalities (Fairburn & Brownell, 2001). As such they can place considerable burdens on the health care system. Eating disorders are at 15th place among the top 20 causes of disability in Australian women measured in years lost due to disability (Vos *et al.*, 2001). Similar rates probably apply in the UK.

In an Australian burden of mental diseases study (Vos *et al.*, 2001), the estimated average duration for anorexia and bulimia nervosa was eight and five years, respectively. These assumptions were based on follow-up studies reporting 24 per cent persistence of anorexia nervosa after 10 to 15 years and 20 per cent persistence of bulimia nervosa after five to 10 years (Strober *et al.*, 1997; Keel & Mitchell, 1997). Anorexia nervosa has the highest mortality rate for any psychiatric condition from the effects of starvation or by committing suicide. At 10-year follow-up the standardised mortality ratio was six per cent, at 20-year follow-up the mortality rate was estimated to be 13 to 20 per cent (Howlett *et al.*, 1995). The annualised mortality rate for individuals with anorexia nervosa was found to be 0.56 per cent in a meta-analysis (Sullivan, 1995) and it was not elevated in bulimia (Nielsen *et al.*, 1998). Very little is known about the mortality associated with BED and EDNOS, although the obesity common in BED is expected to increase the mortality risk (Crow & Peterson, 2003).

Physical complications and mortality in these illnesses are well recognised, but other social, occupational and economic costs and the negative impact on quality of life (Keilen *et al.*, 1994) have received far less attention. The chronic nature of eating disorders and the numerous co-morbidities and complications suggest that people with eating disorders need multi-dimensional treatment and are high consumers of medical and social care. However, a comprehensive study of health or social services use of these individuals has not been carried out either in the UK or internationally (Garvin, 2001). Only a limited literature exists about the broader costs of eating disorders in the health care system and this research evidence indicates significant economic burden posed by eating disorders.

2.6.1 Primary care

Studies from the US and continental Europe suggest that only a fraction of people with eating disorders receive specialised treatment for their eating disorders. For example, in a large sample of female primary care and obstetric gynecology attendees in the US fewer than one in 10 cases with bulimia nervosa or BED were recognised by the physician (Johnson *et al.*, 2001). In the Netherlands, on average, only 40 per cent of the community cases of anorexia nervosa are detected by general practitioners and 79 per cent of these patients are referred on for mental health care (Hoek, 2003). In the case of bulimia nervosa, only a small subgroup, an average 11 per cent of the community cases, are detected in primary care and 51 per cent of these cases are referred to secondary care. A general practitioner with a list of 2000 people could expect to have one or two patients with anorexia nervosa and 18 patients with bulimia nervosa (Hoek, 1991). Importantly, the poor detection rates for eating disorders do not suggest that these patients avoid their general practitioners. Indeed, over the five years prior to the diagnosis of the eating disorder, these individuals consult their general practitioners significantly more frequently than do people without an eating disorder (Ogg *et al.*, 1997). In these earlier consultations, patients typically present with psychological, gastro-intestinal or gynaecological complaints prompted by symptoms of the eating disorder or its complications. These findings suggest that there are high levels of hidden eating disorder morbidity at primary care level leading to a considerable underestimate of costs, and greatly emphasise the importance of primary care in the detection and early treatment of eating disorders.

In the UK, an epidemiological study using the general practice research database found similar figures for referrals, 80 per cent of cases of anorexia nervosa and 60 per cent of cases of bulimia nervosa were referred on to secondary care, the majority to psychiatrists. The study also revealed that general practitioners tend to prescribe laxatives or diuretics for 27 of 100 people with the diagnosis of bulimia nervosa and psychotropic medication in 45 per cent of the eating disorders cases (Turnbull *et al.*, 1996) It should also be noted that many GPs may fail to consider an eating disorder as possible diagnosis in children presenting with typical eating disorder features (Bryant-Waugh *et al.*, 1992). The only calculation of the total cost of eating disorders in primary care was done based on the Third National Survey of Morbidity in General Practice which found that 1/1000 females and 0.6/1000 males consulted their general practitioner for anorexia nervosa (no data for bulimia nervosa, EDNOS or BED were available) in one year (Office of Health Economics, 1994). Applying these rates to the

UK populations of 1990 suggest that approximately 47,000 individuals consult their GP with anorexia nervosa each year, which yields an estimated cost of £580,000 for anorexia nervosa consultations in primary care in 1991 prices (Office of Health Economics, 1994).

2.6.2 Secondary and tertiary care

A recent North American study analysing a national insurance claim database found that specialist eating disorder treatment provision is rare and eating disorders usually remain undetected or undertreated especially in the case of men (Striegel-Moore, 2000). A UK study of patients with anorexia nervosa revealed that under-diagnosis is common. Some patients may spend months or years in non-specialist units posing enormous extra costs for the NHS (Howlett, 1995). The NICAPS study (O'Herlihy et al., 2001) has shown that more beds were occupied by young people with eating disorders than any other diagnostic group, with the same number of patients with eating disorders in specialist eating disorders services being found as in non-specialist psychiatric units. In all, there was a total of 22.2 per cent of the inpatient population with a diagnosis of an eating disorder.

In the US as in the UK, outpatient treatment is the norm with low hospitalisation rates for eating disorders. Striegel-Moore (2000) reviewed costs for the disorders in the US. The average numbers of outpatient episodes are 17, 15.6 and 13.7 for anorexia nervosa, bulimia nervosa and EDNOS, respectively. Only 21.5 per cent of women with anorexia nervosa are hospitalised per year with an average length of stay in the US of 26 days, and very much lower hospitalisation rates were found for bulimia nervosa and EDNOS. Mean annual treatment (outpatient and inpatient) costs for female patients were $6,045 for anorexia nervosa, $2,962 for bulimia nervosa and $3,207 for EDNOS. These costs of treating eating disorders were compared with treatment costs of schizophrenia and obsessive-compulsive disorder (OCD). The mean treatment cost for anorexia nervosa was significantly higher than the mean cost for schizophrenia, but mean treatment cost for bulimia nervosa was significantly lower than for schizophrenia. Treatment costs for any eating disorder were much greater than that of OCD. These cost estimates are likely to represent an underestimate of the true costs of these illnesses since costs were calculated based on diagnostic codes (Crow & Peterson, 2003).

In the UK in 1985 an estimated 25,748 bed days were allocated to inpatient treatment of women and girls with anorexia nervosa (Hospital Inpatient Enquiry) with the average length of 21.5 days per episode. Only a fraction of the medication costs were estimated in the same study. There are no more recent UK estimates about inpatient treatment, other medication, outpatient treatment and psychotherapy costs, and no data are available for bulimia nervosa, EDNOS or BED. When looking at the organisation of eating disorders care in the UK, it is important to mention the significant role of private providers even though they are acknowledged as being a more expensive way to contract with providers (Brown, 1997).

The most recent estimate of the health care costs of eating disorders comes from Germany. Krauth et al. (2002) calculated that the health care costs of anorexia nervosa for the year 1998 amounts to 64.9 million euros and that of bulimia nervosa to 9.8 million euros without the costs of primary care, outpatient care (including psychotherapy) and pharmaceuticals. The estimated hospitalisation cost of 12,800 euros per patient with anorexia nervosa was found to be much higher than the hospitalisation cost of 3600 euros for an average patient with bulimia nervosa (Krauth *et al.*, 2002). However, it is worth mentioning that in Germany the threshold for inpatient admission for anorexia nervosa is probably much lower than in the NHS in the UK if not in the private sector.

The cost of managing physical and dental complications (such as infertility, osteoporosis and reconstructive dentistry) in secondary care has not been quantified but may be considerable.

2.6.3 Non-health care burden

Eating disorders have a substantial impact on social functioning, including occupational and educational impairment. These disorders are the most common at an age when people are in secondary school, in higher education or at the beginning of their working careers. Eating disorders often result in lost productivity due to the inability of people to work or premature death. The lost productivity costs of anorexia nervosa were estimated to be 130.5 million euros (inability to work: eight million euros, death: 122.5 million euros) for the 82 million German population in the year 1998. The same figure for the indirect economic burden of bulimia nervosa was 113.9 million euros (inability to work: 1.7 million euros, death: 112.2 million euros) (Krauth *et al.*, 2002).

The average duration of an episode of anorexia nervosa is six years (Herzog *et al.*, 1997) and the family are usually the main carers for most of the duration of the illness. A recent UK pilot study found that carers of anorexic patients reported similar experiences in terms of the difficulties experienced to those of carers of adults with psychosis, but had significantly higher level of psychological distress (Treasure *et al.*, 2001). The burden of caregiving has never been examined in economic terms.

These estimates suggest that the broader social costs of eating disorders may be even more substantial than their health care costs, and that early diagnosis, prevention of chronicity and appropriate and cost-effective treatments may greatly reduce the broad economic burden of eating disorders.

2.7 The treatment and management of eating disorders in the NHS

Until the last few decades of the 20th century, in the UK, general physicians generally managed anorexia nervosa. Treatment consisted of bed rest, often in a side room of a general medical ward. A few psychiatrists started to take an interest in the condition from the middle of the 20th century. Dally and Sargant used physical methods of treatment such as insulin and chlorpromazine (Dally, 1969). Then two academic psychiatrists, Professor Arthur Crisp and Professor Gerald Russell, took an interest in the condition initially with a particular interest in the endocrine and metabolic aspects. They developed specialised units, which were replicated across the UK and the world and trained most of the current generation of psychiatrists working in eating disorder services. Skilled, supportive nursing was the cornerstone of such units and over time more specific forms of psychotherapy were developed. At the Maudsley Hospital, for example, there was a particular interest in family therapy.

The description of bulimia nervosa by Gerald Russell in 1979 was a landmark event. An explosion of research followed this into both psychotherapeutic and physical (antidepressants and appetite suppressants) treatments. The most widely researched treatment has been cognitive behaviour therapy developed by Chris Fairburn.

At the present time, there are wide variations in the provision of eating disorder services and models of service delivery throughout the UK. Services range from 'generic', in which outpatient therapies are provided by community mental health teams, backed up by psychiatric admission, to variable models of specialist eating disorder service. These latter vary widely in staffing, service configuration and therapeutic interventions offered. At the more modest end of the spectrum, an outpatient-only service may offer therapeutic input, but little in the way of medical assessment or management, responsibility for which remains with primary care. More fully comprehensive models are organised around intensive day-patient provision, an inpatient unit, or both. Many of the better-funded resources function as tertiary services, serving a large (on occasions, national) catchment area.

Children and younger adolescents (up to the age of 16) are generally treated in generic child and adolescent mental health services (CAMHS) supported as required by paediatric services. Where inpatient treatment is thought necessary, children and adolescents are admitted either to paediatric wards often with CAMHS liaison, to 'general-purpose' children's or adolescent units, or to private-sector specialist eating disorder services, funded by the NHS.

Where young people are admitted to paediatric medical wards, appropriate communication with CAMHS staff is crucial. The care plan should be agreed between the medical and mental health services and appropriately co-ordinated. There are very few specialist eating disorder inpatient services for this age group in the NHS and none with a comprehensive range of out, day and inpatient provision. Many services attempt to avoid inflexible age boundaries, preferring to take into account the young person's developmental level and whether they are in full-time education or living at home with parents when deciding the appropriate service for them.

Ensuring appropriate communication and handover across transitional boundaries is a particular challenge for those treating children and adolescents. Some services offer combined adolescent/adult treatment, which offer experience in the management of eating disorders, but need to ensure developmentally appropriate therapeutic intervention and social support. In many parts of the country, the potential advantage of specialist inpatient treatment may be offset by the disadvantages of treatment a long way from home, with problems posed for therapeutic involvement of the family, maintaining educational and social contacts and most importantly, ensuring continuity of care post-discharge.

2.7.1 Pharmacological treatment

Pharmacotherapy has not been the treatment of first choice for eating disorders, but it has been used as an adjunct to psychological therapies or to treat physical or co-morbid psychological problems. In anorexia nervosa, medication has to date been disappointing in influencing the core symptoms of the disorder, promoting weight gain or reducing associated mood disturbance (Treasure & Schmidt, 2001). Where modest improvements have been reported, consideration of unwanted effects (e.g. in prolonging the QT cardiac interval), have led researchers to conclude that drugs confer little advantage when added to standard treatment (e.g. Vandereycken, 1984). In bulimia nervosa and binge eating disorder, whilst drugs are not the first option, there is some evidence that antidepressants, particularly selective serotonin reuptake inhibitors (SSRIs) contribute to the cessation of binge eating and purging. As endogenous opiates play a role in the hypothalamic regulation of hunger and satiety, a few trials have been conducted with opiate antagonists.

2.7.2 Psychological interventions

Choosing the most effective treatment approach for someone with an eating disorder should take account of a number of variables, including physical and psychological risk, motivation, social support, comorbidity, and age. Often and particularly in anorexia nervosa, treatment planning will require co-ordinated, multidisciplinary, physical, psychological and service interventions. Psychological interventions are, however, considered to be crucial in addressing the core attitudes that underlie these disorders and in influencing the longer-term outcomes. The nature of the psychological therapies chosen will be influenced by patient preference, their motivation, the nature of associated psychological features and their age or stage of development. Some will prefer a non-verbal projective therapy, using art, drama or music. Younger patients in particular or those who are dependent on relatives or carers are seen as often requiring family or systemic therapy. Of the individual therapies, cognitive behaviour therapy (CBT) is the best researched, though the evidence base in bulimia nervosa and binge eating disorder (BED) is far larger than in anorexia nervosa. The evidence base for other psychological therapies such as supportive psychotherapy and interpersonal psychotherapy (IPT) is growing, while more specialised therapies such as cognitive analytic therapy (CAT) and dialectical behaviour therapy (DBT) have been considered in complex cases, and for DBT those complicated by repeated self-harm (Treasure & Schmidt, 2003).

2.7.3 Service-level interventions

Decisions about the right treatment setting in which to manage a person with an eating disorder currently depend on the nature of the disorder, the level of risk, physical and psychological complications and patient preference. Within the NHS currently, the availability of different models of service is a major consideration with patients and referrers sometimes having to weigh up the advantages of a locally accessible service with those of a more comprehensive service at some geographical distance. In general, those with bulimia nervosa and binge eating disorder will be treated on an outpatient basis either in primary care or secondary services. Those with anorexia nervosa will generally be treated in secondary care, the choice of in, out, or day patient provision depending on the above considerations. Most will have a trial of outpatient intervention first. A stepped-care model in which patients move up from secondary to tertiary care subject to locally agreed protocols makes clinical sense, but there is at present little evidence to guide decisions about service setting. There is also considerable debate over the requirement for some or all of people with eating disorders to be treated in specialist eating disorder services. In general the current practice would seem to favour the treatment of the large majority of adult patients with anorexia within specialist eating disorder services, whereas such specialist services may only be needed for patients with severe forms of bulimia nervosa. However, irrespective of the service setting (specialist secondary or tertiary, or generalist) the key aim of this guideline will be to ensure that as far the evidence allows, effective treatments should be provided. Whatever the service, the setting should be age-appropriate, with the social, and educational needs of children and adolescents requiring particular attention in order to avoid the development of secondary handicaps. Inpatient management will require comprehensive physical and psychological management; currently a number of models exist from medical admission with psychiatric/psychological liaison to psychiatric admission with medical supervision. Children, in particular are often admitted to general medical (paediatric) services.

2.7.4 Primary–secondary care interface

Many patients with eating disorders will require treatment for a considerable time, often for a number of years. During this time, they may require treatment in primary care, secondary and on occasions, tertiary care services. The boundary between primary and secondary care is one of a number of interfaces that need to be managed effectively. Others include the interface between medical and psychiatric services, between inpatient and outpatient services, and for adolescents, between Child and Adolescent Mental Health Services (CAMHS) and adult services. It is particularly important for effective management that communication is good and that areas of responsibility are clear. Sometimes, for example a patient may be receiving psychological therapy from a secondary care service, but responsibility for physical monitoring may remain with primary care. Clear treatment protocols will ensure smooth management across these interfaces.

2.7.5 Physical health care

Patients with eating disorders always require assessment of their physical health and any associated risk as part of a comprehensive assessment. This should also be reviewed as treatment progresses. Physical complications can be classified as follows:

- The complications of starvation (chiefly in anorexia nervosa)

- The consequences of purging behaviours (including dental complications)

- The complications of associated physical conditions (such as diabetes or pregnancy)

- The complications of excessive exercise

- Physical aspects of stunted or incomplete development (in younger people); the main effects being on skeletal growth and the reproductive system

- Physical complications of dietary imbalance (e.g. a high fibre, low fat diet)

- Physical complications of refeeding or restoration of normal diet.

Many of these may have effects on a number of systems within the body. In any treatment plan, it must be clear who is taking responsibility for physical assessment and how any risk identified is to be managed. This often involves effective communication between primary and secondary care services (see Section 2.7.4).

2.7.6 The relationship of the evidence base for adults to that for children and adolescents.

In the absence of a strong body of treatment research in the child and adolescent literature, it is tempting to extrapolate from adult findings, but the validity and limitations of doing so requires careful consideration. A key argument in favour of extrapolating from adult findings is that adolescence is a developmental stage that is not defined merely by age. It can be argued that many young adults with eating disorders are still in the throes of addressing the challenges of adolescence and indeed developmental difficulties have been thought to underlie the aetiology of anorexia nervosa in particular (e.g. Crisp, 1995). A second argument is that the essential features of anorexia nervosa and bulimia nervosa are consistent across the age spectrum – both in terms of characteristic behaviours (dieting, binge eating, purging), specific psychopathology (over-evaluation of the self in terms of weight and shape) and non-specific features (low self-esteem, perfectionism, poor interpersonal confidence). Thirdly some of the literature reports combined adolescent/adult case series without separate analysis. Finally some of the treatments that have been found to be effective in adult eating disorders (e.g. CBT and antidepressants) are effective in the treatment of adolescents with other conditions (particularly depression).

There are, however, a number of reservations about extrapolating from adult findings. In younger patients, the disorders less commonly fall neatly into the ICD10 or DSM-IV categories; that is to say, atypical forms are more commonly diagnosed. Some clinical eating disturbances seen in childhood and early adolescence currently classified as atypical eating disorders may not have much in common with the adult category of EDNOS. As treatments for EDNOS are poorly developed in adults, there are few findings in any case to draw on. The *treatment aims*, particularly in anorexia nervosa are often different in childhood and adolescence, because of the different physical issues involved, i.e. where the onset is before growth and development are complete, treatment needs to address the completion of puberty and growth. Unlike the treatment of adults with anorexia nervosa where recovery usually involves returning to a premorbid healthy physical state, in younger patients it is more a question of coming to terms with a new physical state. In terms of weight targets this involves 'constantly moving the goal posts' as healthy weight is recalculated with the attainment of greater height. All this might indicate a need for a longer duration of treatment for younger cases, whilst a shorter duration of illness before treatment might argue for the opposite.

When considering the literature on pharmacotherapy, one should be aware of differences in the pharmacodynamics and pharmacokinetics in children. In general the latter means that children and adolescents require higher doses of drugs per kg body weight to attain similar blood levels and therapeutic effect, owing to children's more rapid metabolism by the liver and clearance by the kidney.

Irrespective of any consideration of aetiological variables, parents will usually need to be involved in the management of younger patients. This is especially so if they are at risk and parental involvement is likely to reduce the risk. Both anorexia nervosa and bulimia nervosa require aspects of behavioural management and parents will need to be involved if management of these is to be effective; at a practical level, parents usually have a role in shopping for food, meal planning, and managing meal times. The involvement of siblings is generally regarded as beneficial, for the sibling if not for the patient, as this provides an opportunity for them to express fears or guilt and to dispel any false ideas about the nature of the condition, its likely causes and prognosis.

Additional attention will need to be given to the different social and educational needs of this age group in treatment, particularly when treated in hospital.

In addition, carers and parents of adolescents have identified a lack of and need for support, involvement and education about eating disorders for themselves (Kopec-Schrader *et al.*, 1993; Haigh & Treasure, 2003).

2.8 Assessment

Eating disorders may present to the NHS in primary care or to a range of tertiary medical services including mental health, gastroenterology, endocrinology and reproductive medicine. Some patients will volunteer symptoms of eating pathology and disclose the characteristic behaviours, or a relative or other carer will report them (particularly in childhood and adolescence). Others will present with the symptoms of physical or psychological complications either because they are unaware that they are symptoms of an eating disorder, or because they do not wish to reveal it. A most important step in the identification of eating disorders, therefore, is to be open to the possibility of the disorder (see Section 5.1).

Assessment encompasses making a diagnosis and eliciting the necessary information to prepare a care plan, including the assessment of severity and risk. The details of assessment methods are provided in the primary care chapter (Sections 5.2.4.1, 5.2.4.2). Wherever assessment takes place however, some common principles apply:

● Keeping an open mind

● Maintaining a supportive, non-judgmental approach

● Focusing on engagement (see Section 2.9)

● Assessing risk (see Sections 6.4.3, 7.5)

● The patient's right to confidentiality (see Section 2.11.2).

As eating disorders are commonly characterised by ambivalence, assessment should not be seen in isolation from treatment, as the patient's first impressions of services may have a powerful impact on their willingness to consider referral to secondary care and subsequently accept treatment. Specialist eating disorder services are increasingly adopting a motivational approach to assessment and induction into treatment

(Bauer & Treasure, 2003). Throughout this guideline, reference is often made to the comprehensive assessment of physical, psychological and social needs. This should be taken as a general indication as to the content of a comprehensive assessment which will vary form person to person but will often include:

- Current and past physical health and treatment

- Cognitive capacities

- Any present physical disabilities

- A historical and current assessment of family and interpersonal relationships

- Mental state and personality factors

- Social circumstances and supports

- Occupational and social functioning

- Educational and vocational needs.

2.8.1 Clinical practice recommendations

2.8.1.1 Assessment of people with eating disorders should be comprehensive and include physical, psychological and social needs, and a comprehensive assessment of risk to self. (C)

2.8.1.2 The level of risk to the patient's mental and physical health should be monitored as treatment progresses because it may increase – for example following weight change or at times of transition between services in cases of anorexia nervosa. (C)

2.8.1.3 Health care professionals assessing children and adolescents with eating disorders should be alert to indicators of abuse (emotional, physical and sexual) and should remain so throughout treatment. (C)

2.8.1.4 The right to confidentiality of children and adolescents with eating disorders should be respected. (C)

2.8.1.5 Health care professionals working with children and adolescents with eating disorders should familiarise themselves with national guidelines and their employers' policies in the area of confidentiality. (C)

2.9 Engagement, consent and the therapeutic alliance

Many people presenting to NHS services are ambivalent about revealing their symptoms and behaviours and are uncertain about or indeed actively opposed to treatment. There are a number of reasons for this ambivalence. Firstly, the patient may believe that they will be criticised or treated unsympathetically. This belief may be based in guilt about engaging in vomiting or binge eating, or a belief that they will be expected to exert control over these maladaptive behaviours. Alternatively they may have heard about the negative treatment experiences of others (see Section 2.10), or fear compulsory treatment. Anorexia nervosa in particular is sometimes perceived by the patient as a valued life-style choice or the only possible way for them to live. Many will fear the effects of treatment; someone with anorexia nervosa may believe that treatment will make them fat, whilst a patient with bulimia nervosa may fear that stopping vomiting will render them vulnerable to impulsive binge eating without recourse to compensatory purging.

A style of empathic engagement is helpful, therefore, in addressing patient anxieties, but probably also has an important bearing on treatment outcome. Although considerable attention may be necessary to address the physical complications of eating disorders, these interventions rarely address the core attitudes and behaviours underlying the disorders, which are generally addressed by psychological therapies. As in the treatment of any disorder, effective psychological therapy requires engagement in a therapeutic relationship and agreement about treatment aims. Whilst a forceful approach may result in a degree of weight gain in anorexia nervosa, clinicians are increasingly drawing attention to the importance of engagement and positive motivation if short-term gains are to be maintained in the long term, whatever the treatment setting (Ward *et al.*, 1996).

In most cases for adults treatment is offered on the basis of fully informed consent. In rare cases, almost exclusively of anorexia nervosa, this is not possible. Anorexia nervosa strikes at one of the core aspects of being an autonomous individual, the capacity to care for oneself and maintain health and safety. The Department of Health has recognised that a patient with anorexia nervosa who is unable to appreciate his or her failing condition may not be able to comprehend and make use of relevant information and as a result may lack the capacity to make a valid treatment decision (Department of Health, 2001). It is good practice, however, whether treatment is provided on a formal or informal basis to develop a therapeutic alliance, attempt to promote positive motivation and engage in informal treatment as soon as the physical and psychological state of the patient give confidence that informal treatment is likely to be effective.

Similar principles apply to the treatment of children and adolescents. The transition from childhood to adulthood can, however, cause confusion about rights and responsibilities. Potential additional difficulties arise from the need to inform parents and carers about risks, but maintain, as far as possible, the young person's right to confidentiality (see Section 2.11). The government specifically addresses issues relating to consent and confidentiality as it relates to this transitional phase. 'Young people aged 16 and 17 are regarded as adults for the purposes of consent to treatment and are, therefore, entitled to the same duty of confidentiality as adults. Children under the age of 16 who have the capacity and understanding to make decisions about their own treatment are also entitled to make decisions about the use and disclosure of information they have provided in confidence (e.g. receiving treatment and counselling that they do not want their parent to know about). However where a competent child is refusing treatment for a life threatening condition, the duty of care would require confidentiality to be breached to the extent of informing those with parental responsibility for the child, who might then be able to provide the necessary consent to the treatment (Department of Health, 2001).

2.10 The patient experience of eating disorders

For patients, the experience of an eating disorder can be complex, ambivalent, and contradictory. Complex, because a range of issues must be untangled and understood on the often long road to recovery; ambivalent, because of the tension between wanting to get better while fearing the implications of recovery; and contradictory because the disordered eating is at once the problem and the solution – a destructive lifestyle that nevertheless keeps the person in control, safe and protected, while offering a dependable and consistent presence in their life.

Nobody just wakes up one day with an eating disorder. These are conditions that develop over time, sometimes over years and often at a point when life changes bring fear and insecurity. Both anorexia nervosa and bulimia nervosa often start with a period of food restriction of some kind, which gradually becomes stricter and stricter. Such restrictions often are reported as generating a sense of euphoria at being in control of one's weight, of feeling superior to others who might be struggling to manage theirs, and of increased confidence and enhanced appearance. Patients report that it is not unusual to feel moments of intense clarity, insight and of feeling more alive than ever. It is also not unusual to feel considerable physical energy, which may be experienced as though activity could be sustained for many hours without food or sleep at least until the food restriction starts to trigger physical and mental side effects. All this may serve to reinforce a person's negative behaviours around food.

At the same time, patients often sense that all of this is somehow not quite right. While recognising that their eating patterns are unhealthy in terms of quality or quantity of food, they may dread eating more for fear of gaining weight or being unable to stop eating once started. They may become increasingly secretive and devious around food and eating – skipping meals, lying about eating, hiding food, eating in secret, discovering ways to get rid of food once eaten, while denying or not acknowledging that there is a problem. Food increasingly comes to dominate thoughts, feelings and actions. Debating the options of what to eat becomes a constant daily struggle, an internal battle, a desperate self-involved fight where even sleep offers little escape. Not eating is somehow so much easier than eating, but for so many this often ends in chaos, binge eating and weight gain.

Self-hatred about appearance, feelings of being bloated and fat and frequent physical pain are common consequences of these behaviours. Starting to eat can worsen these feelings. Even those who don't get caught in the starve/binge cycle frequently lose touch with friends and family and become increasingly alone and isolated because of the difficulty of discussing these feelings for fear that no one could possibly understand. The person may start to be caught between extreme control and the overwhelming fear of descending into complete chaos – knowing that at any time 'giving in' to food is only a step away. If the control slips, the chaos takes over and shame and guilt flow in its wake.

Many of these feelings are common, whether the diagnosis is of anorexia nervosa, bulimia nervosa or binge eating disorder. The person may be aware of a deep underlying despair, a sense of being inherently inferior, unworthy and undeserving of the good things in life, guilty for wanting to try to fulfil their needs. Yet despite constant attempts to deny the problem and the difficulties inherent in loving, needing and self-acceptance, there is, somewhere, an intense desire to be loved, needed and accepted as one is.

The person may reach the point of acknowledging the problem, and turning to someone to ask for help. This is a critical first step towards recovery although the way ahead may still be fraught with problems. A range of questions arise: 'Who is trustworthy – doctor, teacher, nurse, parent, friend, relative …? Who will really listen and take me seriously? Who will see me as a whole person and not just as an illness or a difficult problem? Who will understand that someone really can have these issues with food? What will happen if I 'come clean' and admit to my behaviours? What will a diagnosis mean in terms of the treatment I might be offered? How much control will I retain? And will admitting to a problem blight the landscape of my future career, work prospects, education, relationships?'

For boys and men, there may be added complications since, despite changing attitudes and understanding, eating disorders are still considered primarily a female issue. This can make it even more difficult for men to seek help. For young people, there are often particular questions surrounding confidentiality: 'If I speak to someone at school or my doctor, will they tell my parents?'; with control of treatment: 'Given my age, who will be "in charge"?'; and with the fear of being treated differently to one's peer group: '
You have a problem with food, therefore you cannot be trusted!'' All of these issues, together with low confidence and self-esteem may convince someone that keeping the disorder hidden is the safest option, even if, deep down, they want to move forward. They may just not believe that they are strong enough to do so.

Being given a diagnosis can raise a new set of issues. Treatment in mainstream services can be a postcode lottery with long waiting lists. It can be difficult, if not impossible, to learn about the range of treatment options and services if the GP lacks experience of working with eating disorders. There may be a debate about how best to treat the individual, and treatment may be only available at some distance from family and friends. The time-lag between raising the issue, getting a diagnosis and accessing treatment can leave the person with an eating disorder feeling 'let-down' or rejected and compound feelings of unworthiness after having found the courage to speak out. Any delay also provides an opportunity for 'ambivalence' to creep back in again – the person may then ask: 'Do I really want this treatment anyway?'

Eating disorders present complex challenges and treatment tends to be long-term with the possibility of frequent relapses. Whatever the setting, finding the 'right person' to work with – someone with expert knowledge and particular qualities who will accept and understand the person as 'an individual with a unique experience' rather than as 'a case of pathology' – seems critical to treatment 'success'. Trust is also vitally important when deciding to give up the principal means to cope with life. Getting help with food itself, through dietetic intervention to include assessment, modification, education and monitoring, can also be important particularly with bulimia nervosa. It can be very difficult for an individual to focus on psychological and emotional processes when thoughts are crowded with what one will/won't, can/can't eat, or when the body is in a state of starvation, poor blood sugar control, hormone/neurotransmitter imbalance, etc.

Establishing a structured approach to food and being given permission to 'legalise' foods that have long been forbidden is often vital for the person with bulimia nervosa. Increasing food intake bit by bit, day by day, may be a better approach for an adult with anorexia nervosa than a narrow focus on restoring weight at a speed that only results in feeling completely out of control. Clear and regular communication between clinicians, patient, carers and family is also a vital and often overlooked part of treatment.

For most people, recovery goes through several stages and is characterised by steps forward and steps back. There may be longer-term complications and a sense of an ongoing vulnerability around food long after the main issues have been resolved. During the treatment process, there is often an exchange of views on what constitutes recovery – the patient's understanding may differ significantly from that of the professionals. There can be other issues – views on managing treatment may be at odds, understanding and dealing with the expectations of others can be very hard at times, particularly as those with eating disorders tend to want to please and have a deep internal need for external approval and affirmation. An additional dilemma may occur if the individual senses that the treatment approach is not working, whilst at the same time knowing it might be all that is on offer.

Staying positive and maintaining commitment, learning how to deal with lapses and managing the ambivalence that can flare up with a vengeance throughout recovery will be all too familiar for those who have been through this experience. The path is not always easy. But throughout this time, it is important to stay focused and to know and remember that recovery is possible and there are people who want to help overcome the disorder.

And what about those who want to help the person with an eating disorder – partners, spouses, friends, relatives, colleagues, siblings, parents? It seems that their experience is also one of complexity, ambivalence and contradiction. How can they help you face issues and accept that there is a problem? What role should they play? Where can they get information about treatment approaches and how do they communicate this? How do they deal with the medical professionals? And what about issues of patient confidentiality? Many who have been involved with somebody struggling with eating distress, have reported how desperate and isolated they have felt at times, how they have been 'at their wits end, not knowing where to turn for help'. They will also often speak of their guilt and remorse and feeling of responsibility for the illness; have they caused or contributed to the situation? What could they have done to make things different?

For carers as for sufferers, the expectations of treatment, its duration and impact on those involved, may differ greatly from the actual reality. From the outset, it is important to understand and expect an arduous, challenging and unpredictable journey, with emotions previously controlled and contained, spilling out into the open.

Regardless of their nature, relationships are likely to be permanently changed by the experience of coping with an eating disorder. In the early days when the 'sufferer' is either stuck in denial or does not know how to even admit there is an issue, the impact on relationships can be very negative. Once the issue is out in the open things may change as the 'sufferer' becomes more accepting of care and support, although the road is still pretty rocky at times. Support groups of various kinds can be an important component of the healing process.

A readiness to change and to accept self-responsibility and a real desire for a life where eating does not dominate every moment, are perhaps the true keys to full recovery. The experience of an eating disorder may leave a lifelong mark, however letting go, developing self-acceptance, forgiving events in the past, and dropping feelings of shame can lead to growth and to an end which in so many ways is, of course, only the beginning.

2.10.1 Clinical practice recommendations

2.10.1.1   Health care professionals should acknowledge that many people with eating disorders are ambivalent about treatment. Health care professionals should also recognise the consequent demands and challenges this presents. (C)

2.10.1.2   Patients and, where appropriate, carers should be provided with education and information on the nature, course and treatment of eating disorders. (C)

2.11 The involvement of family members/carers

2.11.1 Involving carers

Eating disorders have a social as well as an individual context. Once 'out in the open', family members and carers are inevitably drawn into the illness and many will want to offer whatever help they can. The UK government has recognised the important role and contribution that carers provide for people with a range of mental health problems and information and guidance is available through a website (www.carers.gov.uk).

2.11.2 Confidentiality

Some patients will be concerned that the involvement of their relatives may breach their rights of confidentiality. Consultations between those with eating disorders and health care professionals are bound by generic rules regarding confidentiality, i.e. that this should only be breached if the patient or others are at significant risk and that a breach of confidentiality is likely to reduce that risk (Department of Health, 2001; GMC, 2003). Furthermore the patient should be informed of any necessary breach of confidentiality. However issues of good practice with regard to confidentiality should not be accepted as an excuse for not listening to or communicating effectively with carers. Carers should be given sufficient information by medical and mental health services in a way that they can readily understand, to help them provide care effectively (Department of Health, 2003). Information from carers is also subject to the same rules of confidentiality as those applied to the individual with the illness.

2.11.3 Information for carers

Carers should be given the opportunity to ask health care professionals about the illness in general and specific risks. The following information might reasonably be expected to be available to them:

Information about eating disorders

- The general causes of an eating disorder

- The general maintaining factors of an eating disorder

- The best strategies to help someone with an eating disorder

- The evidence base for the treatment and management of people with anorexia nervosa

- The prognosis and expected course and outcome of people with eating disorders.

Information about physical risk

- That a physical and psychological risk assessment of the patient is being regularly undertaken

- That they will be informed if the threat to the health and safety of the patient is severe

- The danger signs that should to alert them to physical risk of the patient

- What they should do in the event that they are concerned about the health and safety of the patient and how they can recruit help when necessary.

2.11.4 Carer involvement in treatment

The extent to which the family and/or next of kin need to be involved in treatment relates to age and developmental issues, the severity of the illness and the risk of harm. In general, parents and other family members will be included in the treatment of children and adolescents and in the treatment of adults depending on their wishes and the assessment of risk or severity. In the rare cases where compulsory treatment is necessary, there is a statutory role for the next of kin enshrined in the 1983 Mental Health Act legislation.

Therefore, although services should aim to keep treatment confidential they also have to ensure that they practice safely and consider the needs of carers. They have a statutory obligation to let other people know if there are health and safety issues that need to be considered.

2.11.5 Carers' experiences and wishes

A survey of carers (Haigh & Treasure, 2003) and a focus group convened to inform the GDG, revealed a number of common themes:

- Carers are concerned about a perceived variable range of experience and expertise in the management of eating disorders amongst health service professionals.

- They express a need for quality information and effective communication.

- They often express a wish to be included in their relative's 'treatment team'.

- They are concerned about a perceived lack (in many areas) of adequate service provision and many worry about delays in accessing effective services and smooth transition between tiers of care.

The issues raised can be classified as engaging with primary care, experiences of treatment, and issues in aftercare. The carers focus group also made the following observations.

2.11.5.1 Engaging with primary care

- GPs may think issues and symptoms are trivial, partly because they often have little experience of eating disorders.

- A GP's inexperience and lack of training in eating disorders can lead to a delay in diagnosis.

- Pathways between primary and secondary care are slow and fraught with obstacles, including lack of choice.

- There are often difficulties in receiving information and effective communication particularly in relation to the treatment of older adolescents. These relate both to issues of confidentiality, and to problems in communication in the transition between child and adolescent and adult services.

2.11.5.2 Experiences of treatment

- Concern was expressed about the poor response of adolescents to inpatient treatment for a range of reasons.

- Poor communication is common, partly related to shift working in inpatient units. The treatment plan was sometimes poorly explained.

- Carers need information about the disorders, their own rights, and compulsory treatment.

- Siblings need support as well as parents/adult carers.

- Support, for example from relatives support groups, was welcomed.

- Community-based services are preferred to inpatient treatment where this can be managed.

2.11.5.3 Aftercare

- Aftercare provision is often limited and can undermine the benefit of inpatient treatment.

- Responsibility for aftercare is often unclear.

- Co-existing or residual difficulties are often not addressed.

- Little choice is offered.

2.11.5.4 Carer advice

The focus group suggested that improvements could be made in the following areas:

- More training of health service staff is required, particularly for those in general practice including GPs. This would include training in the detection and the features of eating disorders and an understanding of how motivation and ambivalence can affect engagement in treatment.

- Carers should be actively involved in treatment programmes.

- Treatment plans and other information should be provided to carers, including written reference resources.

- Carers should be offered the opportunity to learn from and benefit from the experience and support of others in the same situation.

- Recovered or recovering patients could be used to provide support to patients at an earlier stage of treatment.

- A greater focus on outreach and community services rather than inpatient services is desirable, in order to avoid dislocation from the patient's family and social support.

- A greater uniformity of treatment protocols and approaches, based on the available evidence rather than service constraints is desirable, in order to reduce idiosyncratic practice.

2.11.5.5

In addition to the provision of information, family and carers may be informed of self-help groups and support groups and offered the opportunity to participate in such groups where they exist. (C)

2.12 Stigma

The above review of the experience of eating disorders from the patients' and carers' perspective reveals the disabling nature of these disorders. Those who suffer from eating disorders often carry the added burden of stigmatising attitudes from the lay public and health services staff. These attitudes not only restrict the opportunities for effective treatment, but also confer additional handicaps. The Royal College of Psychiatrists stigma campaign (Cowan & Hart, 1998), followed a survey of the general public which revealed that stigmatising attitudes were based on four beliefs about those with mental health problems, namely:

- Sufferers are thought to be dangerous to others.

- The disorders are thought to be self-inflicted.

- The outcome is thought to be poor.

- It is difficult to communicate with sufferers.

Crisp *et al.* (2000) have indeed shown that those with eating disorders are believed by the general public to be unpredictable, hard to talk to, are different from them, have only themselves to blame and should 'pull themselves together'. Gowers and Shore (1999) have reviewed the part played by these factors in stigmatising those with eating disorders and have argued for improved training of health service staff and greater public education. Crucially, stigma can be reduced by placing the person with an eating disorder at the centre of their treatment and by engaging them in a positive therapeutic relationship (see Section 2.9). This is a key aim of this guideline.

3 Methods used to develop this guideline

3.1 Overview

The development of this guideline drew upon methods outlined by NICE (NICE, 2002; Eccles & Mason, 2001). A team of experts, professionals, and a patient representative, known as the Guideline Development Group (GDG), undertook the development of a patient centred, evidence-based guideline with support from the NCCMH staff. There are five basic steps in the process of developing a guideline:

● Define clinical questions considered important for practitioners and patients.

● Develop criteria for evidence searching and search for evidence.

● Design validated protocols for systematic review and apply to evidence recovered by search.

● Synthesise and (meta-) analyse data retrieved, guided by the clinical questions.

● Answer clinical questions with evidence-based recommendations for clinical practice.

The clinical practice recommendations made by the GDG are therefore derived from the most up-to-date and robust evidence base for the clinical and cost-effectiveness of the treatments and services used in the management of eating disorders. In addition, to ensure a patient and carer focus, their concerns regarding clinical practice have been highlighted and addressed by recommendations agreed by the whole GDG. The evidence-based recommendations are the core of this guideline.

3.2 The Guideline Development Group

The eating disorders GDG consisted of: professionals in psychiatry, clinical psychology, nursing, social work, and general practice; academic experts in psychiatry and psychology; a patient, and a representative from a patient organisation. The carer perspective was provided through focus group discussion with carers; the group was run by the patient on the GDG. The guideline development process was supported by staff from the NCCMH review team, who undertook the clinical and health economics literature searches, reviewed and presented the evidence to the GDG, managed the process, and contributed to the drafting of the guideline.

3.2.1 Guideline Development Group meetings

Twenty-three eating disorders GDG meetings were held between March 2002 and October 2003. During the series of day-long meetings, clinical questions were written, clinical evidence was reviewed and assessed, statements developed and recommendations formulated. At each meeting, all GDG members declared any potential conflict of interests, and patient and carer concerns were routinely discussed as part of a standing agenda.

3.2.2 Topic groups

The GDG divided its workload along clinically relevant lines to simplify the guideline development process by forming smaller topic groups to undertake guideline work in specified areas of clinical practice. Topic groups covered physical management, service-level interventions, and psychological interventions. These groups were designed to efficiently manage the large volume of evidence appraisal prior to presenting it to the GDG as a whole. Each topic group was chaired by a GDG member with expert knowledge of the topic area (one of the healthcare professionals). Topic groups refined the clinical definitions of treatment interventions, identified relevant clinical questions, reviewed and prepared the evidence with the systematic reviewer before presenting it to the GDG as a whole, and helped the GDG to identify further expertise in the topic. Topic group leaders reported the status of the group's work as part of the standing agenda. They also introduced and led the GDG discussion of the evidence review for that topic and assisted the GDG Chair in drafting that Section of the guideline relevant to the work of each topic group.

3.2.3 Patients and carers

The GDG included a patient and representatives of a national patient group. Given their direct experience of services, they gave an integral patient focus to the GDG and the guideline. They contributed as full GDG members to writing the clinical questions, helping to ensure that the evidence addressed their views and preferences, highlighting sensitive issues and terminology associated with eating disorders, and bringing service-user research to the attention of the GDG. They wrote the section on the patient perspective, organised, conducted and reported on the carer focus group contribution, and identified recommendations from the patient and carer perspective.

The carer perspective was provided through a focus group held with carers. The main objective of the group discussion was to discuss carers' views about communication with clinicians and other professionals, including guidance on responsibility and expectations of clinicians, carers, and people with eating disorders; the role of carers in identifying eating disorders and subsequent treatment, and accessing appropriate services. Twelve people, currently caring for someone with anorexia nervosa as a parent or spouse, were recruited by the Eating Disorders Association and the Carers Volunteers Database at the Eating Disorders Research Unit of the Institute of Psychiatry. Geographic distribution of members included Cornwall, the Midlands, East Anglia, south east England and London. Participants were told the purpose of the session, and signed a participant consent form. Discussions were tape-recorded with the full knowledge of the participants, transcribed, and key themes identified.

3.2.4 Special advisors

Special advisors who had specific expertise in one or more aspects of the treatment and management of eating disorders were invited to assist the GDG, to comment on specific aspects of the developing guideline and to present evidence and observations on areas of their expertise to the GDG. Appendix 2 lists those who agreed to act as special advisors.

3.2.5 National and international experts

National and international experts in eating disorders research were identified through the literature search and through the experience of the GDG members. These experts were invited to recommend unpublished or soon-to-be published studies in order to ensure that the most recent evidence on the management of eating disorders was included in the development of the guideline. They informed the group about completed trials at the pre-publication stage, systematic reviews in the process of being published, studies relating to the cost-effectiveness of treatment, and trial data if the GDG could be provided with full access to the complete trial report. Appendix 5 lists researchers who were contacted.

3.3 Clinical questions

Clinical questions were used to guide the identification and interrogation of the evidence base relating to the use of psychological interventions, service-level interventions, and physical interventions in the treatment and management of eating disorders. The GDG necessarily had to limit the number of questions to those they regarded as important. Questions were developed for each clinical topic area. Appendix 6 lists the clinical questions.

3.4 Systematic clinical literature review strategies

The aim of the clinical literature review was to systematically identify and synthesise relevant evidence from the literature in order to answer specific clinical questions developed by the GDG. Thus, clinical practice recommendations are evidence-based, where possible, and if evidence is not available, gaps are identified where future research is needed.

3.4.1 Methodology

A stepwise, hierarchical approach was taken to locating and presenting evidence to the GDG. The NCCMH review team had developed this process based on advice from the National Guidelines Support and Research Unit (NICE) and after considering recommendations from a range of other sources. These included:

- Centre for Clinical Policy and Practice of the New South Wales Health Department (Australia)

- Clinical Evidence Online

- Cochrane Collaboration

- New Zealand Guideline Group

- NHS Centre for Reviews and Dissemination

- Oxford Centre for Evidence-Based Medicine

- Scottish Intercollegiate Guidelines Network (SIGN)

- United States Agency for Health Research and Quality

- Oxford Systematic Review Development Programme.

3.4.2 The review process

3.4.2.1   Questions of treatment efficacy

For questions related to the efficacy of treatment, the initial evidence base was formed from high-quality, recently published or updated randomised controlled trials (RCTs) that addressed at least one of the clinical questions developed by the GDG. Systematic reviews were selected on predetermined quality criteria. Further searches for new RCTs were undertaken. New RCTs meeting inclusion criteria set by the GDG were incorporated into existing systematic reviews and fresh analyses performed. If no systematic reviews were available, the review team located all relevant high quality RCTs for review and, where appropriate, meta-analysis. The review process is illustrated in Flowchart 1 overleaf.

Although there are a number of difficulties with the use of RCTs in the evaluation of interventions in mental health, some of which also apply to the use of RCTs in any health research, the RCT remains the most important method for establishing efficacy. However, in some cases it was not possible to identify high-quality systematic reviews or a substantial body of RCTs that directly addressed a clinical question. In this situation, an informal consensus process was adopted (see Section 3.4.7). Future guidelines on the treatment and management of eating disorders will be able to update and extend the usable evidence base starting from the evidence collected, synthesised and analysed for this guideline.

3.4.2.2   Questions of diagnosis and prognosis

For questions related to diagnosis and prognosis, the initial evidence base was formed from studies with the most appropriate and reliable design to answer the particular question (i.e, diagnosis – cross sectional studies; prognosis – cohort studies of representative patients). The review process was similar to that described for questions of efficacy. The main difference concerned the study search filter and the criteria used to assess methodological quality. In situations where it was not possible to identify high-quality systematic reviews or a substantial body of appropriately designed studies that directly addressed a clinical question, an informal consensus process was adopted (see Section 3.4.7).

Flowchart 1: Eating disorders Guideline Review Process

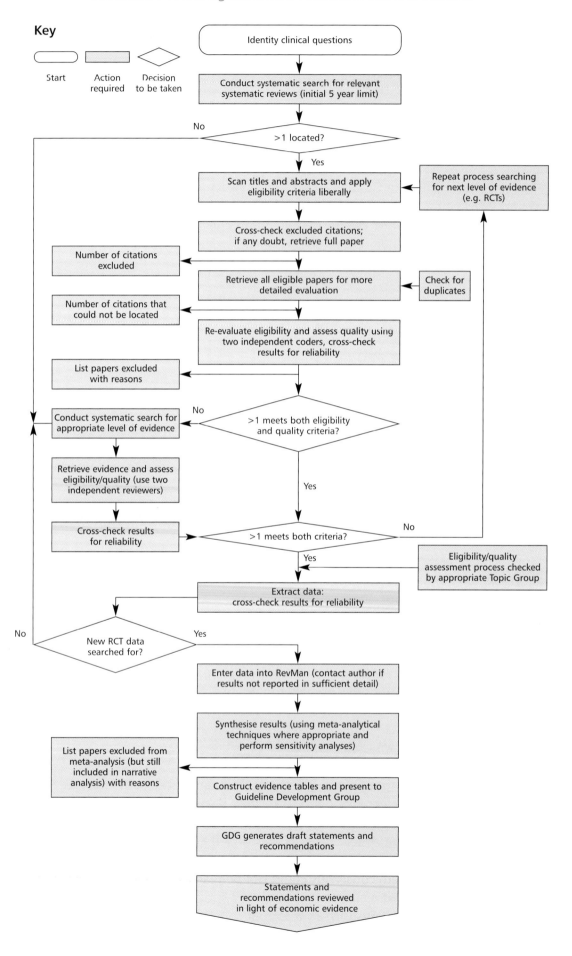

Key

Start | Action required | Decision to be taken

- Identity clinical questions
- Conduct systematic search for relevant systematic reviews (initial 5 year limit)
- >1 located? — No / Yes
- Scan titles and abstracts and apply eligibility criteria liberally
- Repeat process searching for next level of evidence (e.g. RCTs)
- Cross-check excluded citations; if any doubt, retrieve full paper
- Number of citations excluded
- Retrieve all eligible papers for more detailed evaluation
- Check for duplicates
- Number of citations that could not be located
- Re-evaluate eligibility and assess quality using two independent coders, cross-check results for reliability
- List papers excluded with reasons
- >1 meets both eligibility and quality criteria? — No / Yes
- Conduct systematic search for appropriate level of evidence
- Retrieve evidence and assess eligibility/quality (use two independent reviewers)
- Cross-check results for reliability
- >1 meets both criteria? — Yes / No
- Eligibility/quality assessment process checked by appropriate Topic Group
- Extract data: cross-check results for reliability
- New RCT data searched for? — No / Yes
- Enter data into RevMan (contact author if results not reported in sufficient detail)
- Synthesise results (using meta-analytical techniques where appropriate and perform sensitivity analyses)
- List papers excluded from meta-analysis (but still included in narrative analysis) with reasons
- Construct evidence tables and present to Guideline Development Group
- GDG generates draft statements and recommendations
- Statements and recommendations reviewed in light of economic evidence

3.4.3 Search strategies

In conducting the review, the team systematically searched the literature for all English-language systematic reviews relevant to the eating disorders scope that were published or updated after 1995.

Search filters developed by the review team consisted of a combination of subject heading and free-text phrases. A general filter was developed for eating disorders along with more specific filters for each clinical question. In addition, filters were developed for RCTs and for other appropriate research designs. (The search filters can be found in Appendix 8.)

Electronic searches were made of the major bibliographic databases (MEDLINE, EMBASE, PsycINFO, CINAHL), in addition to the Cochrane Database of Systematic Reviews, the NHS R&D Health Technology Assessment database, Evidence-Based Mental Health and Clinical Evidence (Issue 5).

Ineligible articles were excluded, and a second independent reviewer crosschecked these for relevance. The remaining references were acquired in full and re-evaluated for eligibility. The most recently published reviews that appropriately addressed a clinical question were selected. For each systematic review used, a search was made for new studies, and the papers for these and for existing studies, were retrieved.

The search for further evidence included research published after each review's search date, in-press papers identified by experts, and reviewing reference lists and recent contents of selected journals. All reports that were retrieved but later excluded are listed with reasons for exclusion in the appropriate evidence table. Where no relevant systematic reviews were located, the review team asked the GDG to decide whether a fresh systematic review should be undertaken. Eligible reviews were critically appraised for methodological quality and the reliability of this procedure was confirmed by parallel independent assessment. The eligibility/quality assessment was tested on a representative sample of papers. (Appendix 10 provides the quality checklist.)

3.4.4 Synthesising the evidence

Where possible, outcome data were extracted directly from all eligible studies that met the quality criteria into Review Manager 4.2 (Cochrane Collaboration, 2003). Meta-analysis was then used to synthesise the evidence where appropriate using Review Manager. If necessary, reanalyses of the data or sensitivity analyses were used to answer clinical questions not addressed in the original studies or reviews. Where meta-analysis was not appropriate and/or possible, the reported results from each primary-level study were entered into the Access database. Evidence tables were used to summarise general information about each study. Consultation was used to overcome difficulties with coding. Data from studies included in existing systematic reviews were extracted independently by one reviewer directly into Review Manager and crosschecked with the existing data set. Two independent reviewers extracted data from new studies, and disagreements were resolved by discussion. Where consensus could not be reached, a third reviewer resolved the disagreement. Masked assessment (i.e. blind to the journal from which the article comes, the authors, the institution, and the magnitude of the effect) was not used since it is unclear that doing so reduces bias (Jadad *et al.*, 1996; Berlin, 1997).

3.4.5 Presenting the data to the GDG

Where possible, the GDG was given a graphical presentation of the results using forest plots generated with the Review Manager software. Each forest plot displayed the effect size and confidence interval (CI) for each study as well as the overall summary statistic. The graphs were organised so that the display of data in the area to the left of the 'line of no effect' indicated a 'favourable' outcome for the treatment in question. Dichotomous outcomes were presented as relative risks (RR) and the associated 95 per cent CI (see Figure 1). A relative risk (or risk ratio) is the ratio of the treatment event rate to the control event rate. A RR of 1 indicates no difference between treatment and control. In Figure 1, the overall RR of 0.73 indicates that the event rate (i.e. non-remission rate) associated with intervention A is about three-quarters of that with the control intervention, or in other words, intervention A reduces non-remission rates by 27 per cent. In addition, the CI around the RR does not cross the 'line of no effect' indicating that this is a statistically significant effect. The CI shows with 95 per cent certainty the range within which the true treatment effect should lie.

All dichotomous outcomes were calculated on an intention-to-treat basis (i.e. a 'once-randomised-always-analyse' basis). This assumes that those participants who ceased to engage in the study – from whatever group – had an unfavourable outcome (with the exception of the outcome of 'death'). The Number Needed to Treat (NNT) or the Number Needed to Harm (NNH) was reported for each statistically significant outcome where the baseline risk (i.e., control group event rate) was similar across studies. In addition, NNTs calculated at follow-up were only reported where the length of follow-up was similar across studies. When length of follow-up or baseline risk varies (especially with low risk), the NNT is a poor summary of the treatment effect (Deeks, 2002).

Figure 1. Example of a forest plot displaying dichotomous data

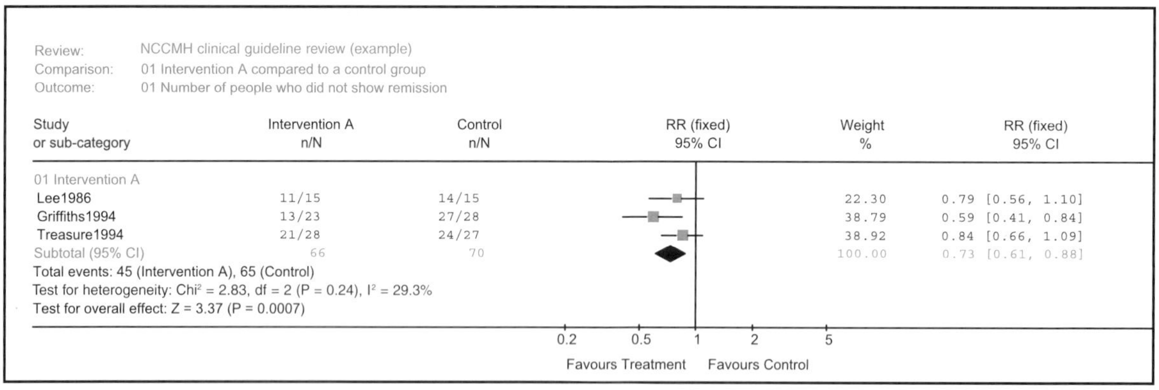

Figure 2. Example of a forest plot displaying continuous data

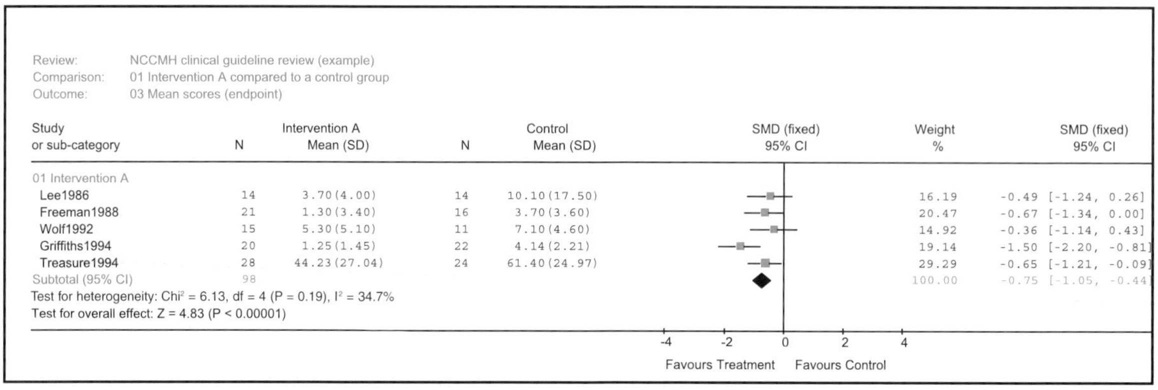

Both the I^2 test of heterogeneity and the chi-squared test of heterogeneity ($p <0.10$) were used, as well as visual inspection of the forest plots, to look for the possibility of heterogeneity. I^2 describes the proportion of total variation in study estimates that is due to heterogeneity (Higgins & Thompson, 2002). An I^2 of less than 30 per cent was taken to indicate mild heterogeneity and a fixed effects model was used to synthesise the results. An I^2 of more than 50 per cent was taken as notable heterogeneity. In this case an attempt was made to explain the variation. If studies with heterogeneous results were found to be comparable, a random effects model was used to summarise the results (DerSimonian & Laird, 1986). In the random effects analysis, heterogeneity is accounted for both in the width of CIs and in the estimate of the treatment effect. With decreasing heterogeneity the random effects approach moves asymptotically towards a fixed effects model. An I^2 of 30 to 50 per cent was taken to indicate moderate heterogeneity. In this case, both the chi-squared test of heterogeneity and a visual inspection of the forest plot was used to decide between a fixed and random effects model.

To explore the possibility that the results entered into each meta-analysis suffered from publication bias, data from included studies were entered, where there was sufficient data, into a funnel plot. Asymmetry of the plot was taken to indicate possible publication bias and investigated further.

3.4.6 Forming and grading the statements and recommendations

The evidence tables and forest plots formed the basis for developing clinical statements and recommendations. For intervention studies, the statements were classified according to an accepted hierarchy of evidence. Recommendations were then graded A to C based on the level of associated evidence (see Table 1 overleaf). Key priorities for implementation are denoted by an asterisk following the grade.

In order to facilitate consistency in generating and drafting the clinical statements the GDG utilised a statement decision tree (see Flowchart 2). The flowchart was designed to assist with, but not replace clinical judgement.

Where a statistically significant summary statistic (effect size; ES) was obtained (after controlling for heterogeneity), the GDG considered whether this finding was of clinical significance (i.e. likely to be of benefit to patients) taking into account the trial population, nature of the outcome and size of the effect. On the basis of this consideration the ES was characterised as 'clinically significant' or not. A further consideration was made about the strength of the evidence by examining the CI surrounding the ES. For level I evidence, where the ES was judged to be clinically significant and had a CI entirely within a clinical relevant range, the result was characterised as 'strong evidence' (S1, Flowchart 2). For non-level I evidence or in situations where the upper/lower bound of the CI was not clinically significant, the result was characterised as 'limited evidence' (S2). Where an ES was statistically significant, but not clinically significant and the CI excluded values judged to be clinically important, the result was characterised as 'unlikely to be clinically significant' (S3). Alternatively, if the CI included clinically important values, the result was characterised as 'insufficient to determine clinical significance' (S6).

Table 1: Hierarchy of evidence and recommendations grading scheme

Level	Type of evidence	Grade	Evidence
I	Evidence obtained from a single randomised controlled trial or a meta-analysis of randomised controlled trials	A	At least one randomised controlled trial as part of a body of literature of overall good quality and consistency addressing the specific recommendation (evidence level I) without extrapolation
IIa	Evidence obtained from at least one well-designed controlled study without randomisation	B	Well-conducted clinical studies but no randomised clinical trials on the topic of recommendation (evidence levels II or III); or extrapolated from level I evidence
IIb	Evidence obtained from at least one other well-designed quasi-experimental study		
III	Evidence obtained from well-designed non-experimental descriptive studies, such as comparative studies, correlation studies and case-control studies		
IV	Evidence obtained from expert committee reports or opinions and/or clinical experiences of respected authorities	C	Expert committee reports or opinions and/or clinical experiences of respected authorities (evidence level IV) or extrapolated from level I or II evidence. This grading indicates that directly applicable clinical studies of good quality are absent or not readily available

Adapted from Eccles, M. & Mason, J. (2001), *How to develop cost-conscious guidelines. Health Technology Assessment 5* (16).

Flowchart 2: Guideline Statement Decision Tree

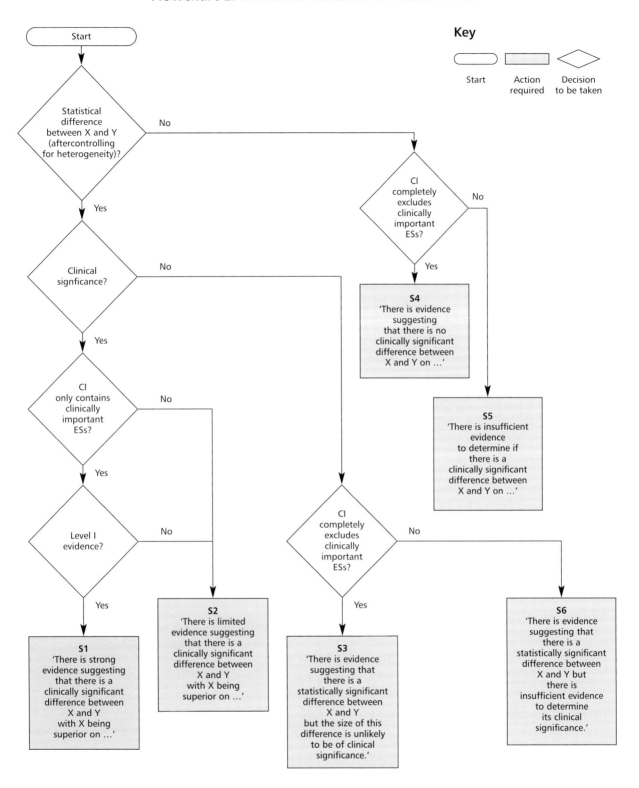

Key

Start — Action required — Decision to be taken

Start

Statistical difference between X and Y (aftercontrolling for heterogeneity)?

No → **CI completely excludes clinically important ESs?**

No → **S5** 'There is insufficient evidence to determine if there is a clinically significant difference between X and Y on …'

Yes → **S4** 'There is evidence suggesting that there is no clinically significant difference between X and Y on …'

Yes → **Clinical signficance?**

No → **CI completely excludes clinically important ESs?**

No → **S6** 'There is evidence suggesting that there is a statistically significant difference between X and Y but there is insufficient evidence to determine its clinical significance.'

Yes → **S3** 'There is evidence suggesting that there is a statistically significant difference between X and Y but the size of this difference is unlikely to be of clinical significance.'

Yes → **CI only contains clinically important ESs?**

No → **S2** 'There is limited evidence suggesting that there is a clinically significant difference between X and Y with X being superior on …'

Yes → **Level I evidence?**

No → **S2** 'There is limited evidence suggesting that there is a clinically significant difference between X and Y with X being superior on …'

Yes → **S1** 'There is strong evidence suggesting that there is a clinically significant difference between X and Y with X being superior on …'

Where a non-statistically significant ES was obtained, the GDG reviewed the trial population, nature of the outcome, size of the effect and, in particular, the CI surrounding the result. If the CI was narrow and excluded a clinically significant ES, this was seen as indicating evidence of 'no clinically significant difference' (S4), but where the CI was wide this was seen as indicating 'insufficient evidence' to determine if there was a clinically significant difference or not (S5).

Once all evidence statements relating to a particular clinical question were finalised and agreed by the GDG, the associated recommendations were produced and graded. Grading the recommendations allowed the GDG to distinguish between the level of evidence and the strength of the associated recommendation. It is possible that a statement of evidence would cover only one part of an area in which a recommendation was to be made or would cover it in a way that would conflict with other evidence. In order to produce more comprehensive recommendations suitable for people in England and Wales, the GDG had to extrapolate from the available evidence. This led to a weaker level of recommendation (i.e. B, as data were based upon level I evidence). It is important to note that the grading of the recommendation is not a reflection of its clinical significance or relevance.

A number of issues relating to the study of eating disorders (see Section 3.4.8) meant that the outcomes available for analysis were classified as primary or secondary. When making recommendations, the primary outcomes were given more weight during the decision process.

The process also allowed the GDG to moderate recommendations based on factors other than the strength of evidence. Such considerations include the applicability of the evidence to people with eating disorders, economic considerations, values of the development group and society, or the group's awareness of practical issues (Eccles *et al.*, 1998).

3.4.7 Method used to answer a clinical question in the absence of appropriately designed, high-quality research

Where it was not possible to identify at least one appropriately designed study or high-quality systematic review, or where the GDG was of the opinion (on the basis of previous searches or their knowledge of the literature) that there was unlikely to be appropriately designed primary-level research that directly addressed the clinical question, an informal consensus process was adopted. This process focused on those questions that the GDG considered a priority.

The starting point for this process of informal consensus was that a member of the topic group identified, with help from the systematic reviewer, a narrative review that most directly addressed the clinical question. Where this was not possible a new review of the recent literature was initiated.

This existing narrative review or new review was used as a basis for identifying lower levels of evidence relevant to the clinical question. This was then presented for discussion to the GDG. On the basis of this, additional information was sought and added to the information collected. This may include studies that did not directly address the clinical question but were thought to contain relevant data. This led to the development of an initial draft report that addressed the following issues:

● A description of what is known about the issues concerning the clinical question.

● A brief review of the existing evidence, including RCTs, non-randomised controlled studies, cohort studies and other studies that help answer the question.

● The summary of the evidence so far obtained. This was then presented in narrative form to the GDG and further comments were sought about the evidence and its perceived relevance to the clinical question.

● If, during the course of preparing the report, a significant body of primary-level studies (of appropriate design to answer the question) were identified, a full systematic review was done.

● At this time, subject possibly to further reviews of the evidence, a series of statements that directly addressed the clinical question were developed.

● Following this, on occasions and as deemed appropriate by the development group, the report was then sent to appointed experts outside of the GDG for peer review and comment. The information from this process was then fed back to the GDG for further discussion of the statements.

● Recommendations were then developed and could also be sent for further external peer review.

● After this final stage of comment, the statements and recommendations were again reviewed and agreed upon by the GDG.

3.4.8 Issues concerning research on eating disorders

Studying the treatment of eating disorders presents certain particular challenges. First, since psychological treatments have a major role in their management, the methods needed to evaluate psychotherapeutic treatments have to be adopted. Some of these are mentioned in the national clinical practice guideline on schizophrenia (Kendall et al., 2003) including the need for some degree of standardisation of the psychological treatment provided (usually in the form of a treatment manual) and the importance of quality assessment and control. Additional refinements have been included in some eating disorder studies including the use of 'dismantling' research designs to identify the active components of psychological treatments (e.g. Fairburn et al., 1991, 1993); studies of the mediators of psychological treatments, a stage towards the identification of their mechanism of action (e.g. Wilson et al., 2002); fine-grain comparisons of different ways of implementing specific psychotherapeutic procedures (e.g. Bulik et al., 1998); and 'effectiveness' studies of simplified psychological treatments designed for general dissemination (e.g. Carter & Fairburn, 1998).

The second challenge is the measurement of outcome. Eating disorders affect many aspects of functioning including behaviour (e.g. eating habits), attitudes and values (e.g. the evaluation of shape and weight), psychosocial functioning (e.g. levels of depression and anxiety; interpersonal functioning) and physical health (e.g. body weight, serum electrolytes) (Fairburn & Harrison, 2003). It is also usual for there to be comorbidity with Axis I and II disorders co-existing with the eating disorder (Bulik, 2002). Therefore, most treatment studies employ a range of different outcome measures to determine whether the treatments studied affect all or part of the psychopathology present. Having said this, there are accepted primary outcome variables that treatments must influence if they can be said to have an impact on the core eating disorder. For anorexia nervosa, the primary outcome variable is body weight adjusted for height, usually represented as the BMI or the percentage of expected weight for the person's age, height and sex. For bulimia nervosa the comparable variable is the frequency of binge eating and 'purging' (self-induced vomiting or the use of laxatives to influence body shape or weight); that is, the frequency of these forms of behaviour over a set period of time (usually one or four weeks). In addition, it is now established practice to report the proportion of participants who no longer practise the behaviour (sometime referred to as the 'abstinence' rates). For binge eating disorder the primary outcome variable is the frequency of binge eating, represented as for bulimia nervosa. An important point to note is that the frequency of binge eating and purging is skewed rather than being normally distributed so these data have to be transformed prior to analysis. However, because most reports give uncorrected means and standard deviations, the GDG gave less weight to frequency data than abstinence rates when making recommendations.

The third challenge is determining whether treatment effects persist over time. Anorexia nervosa and bulimia nervosa tend to run a chronic course so short-lived treatment effects are of limited clinical significance. Thus it has become established research practice to follow-up patients following the end of treatment to see whether any changes last, and with interventions that are known to be associated with a high rate of relapse (e.g. inpatient treatment of anorexia nervosa) there have been attempts to develop and evaluate subsequent 'relapse prevention' strategies (e.g. Kaye *et al.*, 2001; Pike *et al.*, 2003).

The fourth challenge is largely peculiar to research on the treatment of anorexia nervosa. It is exceptionally difficult recruiting cases for treatment studies. This is for a number of reasons. First, anorexia nervosa is uncommon. Second, it can be life-threatening with the result that it is not ethical to recruit certain patients. And third, patients with anorexia nervosa are notoriously reluctant to have treatment and this reluctance can be magnified if the clinician raises the possibility of taking part in a research trial. For these reasons the few studies of the treatment of anorexia nervosa have mostly involved small numbers of patients. As a result it is difficult to draw robust evidence-based conclusions about the treatment of the disorder.

3.5 Health economics review strategies

The aim of the health economics review was to contribute to the guideline development process. Data on the economic burden of eating disorders and evidence of cost-effectiveness of the different treatment options for eating disorders were collected and assessed in order to help the decision-making process. See Chapter 9, Health Economics Evidence, for the detailed review strategies.

3.6 Stakeholder contributions

Professionals, patients, and companies have contributed to and commented on the eating disorders guideline at key stages in its development. Stakeholders for this guideline include:

- Patient/carer stakeholders: the national patient and carer organisations that represent people whose care is described in this guideline

- Professional stakeholders: the national organisations that represent healthcare professionals who are providing services to patients

- Commercial stakeholders: the companies that manufacture medicines used in the treatment of eating disorders

- Primary Care Trusts

- Department of Health and Welsh Assembly Government.

Stakeholders have been involved in the guideline's development at the following points:

- Commenting on the initial scope of the guideline with patient organisation stakeholders attending a briefing meeting held by NICE

- Contributing lists of evidence to the GDG

- Commenting on the first and second drafts of the guideline.

3.7 Validation of this guideline

This guideline has been validated through two consultation exercises. The first consultation draft was submitted to the NICE Guidelines Review Panel, and circulated to stakeholders, special advisors, and other reviewers nominated by GDG members.

After taking into account comments from stakeholders, the NICE Guidelines Review Panel, a number of health authority and trust representatives and a wide range of national and international experts from this round of consultation, the GDG responded to all comments and prepared a final consultation draft which was submitted to NICE, circulated to all stakeholders for final comments and posted on the website for public consultation. The final draft was then submitted to the NICE Guidelines Review Panel for review prior to publication.

4 Summary of recommendations

Anorexia nervosa

- Most adults with anorexia nervosa should be managed on an outpatient basis with psychological treatment provided by a service that is competent in giving that treatment and assessing the physical risk of people with eating disorders.

- People with anorexia nervosa requiring inpatient treatment should normally be admitted to a setting that can provide the skilled implementation of refeeding with careful physical monitoring (particularly in the first few days of refeeding) and in combination with psychosocial interventions.

- Family interventions that directly address the eating disorder should be offered to children and adolescents with anorexia nervosa.

Bulimia nervosa

- As a possible first step, patients with bulimia nervosa should be encouraged to follow an evidence-based self-help programme.

- As an alternative or additional first step to using an evidence-based self-help programme, adults with bulimia nervosa may be offered a trial of an antidepressant drug.

- Cognitive behaviour therapy for bulimia nervosa (CBT-BN), a specifically adapted form of CBT, should be offered to adults with bulimia nervosa. The course of treatment should be for 16 to 20 sessions over four to five months.

- Adolescents with bulimia nervosa may be treated with CBT-BN, adapted as needed to suit their age, circumstances, level of development, and including the family as appropriate.

Atypical eating disorders

- In the absence of evidence to guide the management of atypical eating disorders (also known as eating disorders not otherwise specified) other than binge eating disorder, it is recommended that the clinician considers following the guidance on the treatment of the eating problem that most closely resembles the individual patient's eating disorder.

- Cognitive behaviour therapy for binge eating disorder (CBT-BED), a specifically adapted form of CBT, should be offered to adults with binge eating disorder.

For all eating disorders

●   Family members including siblings should normally be included in the treatment of children and adolescents with eating disorders. Interventions may include sharing of information, advice on behavioural management and facilitating communication.

The following guidance is evidence-based. All evidence was classified according to a accepted hierarchy of evidence that was originally adapted from the US Agency for Healthcare Policy and Research Classification. Recommendations were then graded A to C based on the level of associated evidence. This grading scheme is based on a scheme formulated by the Clinical Outcomes Group of the NHS Executive (1996) and is described in Section 3.4.6; a summary of the evidence on which the guidance is based is provided in Chapters 5 through 8.

4.1 Introduction

This guideline makes recommendations for the identification, treatment and management of anorexia nervosa, bulimia nervosa, and atypical eating disorders (including binge eating disorder) in primary, secondary and tertiary care.

4.2 Care across all conditions

4.2.1 Assessment and co-ordination of care

4.2.1.1   Assessment of people with eating disorders should be comprehensive and include physical, psychological and social needs, and a comprehensive assessment of risk to self. (C)

4.2.1.2   The level of risk to the patient's mental and physical health should be monitored as treatment progresses because it may change – for example following weight change or at times of transition between services in cases of anorexia nervosa. (C)

4.2.1.3   For people with eating disorders presenting in primary care, GPs should take responsibility for the initial assessment and the initial co-ordination of care. This includes the determination of the need for emergency medical or psychiatric assessment. (C)

4.2.1.4   Where management is shared between primary and secondary care, there should be clear agreement amongst individual health care professionals on the responsibility for monitoring patients with eating disorders. This agreement should be in writing (where appropriate using the care programme approach) and should be shared with the patient and, where appropriate, their families and carers. (C)

4.2.2 Providing good information and support

4.2.2.1   Patients and, where appropriate, carers should be provided with education and information on the nature, course and treatment of eating disorders. (C)

4.2.2.2   In addition to the provision of information, family and carers may be informed of self-help groups and support groups and offered the opportunity to participate in such groups where they exist. (C)

4.2.2.3   Health care professionals should acknowledge that many people with eating disorders are ambivalent about treatment. Health care professionals should also recognise the consequent demands and challenges this presents. (C)

4.2.3 Getting help early

There can be serious long-term consequences to a delay in obtaining treatment.

4.2.3.1   People with eating disorders should be assessed and receive treatment at the earliest opportunity. (C)

4.2.3.2   Whenever possible patients should be engaged and treated before reaching severe emaciation. This requires both early identification and intervention. Effective monitoring and engagement of patients at severely low weight or with falling weight should be a priority. (C)

4.2.4 Management of physical aspects

4.2.4.1   Where laxative abuse is present, patients should be advised to gradually reduce laxative use and informed that laxative use does not significantly reduce calorie absorption. (C)

4.2.4.2   Treatment of both subthreshold and clinical cases of an eating disorder in people with diabetes is essential because of the greatly increased physical risk in this group. (C)

4.2.4.3   People with Type 1 diabetes and an eating disorder should have intensive regular physical monitoring because they are at high-risk of retinopathy and other complications. (C)

4.2.4.4   Pregnant women with eating disorders require careful monitoring throughout the pregnancy and in the post-partum period. (C)

4.2.4.5   Patients who are vomiting should have regular dental reviews. (C)

4.2.4.6   Patients who are vomiting should be given appropriate advice on dental hygiene, which should include avoiding brushing after vomiting, rinsing with a non-acid mouthwash after vomiting, and reducing an acid oral environment (for example, limiting acidic foods). (C)

4.2.4.7   Health care professionals should advise people with eating disorders and osteoporosis or related bone disorders to refrain from physical activities that significantly increase the likelihood of falls. (C)

4.2.5 Additional considerations for children and adolescents

4.2.5.1   Family members including siblings, should normally be included in the treatment of children and adolescents with eating disorders. Interventions may include sharing of information, advice on behavioural management and facilitating communication. (C)

4.2.5.2   In children and adolescents with eating disorders, growth and development should be closely monitored. Where development is delayed or growth stunted despite adequate nutrition, paediatric advice should be sought. (C)

4.2.5.3   Health care professionals assessing children and adolescents with eating disorders should be alert to indicators of abuse (emotional, physical and sexual) and should remain so throughout treatment. (C)

4.2.5.4   The right to confidentiality of children and adolescents with eating disorders should be respected. (C)

4.2.5.5   Health care professionals working with children and adolescents with eating disorders should familiarise themselves with national guidelines and their employers' policies in the area of confidentiality. (C)

4.3 Identification and screening of eating disorders in primary care and non-mental health settings

4.3.1.1   Target groups for screening should include young women with low body mass index (BMI) compared with age norms, patients consulting with weight concerns who are not overweight, women with menstrual disturbances or amenorrhoea, patients with gastrointestinal symptoms, patients with physical signs of starvation or repeated vomiting and children with poor growth. (C)

4.3.1.2   When screening for eating disorders one or two simple questions should be considered for use with specific target groups (for example, 'Do you think you have an eating problem?' and 'Do you worry excessively about your weight?') (C)

4.3.1.3   Young people with Type 1 diabetes and poor treatment adherence should be screened and assessed for the presence of an eating disorder. (C)

4.4 Anorexia nervosa

4.4.1 Management of anorexia nervosa in primary care

4.4.1.1   In anorexia nervosa, although weight and body mass index (BMI) are important indicators of physical risk they should not be considered the sole indicators (as on their on they are unreliable in adults and especially in children). (C)

4.4.1.2   In assessing whether a person has anorexia nervosa, attention should be paid to the overall clinical assessment (repeated over time), including rate of weight loss, growth rates in children, objective physical signs and appropriate laboratory tests. (C)

4.4.1.3   Patients with enduring anorexia nervosa not under the care of a secondary care service should be offered an annual physical and mental health review by their GP. (C)

4.4.2 Psychological interventions for anorexia nervosa

The delivery of psychological interventions should be accompanied by regular monitoring of a patient's physical state including weight and specific indicators of increased physical risk.

Common elements of the psychological treatment of anorexia nervosa

4.4.2.1   Therapies to be considered for the psychological treatment of anorexia nervosa include cognitive analytic therapy (CAT), cognitive behaviour therapy (CBT), interpersonal psychotherapy (IPT), focal psychodynamic therapy and family interventions focused explicitly on eating disorders. (C)

4.4.2.2   Patient and, where appropriate, carer preference should be taken into account in deciding which psychological treatment is to be offered. (C)

4.4.2.3   The aims of psychological treatment should be to reduce risk, encourage weight gain, healthy eating, and reduce other symptoms related to an eating disorder, and to facilitate psychological and physical recovery. (C)

Outpatient psychological treatments in first episode and later episodes

4.4.2.4   Most people with anorexia nervosa should be managed on an outpatient basis with psychological treatment (with physical monitoring) provided by a health care professional competent to give it and to assess the physical risk of people with eating disorders. (C)

4.4.2.5   Outpatient psychological treatment and physical monitoring for anorexia nervosa should normally be of at least six months' duration. (C)

4.4.2.6   For patients with anorexia nervosa, if during outpatient psychological treatment there is significant deterioration, or the completion of an adequate course of outpatient psychological treatment does not lead to any significant improvement, more intensive forms of treatment (for example, a move from individual therapy to combined individual and family work or day care, or inpatient care) should be considered. (C)

4.4.2.7   Dietary counselling should not be provided as the sole treatment for anorexia nervosa. (C)

Psychological aspects of inpatient care

4.4.2.8   For inpatients with anorexia nervosa, a structured symptom-focused treatment regimen with the expectation of weight gain should be provided in order to achieve weight restoration. It is important to carefully monitor the patient's physical status during refeeding. (C)

4.4.2.9   Psychological treatment should be provided which has a focus both on eating behaviour and attitudes to weight and shape, and wider psychosocial issues with the expectation of weight gain. (C)

4.4.2.10   Rigid inpatient behaviour modification programmes should not be used in the management of anorexia nervosa. (C)

Post-hospitalisation psychological treatment

4.4.2.11   Following inpatient weight restoration people with anorexia nervosa should be offered outpatient psychological treatment that focuses both on eating behaviour and attitudes to weight and shape, and wider psychosocial issues with regular monitoring of both physical and psychological risk. (C)

4.4.2.12   The length of outpatient psychological treatment and physical monitoring following inpatient weight restoration should typically be at least 12 months. (C)

Additional considerations for children and adolescents with anorexia nervosa

4.4.2.13   Family interventions that directly address the eating disorder should be offered to children and adolescents with anorexia nervosa. (B)

4.4.2.14   Children and adolescents with anorexia nervosa should be offered individual appointments with a health care professional separate from those with their family members or carers. (C)

4.4.2.15   The therapeutic involvement of siblings and other family members should be considered in all cases because of the effects of anorexia nervosa on other family members. (C)

4.4.2.16   In children and adolescents with anorexia nervosa the need for inpatient treatment and the need for urgent weight restoration should be balanced alongside the educational and social needs of the young person. (C)

4.4.3 Pharmacological interventions for anorexia nervosa

There is a very limited evidence base for the pharmacological treatment of anorexia nervosa. A range of drugs may be used in the treatment of comorbid conditions but caution should be exercised in their use given the physical vulnerability of many people with anorexia nervosa.

4.4.3.1   Medication should not be used as the sole or primary treatment for anorexia nervosa. (C)

4.4.3.2   Caution should be exercised in the use of medication for comorbid conditions such as depressive or obsessive-compulsive features as they may resolve with weight gain alone. (C)

4.4.3.3   When medication is used to treat people with anorexia nervosa, the side effects of drug treatment (in particular, cardiac side effects) should be carefully considered because of the compromised cardiovascular function of many people with anorexia nervosa. (C)

4.4.3.4   Health care professionals should be aware of the risk of drugs that prolong the QTc interval on the ECG; for example, antipsychotics, tricyclic antidepressants, macrolide antibiotics, and some antihistamines. In patients with anorexia nervosa at risk of cardiac complications, the prescription of drugs with side effects that may compromise cardiac function should be avoided. (C)

4.4.3.5   If the prescription of medication that may compromise cardiac functioning is essential, ECG monitoring should be undertaken. (C)

4.4.3.6   All patients with a diagnosis of anorexia nervosa should have an alert placed in their prescribing record concerning the risk of side effects. (C)

4.4.4 Physical management of anorexia nervosa

Anorexia nervosa carries considerable risk of serious physical morbidity. Awareness of the risk, careful monitoring and, where appropriate, close liaison with an experienced physician are important in the management of the physical complications of anorexia nervosa.

Managing weight gain

4.4.4.1   In most patients with anorexia nervosa an average weekly weight gain of 0.5 to 1 kg in inpatient settings and 0.5 kg in outpatient settings should be an aim of treatment. This requires about 3500 to 7000 extra calories a week. (C)

4.4.4.2   Regular physical monitoring, and in some cases treatment with a multi-vitamin/multi-mineral supplement in oral form is recommended for people with anorexia nervosa during both inpatient and outpatient weight restoration. (C)

4.4.4.3   Total parenteral nutrition should not be used for people with anorexia nervosa, unless there is significant gastrointestinal dysfunction. (C)

Managing risk

4.4.4.4   Health care professionals should monitor physical risk in patients with anorexia nervosa. If this leads to the identification of increased physical risk, the frequency and the monitoring and nature of the investigations should be adjusted accordingly. (C)

4.4.4.5   People with anorexia nervosa and their carers should be informed if the risk to their physical health is high. (C)

4.4.4.6   The involvement of a physician or paediatrician with expertise in the treatment of physically at-risk patients with anorexia nervosa should be considered for all individuals who are physically at risk. (C)

4.4.4.7   Pregnant women with either current or remitted anorexia nervosa may need more intensive prenatal care to ensure adequate prenatal nutrition and fetal development. (C)

4.4.4.8   Oestrogen administration should not be used to treat bone density problems in children and adolescents as this may lead to premature fusion of the epiphyses. (C)

Feeding against the will of the patient

4.4.4.9   Feeding against the will of the patient should be an intervention of last resort in the care and management of anorexia nervosa. (C)

4.4.4.10   Feeding against the will of the patient is a highly specialised procedure requiring expertise in the care and management of those with severe eating disorders and the physical complications associated with it. This should only be done in the context of the Mental Health Act 1983 or Children Act 1989. (C)

4.4.4.11   When making the decision to feed against the will of the patient the legal basis for any such action must be clear. (C)

4.4.5 Service interventions for anorexia nervosa

The following section considers those aspects of the service system relevant to the treatment and management of anorexia nervosa.

4.4.5.1   Most people with anorexia nervosa should be treated on an outpatient basis. (C)

4.4.5.2   Where inpatient management is required, this should be provided within reasonable travelling distance to enable the involvement of relatives and carers in treatment, to maintain social and occupational links and to avoid difficulty in transition between primary and secondary care services. This is particularly important in the treatment of children and adolescents. (C)

4.4.5.3   Inpatient treatment should be considered for people with anorexia nervosa whose disorder is associated with high or moderate physical risk. (C)

4.4.5.4   People with anorexia nervosa requiring inpatient treatment should be admitted to a setting that can provide the skilled implementation of refeeding with careful physical monitoring (particularly in the first few days of refeeding) and in combination with psychosocial interventions. (C)

4.4.5.5   Inpatient treatment or day patient treatment should be considered for people with anorexia nervosa whose disorder has not improved with appropriate outpatient treatment, or for whom there is a significant risk of suicide or severe self-harm. (C)

4.4.5.6   Health care professionals without specialist experience of eating disorders, or in situations of uncertainty, should consider seeking advice from an appropriate specialist when contemplating a compulsory admission for a patient with anorexia nervosa regardless of the age of the patient. (C)

4.4.5.7   Health care professionals managing patients with anorexia nervosa, especially that of the binge purging sub-type, should be aware of the increased risk of self-harm and suicide, particularly at times of transition between services or service settings. (C)

4.4.6 Additional considerations for children and adolescents

4.4.6.1   Health care professionals should ensure that children and adolescents with anorexia nervosa who have reached a healthy weight have the increased energy and necessary nutrients available in the diet to support further growth and development. (C)

4.4.6.2   In the nutritional management of children and adolescents with anorexia nervosa, carers should be included in any dietary education or meal planning. (C)

4.4.6.3   Admission of children and adolescents with anorexia nervosa should be to age-appropriate facilities (with the potential for separate children and adolescent services), which have the capacity to provide appropriate educational and related activities. (C)

4.4.6.4   When a young person with anorexia nervosa refuses treatment that is deemed essential, consideration should be given to the use of the Mental Health Act 1983 or the right of those with parental responsibility to override the young person's refusal. (C)

4.4.6.5   Relying indefinitely on parental consent to treatment should be avoided. It is recommended that the legal basis under which treatment is being carried out should be recorded in the patient's case notes, and this is particularly important in the case of children and adolescents. (C)

4.4.6.6   For children and adolescents with anorexia nervosa, where issues of consent to treatment are highlighted, health care professionals should consider seeking a second opinion from an eating disorders specialist. (C)

4.4.6.7   If the patient with anorexia nervosa and those with parental responsibility refuse treatment, and treatment is deemed to be essential, legal advice should be sought in order to consider proceedings under the Children Act 1989. (C)

4.5 Bulimia nervosa

4.5.1 Psychological interventions for bulimia nervosa

4.5.1.1   As a possible first step, patients with bulimia nervosa should be encouraged to follow an evidence-based self-help programme. (B)

4.5.1.2   Health care professionals should consider providing direct encouragement and support to patients undertaking an evidence-based self-help programme as this may improve outcomes. This may be sufficient treatment for a limited subset of patients. (B)

4.5.1.3   Cognitive behaviour therapy for bulimia nervosa (CBT-BN), a specifically adapted form of cognitive behaviour therapy, should be offered to adults with bulimia nervosa. The course of CBT-BN should normally be of 16 to 20 sessions over four to five months. (A)

4.5.1.4   Adolescents with bulimia nervosa may be treated with CBT-BN adapted as needed to suit their age, circumstances, level of development and including the family as appropriate. (C)

4.5.1.5   When people with bulimia nervosa have not responded to or do not want CBT, other psychological treatments should be considered. (B)

4.5.1.6   Interpersonal psychotherapy should be considered as an alternative to cognitive behaviour therapy, but patients should be informed it takes eight to 12 months to achieve results comparable to cognitive behaviour therapy. (B)

4.5.2 Pharmacological interventions for bulimia nervosa

4.5.2.1   As an alternative or additional first step to using an evidence-based self-help programme, adults with bulimia nervosa may be offered a trial of an antidepressant drug. (B)

4.5.2.2   Patients should be informed that antidepressant drugs can reduce the frequency of binge eating and purging, but the long-term effects are unknown. Any beneficial effects will be rapidly apparent. (B)

4.5.2.3   Selective serotonin reuptake inhibitors (SSRIs) (specifically fluoxetine) are the drugs of first choice for the treatment of bulimia nervosa in terms of acceptability, tolerability and reduction of symptoms. (C)

4.5.2.4   For people with bulimia nervosa, the effective dose of fluoxetine is higher than for depression (60 mg daily). (C)

4.5.2.5   No drugs, other than antidepressants, are recommended for the treatment of bulimia nervosa. (B)

4.5.3 Management of physical aspects of bulimia nervosa

Patients with bulimia nervosa can experience considerable physical problems as a result of a range of behaviours associated with the condition. Awareness of the risks and careful monitoring should be a concern of all health care professionals working with people with this disorder.

4.5.3.1   Patients with bulimia nervosa who are vomiting frequently or taking large quantities of laxatives (and especially if they are also underweight) should have their fluid and electrolyte balance assessed. (C)

4.5.3.2   When electrolyte disturbance is detected, it is usually sufficient to focus on eliminating the behaviour responsible. In the small proportion of cases where supplementation is required to restore the patient's electrolyte balance oral rather than intravenous administration is recommended, unless there are problems with gastro intestinal absorption. (C)

4.5.4 Service interventions for bulimia nervosa

The great majority of patients with bulimia nervosa can be treated as outpatients. There is a very limited role for the inpatient treatment of bulimia nervosa. This is primarily concerned with the management of suicide risk or severe self-harm.

4.5.4.1   The great majority of patients with bulimia nervosa should be treated in an outpatient setting. (C)

4.5.4.2   For patients with bulimia nervosa who are at risk of suicide or severe self-harm, admission as an inpatient or a day patient or the provision of more intensive outpatient care, should be considered. (C)

4.5.4.3   Psychiatric admission for people with bulimia nervosa should normally be undertaken in a setting with experience of managing this disorder. (C)

4.5.4.4   Health care professionals should be aware that patients with bulimia nervosa who have poor impulse control, notably substance misuse, may be less likely to respond to a standard programme of treatment. As a consequence treatment should be adapted to the problems presented. (C)

4.5.5 Additional considerations in children and adolescents

4.5.5.1   Adolescents with bulimia nervosa may be treated with CBT-BN adapted as needed to suit their age, circumstances and level of development and including the family as appropriate. (C)

4.6 Treatment and management of atypical eating disorders including binge eating disorder

4.6.1 General treatment of atypical eating disorders

4.6.1.1   In the absence of evidence to guide the management of atypical eating disorders (eating disorders not otherwise specified) other than binge eating disorder, it is recommended that the clinician considers following the guidance on the treatment of the eating problem that most closely resembles the individual patient's eating disorder. (C)

4.6.2 Psychological treatments for binge eating disorder

4.6.2.1   As a possible first step, patients with binge eating disorder should be encouraged to follow an evidence-based self-help programme. (B)

4.6.2.2   Health care professionals should consider providing direct encouragement and support to patients undertaking an evidence-based self-help programme as this may improve outcomes. This may be sufficient treatment for a limited subset of patients. (B)

4.6.2.3   Cognitive behaviour therapy for binge eating disorder (CBT-BED), a specifically adapted form of CBT, should be offered to adults with binge eating disorder. (A)

4.6.2.4   Other psychological treatments (interpersonal psychotherapy for binge eating disorder, and modified dialectical behaviour therapy) may be offered to adults with persistent binge eating disorder. (B)

4.6.2.5   Patients should be informed that all psychological treatments for binge eating disorder have a limited effect on body weight. (A)

4.6.2.6   When providing psychological treatments for patients with binge eating disorder, consideration should be given to the provision of concurrent or consecutive interventions focusing on the management of comorbid obesity. (C)

4.6.2.7   Suitably adapted psychological treatments should be offered to adolescents with persistent binge eating disorder. (C)

4.6.3 Pharmacological interventions for binge eating disorder

4.6.3.1   As an alternative or additional first step to using an evidence-based self-help programme, consideration should be given to offering a trial of a SSRI antidepressant drug to patients with binge eating disorder. (B)

4.6.3.2   Patients with binge eating disorders should be informed that SSRIs can reduce binge eating, but the long-term effects are unknown. Antidepressant drugs may be sufficient treatment for a limited subset of patients. (B)

4.7 Research recommendations

The following research recommendations have been identified to address gaps in the evidence base:

- Adequately powered efficacy studies of specific treatments and services for people with anorexia nervosa are required.

- Efficacy studies of the treatment for atypical eating disorders (eating disorders not otherwise specified) are required.

- Efficacy studies of the treatment of adolescents with bulimia nervosa and non-responders to cognitive behaviour therapy are required.

- Effectiveness studies of the treatment of bulimia nervosa in adults are required.

- Patient and carer satisfaction is an important outcome and may influence treatment approaches. It should be considered a routine outcome in research.

- Further research is needed to assess the validity of screening instruments in primary care.

5 Identification of eating disorders in primary care

5.1 Introduction

Although new cases of clinical anorexia nervosa are not a common occurrence in primary care (an average GP list of 1900 will have only one or two sufferers), eating disorders including bulimia nervosa and EDNOS reach a prevalence of five per cent in young women. Community studies show that less than half of clinical cases of eating disorders are identified in primary care. Despite this, patients with eating disorders consult more frequently prior to diagnosis with a variety of symptoms, psychological, gynaecological and gastroenterological (Ogg *et al.*, 1997). The difficulties facing primary care clinicians in diagnosis derive in part from illness-related factors, such as ambivalence, denial, secrecy and shame, which make it difficult for sufferers to be open with their doctors. GPs may have little experience with eating disorders, and feel anxious about their management or unsympathetic towards an illness that may appear in part self-inflicted. Patients may report that the problem is not always taken seriously enough if presented at an early stage. Practitioners risk failing to identify eating disorders if they do not consider the fact that these illnesses also occur in groups not traditionally considered to be at risk, such as children, men and those from ethnic minority groups, and lower social classes.

The effective management of anorexia nervosa depends on a full assessment of physical status, psychological features, risk and capacity to consent to treatment. The details of appropriate physical assessment are detailed in Section 5.2.4, but included in the assessment of high physical risk will be an assessment of degree of emaciation (BMI/BMI centile), the presence of purging and any fluid restriction. The rate of weight loss is also an important indicator. In children and younger adolescents, reference to BMI norms is necessary, but it is also of note that children's relatively small fat stores render them at risk with relatively less weight loss. Psychosocial assessment should take account of motivation and social support.

5.1.1 Current practice

Little is known about how eating disorders are actually assessed or managed in primary care. Referrals to secondary care services (including specialist eating disorder centres) vary widely as does the information contained in them. Current practice is not underpinned by an evidence base derived from primary care settings and guidance has largely been extrapolated from secondary or tertiary care settings with experience with more severely ill clinical populations.

5.2 Screening

Early detection and treatment of eating disorders may improve outcomes in eating disorders. General practitioners and other members of the primary care team are in a good position to identify patients with eating problems early. Screening tools may facilitate this process. The most effective screening device probably remains the general practitioner thinking about the possibility of an eating disorder.

It would be impractical for general practitioners to try and screen all their patients for eating disorders, as the prevalence of eating disorders in the general population is low. It might be possible to screen new patients when they register. One or two screening questions could be used to raise the index of suspicion, either verbally during the registration health check or in writing as part of the registration questionnaire.

High-risk groups within the general practice population could be targeted opportunistically. Such groups include young women, patients with a low or high BMI, adolescents consulting with weight concerns, menstrual disturbances or amenorrhoea, gastrointestinal disorders and psychological problems. A brief screening questionnaire could be used for such high-risk groups.

5.2.1 Current practice

Eating disorders may be difficult to detect in primary care settings. Patients may be slow to self-present and many remain undetected by general practitioners (King, 1989; Whitehouse et al., 1992). Adults with eating disorders appear to consult their general practitioner more frequently than controls, presenting particularly with psychological, gastrointestinal and gynaecological problems (Ogg et al., 1997). Consultations of this nature present an opportunity to screen for eating disorders. At present, no formal screening tool for eating disorders is widely used in primary care.

5.2.2 Screening for eating disorders

The aim of screening is to facilitate detection so that treatment can be offered early in the course of the eating disorder.

A systematic review of the literature did not identify a significant body of work in this area, nor were any high quality existing systematic reviews identified. The absence of high quality evidence in this area inevitably limits the conclusions that can be drawn from the review. The relevant studies that were identified are described below.

Existing screening instruments

A range of questionnaires exists of which the Eating Attitudes Test, EAT (Garner & Garfinkel, 1979) is probably the most widely used as a screening tool in epidemiological studies. In addition there are a number of other pencil and paper measures to assess eating disorder psychopathology (e.g. the Eating Disorder Inventory, EDI – Garner et al., 1983). However, these take a long time to administer and may need to be interpreted by specialists. Such instruments may be well suited for evaluating treatment progress in patients with eating disorders, but may not perform well in screening for eating disorders in community samples due to symptom denial and low prevalence (Williams et al., 1982; Carter & Moss, 1984).

Questionnaires of this type may have a role for screening in very high-risk groups in special settings, e.g. in ballet schools, fitness and sports facilities.

They may have occasional application in general practice, when a patient with a probable eating disorder has already been identified.

Several brief screening questionnaires, more suitable for use in community samples, have been developed and evaluated. These include the SCOFF (Morgan *et al.*, 1999), Anstine and Grinenko (2000), the BITE and the BES (Ricca *et al.*, 2000), the EDS-5 (Rosenvinge, 2001), Freund *et al.* (1993), the ESP (Cotton *et al.*, 2003), Ri-BED-8 (Waaddegaard *et al.*, 1999), the EDDS (Stice *et al.*, 2000), the EAT-12 and the EDE-S/Q (Beglin & Fairburn, 1992, 1994). The most promising to date is the SCOFF.

The SCOFF questionnaire (Morgan *et al.*, 1999; Luck *et al.*, 2002; Perry *et al.*, 2002) was developed and validated in the UK. It consists of five questions designed to clarify suspicion that an eating disorder might exist rather than to make a diagnosis. The questions can be delivered either verbally or in written form and there is one study validating the use of the SCOFF in adult women in a general practice population (Luck, 2002). Further research is needed to evaluate the SCOFF questions in general practice populations before they can be recommended for use in primary care.

5.2.3 Clinical summary

A number of brief screening methods have been developed that have some utility in detecting eating disorders. The SCOFF has been shown to be capable of determining cases of eating disorders in adult women in primary care. The place of longer questionnaires (e.g. EAT, EDI, BITE, EDE-Q) may be in further assessment, once index of suspicion has been raised. They may also be useful to facilitate decisions regarding referral to secondary care or other specialist services. Certain clinical presentations should also raise the index suspicion, for example, adolescent girls with concerns about weight, and women consulting with menstrual disturbances, gastrointestinal or psychological symptoms.

5.2.4 Identification

The most important factor in the identification of eating disorders in generalist settings is for the practitioner to consider the possibility of an eating disorder and to be prepared to inquire further in an empathic and non-judgmental manner. The history is paramount and special investigations are not normally required to make a diagnosis.

5.2.4.1   Anorexia nervosa

The first contact with health care services is often made by a worried family member, friend or schoolteacher rather than the patient. Concerns expressed may be related to weight loss, food-related behaviours such as skipping meals, hiding food or adopting a restrictive diet. There may be a change in mood, sleep patterns and increased activity. Typical psychopathological features are fear of gaining weight or becoming fat despite being underweight, disturbance in evaluating or experiencing body weight or shape, undue influence of eating or changes in body weight on self-evaluation and preoccupation with shape or weight-related matters. These features may not all be present, easy to elicit or they may be denied. However, denial of the seriousness of the weight loss or consequences, both physical and psychological is usually present.

Established anorexia nervosa with signs of emaciation is usually obvious. However, patients may present initially in primary care with non-specific physical symptoms such as abdominal pain, bloating, constipation, cold intolerance, light headedness, hair, nail or skin changes. Amenorrhoea, combined with unexplained weight loss, in the population at risk should always prompt further enquiry. Apparent food allergy/intolerance and chronic fatigue syndrome sometimes precede the development of an eating disorder and may cause diagnostic confusion. In children, growth failure may be a presenting feature.

In practice, typical cases should cause little difficulty when the time is taken to explore the history including corroborative information and the patient's attitude to the weight loss. Indeed, diagnosis is often delayed when doctors inadvertently collude by over-investigating and referring to other specialties rather than confronting the possibility of an eating disorder.

Diagnostic criteria

These are outlined in the introduction (see Section 2.1.2).

In children and adolescents under 18, the use of BMI centile charts should be encouraged (Cole, Bellizi *et al.*, 2000) with a cut off less than the 2.4th centile of the reference population indicating underweight.

Centile charts for weight and height are also helpful in showing failure to progress over time.

The list of potential differential diagnoses of weight loss or amenorrhoea is large, but in practice, typical cases should cause little difficulty when the time is taken to explore the history including corroborative information and the patient's attitude to the weight loss. The following factors need to be considered:

● Risk factors – family history of eating disorder, Type 1 diabetes, previously overweight, occupation (e.g. athlete, dancer, model). Although adolescent girls and young women constitute the principal population at risk, it should be remembered that eating disorders also occur in ethnic minorities, men and children.

● Differential diagnosis of weight loss – includes malabsorbtion (e.g. coeliac disease, inflammatory bowel disease), neoplasm, illicit drug use, infection (e.g. TB), autoimmune disease, endocrine disorders (e.g. hyperthyroidism).

● Differential diagnosis of amenorrhoea – includes pregnancy, primary ovarian failure, poly cystic ovary syndrome, pituitary prolactinoma, uterine problems and other hypothalmic causes.

● Psychiatric differential diagnosis – includes depression, obsessive-compulsive disorder, somatisation and, rarely, psychosis.

Initial physical assessment

The rationale for physical assessment is more to determine the presence and severity of emaciation and secondary physical consequences of the anorexia nervosa than to ascertain the primary diagnosis.

It should include as a minimum:

● Height weight and BMI

● Centile charts for age less than 18

● Pulse and blood pressure.

The following may also be helpful to assess the risk of physical instability:

● Core temperature (this is easily done by ear thermometer)

● Examination of peripheries (circulation and oedema)

● Cardiovascular examination including postural hypotension

● Situp/squat test (a test of muscle power) (Robinson, 2003).

Laboratory investigations

Extensive laboratory investigation is not usually required in the diagnosis or assessment of anorexia nervosa in a primary care setting. Many tests remain normal even with extreme weight loss and are a poor guide to physical risk. The diagnosis is always made on the basis of the clinical history.

Investigations

The following would represent a reasonable initial screen in primary care if there are no other indications or diagnostic concerns:

● Full Blood Count, ESR, Urea and Electrolytes, Creatinine, Liver Function Tests, Random Blood Glucose, Urinalysis.

● ECG: This should be considered in all cases and is essential if symptoms/signs of cardiac compromise, bradycardia, electrolyte abnormality or BMI less than 15 kg/m^2. (Or equivalent on centile chart.)

Further tests may be required in more severe cases or to assess complications: Calcium, Magnesium, Phosphate, Serum Proteins, Creatine Kinase (CK or CPK).

Tests that may be needed in the differential diagnosis of amenorrhoea and weight loss:

● Thyroid Function Tests, Follicle Stimulating Hormone, Lutenising Hormone, Prolactin, Chest X-Ray.

A DXA scan may be considered for identification of osteopenia/osteoporosis, which may occur after six to 12 months of amenorrhoea. Although this is not necessarily a primary care level investigation, it has been suggested that it may be helpful in encouraging motivation for change in those not yet ready to accept referral, by demonstrating the real physical consequences of anorexia nervosa.

5.2.4.2   Bulimia nervosa

Identification

The patient with bulimia nervosa is more likely to be older and to consult alone than a patient with anorexia nervosa. There may be a history of previous anorexia nervosa or of unhappiness with previous weight and attempts to diet. Appropriate questioning (see screening section above) may reveal patterns of restriction, binge eating and purging and psychopathology that make the diagnosis clear. Not infrequently, physical symptoms are presented which may be related to or consequences of purging or laxative use. These symptoms, particularly in a young woman should be a 'red flag' in prompting the practitioner to consider further enquiry.

Where the patient does not disclose bulimia nervosa, a range of symptoms may present which should raise the index of suspicion. These include requests for help with weight loss, menstrual disturbance and the physical consequences of vomiting and laxative and diuretic use. Non-specific symptoms may include fatigue, lethargy. Gastrointestinal disorders may be present including bloating, fullness, abdominal pain, irritable bowel syndrome type symptoms, constipation, diarrhoea and rectal prolapse as well as oesophagitis and gastrointestinal bleeding. Oropharyngeal symptoms may include a sore throat, parotid swelling and dental enamel erosion.

Physical examination and investigation

In bulimia nervosa and related conditions, characteristic physical signs have been described (for example, parotid enlargement, Russell's sign (callus formation on the dorsum of the hand) and dental enamel erosion, which are usually manifestations of purging. In practice these are not seen in the majority of patients presenting in primary care with bulimic disorders, although electrolyte abnormalities are reasonably common, so urea and electrolytes should be routinely obtained. These are covered in Section 7.5.2.

5.2.5 Clinical practice recommendations

5.2.5.1   For people with eating disorders presenting in primary care, GPs should take responsibility for the initial assessment and the initial co-ordination of care. This includes the determination of the need for emergency medical or psychiatric assessment. (C)

5.2.5.2   Where management is shared between primary and secondary care, there should be clear agreement amongst individual health care professionals on the responsibility for monitoring patients with eating disorders. This agreement should be in writing (where appropriate using the care programme approach) and should be shared with the patient and, where appropriate, families and carers. (C)

5.2.5.3   Target groups for screening should include young women with low body mass index (BMI) compared with age norms, patients consulting with weight concerns who are not overweight, women with menstrual disturbances or amenorrhoea, people with gastrointestinal symptoms, patients with physical signs of starvation or repeated vomiting, and children with poor growth. (C)

5.2.5.4   When screening for eating disorders one or two simple questions should be considered for use with specific target groups (for example, 'Do you think you have an eating problem?' and 'Do you worry excessively about your weight?'). (C)

5.2.5.5   Young people with Type 1 diabetes and poor treatment adherence should be screened and assessed for the presence of an eating disorder. (C)

5.2.5.6   In anorexia nervosa, although weight and body mass index (BMI) are important indicators of physical risk they should not be considered the sole indicators (as on their own they are unreliable in adults and especially in children). (C)

5.2.5.7   In assessing whether a person has anorexia nervosa, attention should be paid to the overall clinical assessment (repeated over time), including rate of weight loss, growth rates in children, objective physical signs and appropriate laboratory tests. (C)

5.2.5.8   Patients with enduring anorexia nervosa not under the care of secondary care services should be offered an annual physical and mental health review by their general practitioner. (C)

6 Treatment and management of anorexia nervosa

6.1 Introduction

The treatment plan for a patient with anorexia nervosa needs to consider the appropriate service setting, and the psychological and physical management, but unfortunately the research evidence base to guide decision making is very limited. The appropriate setting depends on the assessment of risk and the patient's wishes, but in general the person with anorexia nervosa will initially be treated in a secondary care outpatient service, moving into a day or inpatient setting if required. Although convincing evidence is lacking on the most effective form of psychological therapy, psychological therapy is nevertheless crucial in addressing the underlying behaviours and cognitions. In children and adolescents some family-based psychological intervention is essential. Physical treatments comprise nutritional interventions and psychopharmacological agents. The latter are used to support psychological treatments or for the management of comorbid conditions, rather than being first line treatments.

The treatment options should be discussed fully with the patient in order that he or she can make informed choices. Given the ambivalence inherent in this disorder, engagement and efforts at motivational enhancement may be helpful in maximising adherence to treatment. A small number of patients with anorexia nervosa do not have the capacity to make decisions about their own health and safety and in these cases provision for their admission to hospital and treatment is under the remit of the Mental Health Act 1983 and the Children Act 1989.

6.2 Psychological interventions

6.2.1 Introduction

The earliest models of psychological treatment for anorexia nervosa were psychodynamic in nature, albeit with few attempts to study them systematically (for review see Dare & Crowther, 1995; Herzog & Hartmann, 1997; Kaplan, 2002).

From the 1960s onwards, behaviour therapy for anorexia nervosa became increasingly popular, with many articles reporting on the use of operant conditioning techniques (for review see Bemis *et al.*, 1987; Schmidt, 1989). The basic operant paradigm consisted of isolating patients from social and material reinforcers that were subsequently delivered contingent on weight gain or caloric intake. For a time, this technique became part of many inpatient regimes, because of its efficacy in encouraging weight gain in the short term. However, operant conditioning approaches have been criticised as coercive and controlling (for review see Bemis, 1987), and their influence has waned in recent years.

The seminal – though controversial – work of Minuchin and colleagues (1975) stimulated much interest in the use of family interventions in the treatment of anorexia nervosa. Initially, the rationale for this approach was rooted in the notion that families have a key causal role in the development of anorexia nervosa ('the anorexogenic family'). However, it is now widely agreed that family interventions are best viewed as treatments that mobilise family resources rather than treating family dysfunction, for which there is no empirical evidence (Eisler *et al.*, 2003). The first treatment trial of family therapy was published in 1987 (Russell *et al.*, 1987), studying patients who had undergone a period of weight restoration in a specialist eating disorder inpatient unit prior to starting outpatient psychotherapy. This study showed that in 21 adolescents with a short duration of illness, family therapy was superior to individual supportive counselling in maintaining weight gained. The findings of this study stimulated three further RCTs into different types of family interventions for adolescents with anorexia nervosa (Le Grange *et al.*, 1992; Eisler *et al.*, 2000; Geist *et al.*, 2002). In addition there has been one further comparison of family therapy with individual therapy although the findings are difficult to interpret (Robin *et al.*, 1999). The original Maudsley model of family therapy has since been manualised for therapists (Lock *et al.*, 2001).

A handful of controlled trials, mainly in adults with anorexia nervosa, have evaluated the efficacy of specific individual psychotherapies, such as cognitive behaviour therapy (Channon *et al.*, 1989; Serfaty *et al.*, 2002; Pike *et al.*, in press; MacIntosh *et al.*, submitted); cognitive analytic therapy (Treasure *et al.*, 1995; Dare *et al.*, 2001), focal analytical psychotherapy (Dare *et al.*, 2001) and interpersonal psychotherapy (McIntosh *et al.*, submitted).

More recently there has been interest in the use of motivational interventions in the engagement and treatment of people with anorexia nervosa (Treasure & Ward, 1997; Vitousek *et al.*, 1998), however, RCTs in this area are as yet lacking.

Overall, the body of research into the treatment of anorexia nervosa is small and inconsistent in methodological quality. The conclusions that can be drawn are limited because many studies have no follow-up data, lack the statistical power necessary to detect real effects, and use different study entry criteria and outcome measures.

6.2.2 Current practice

There is wide variability in the availability of psychological therapies for patients with anorexia nervosa. There is no uniform or agreed approach to the psychological treatment or management of anorexia nervosa in adults, either in terms of types of treatment offered, their duration, intensity or the setting in which treatment is provided.

In the treatment of anorexia nervosa in children and adolescents, family interventions are usually offered. These may vary in approach and not all of them will resemble the evidence-based family interventions that have a focus on eating behaviours. Specialist eating disorder services may offer a range of individual psychological therapies including cognitive behaviour therapy, psychodynamic psychotherapy, motivational enhancement therapy and family interventions.

Principles of psychological treatment: engagement

Many people with anorexia nervosa find it hard to acknowledge that they have a problem and are ambivalent about change. This contributes to their reluctance to engage with treatment and services. A precondition for any successful psychological treatment is the effective engagement of the patient in the treatment plan. Health care professionals involved in the treatment of anorexia nervosa should take time to build an empathic, supportive and collaborative relationship with patients and, if applicable, their carers. This should be regarded as an essential element of the care offered. Motivation to change may go up and down over the course of treatment and the therapist needs to remain sensitive to this. Special challenges in the treatment of anorexia nervosa include the highly positive value placed by people with anorexia nervosa on some of their symptoms, and their denial of the potentially life-threatening nature of their disorder.

Aims of psychological interventions

In general, the aims of psychological treatment are to promote weight gain and healthy eating, to reduce other eating disorder related symptoms and to promote psychological recovery. In patients who have just had their weight restored in hospital the maintenance of weight gain is a prominent goal, together with continued healthy eating, the reduction of other eating disorder related symptoms and the promotion of psychological recovery. In patients with enduring anorexia nervosa, psychological treatment may have more modest goals and may focus on improving quality of life and maintaining a stable or safe weight rather than aiming for an optimal weight.

6.2.3 Outpatient psychological treatments (first episode and later episodes)

This section focuses on psychological treatments given as the main or only treatment to patients who present during a first or later episode of anorexia nervosa.

6.2.3.1   Psychological treatments reviewed

The following treatments were included:

● Behaviour therapy (BT)

● Cognitive analytic therapy (CAT)

● Cognitive behaviour therapy (CBT)

● Interpersonal psychotherapy (IPT)

● Family therapy and family interventions

● Psychodynamic psychotherapy

● Psychological treatment not otherwise specified (Psychotherapy NOS).

The Psychological Topic Group established definitions for each treatment (see Glossary). Two members of the Topic Group assessed each study for eligibility and classified each psychological treatment. Where disagreements arose, they were resolved by discussion.

6.2.3.2   Studies considered[2]

The review team conducted a new systematic search for RCTs of outpatient psychological treatments used for the initiation of treatment during the first or later episodes of anorexia nervosa. Eleven small RCTS (Bachar, 1999; Channon, 1989; Crisp, 1991; Dare, 2001; Eisler, 2000; Hall, 1987; McIntosh, submitted; Robin, 1999; Serfaty, 1999; Treasure, 1995; Wallin, 2000) were identified providing data on 459 participants ranging in age from adolescents to young adults.

Full details of studies included in the guideline and reasons for excluding studies are given in Appendix 18.

6.2.3.3   Evidence statements[3]

Due to major differences in the way the main outcomes were reported in each study and the lack of extractable data in several studies, no meta-analysis of results was conducted. The statements in this section relate to adults, except where explicitly stated. For each evidence statement, where necessary, N represents the number of studies and n the total number of participants. The level of evidence (I, IIa, IIb, III, IV) is given after each statement (see Section 3.4.6 for more information about the classification of evidence).

Effect of outpatient psychological treatments given for the treatment of first episodes or later acute episodes upon symptoms (weight gain and/or proportion recovered)

There is limited evidence that family interventions, psychotherapy NOS and focal psychoanalytic psychotherapy provided at tertiary referral centres are superior to 'treatment as usual' in terms of weight gain by end of treatment and post-treatment follow-up (n = 174; Crisp, 1991; Dare, 2001). I

There is limited evidence that both family interventions and focal psychoanalytic psychotherapy given at a tertiary referral centre are superior to 'treatment as usual' in terms of the proportion of people recovered by end of treatment (n = 84; Dare, 2001). I

There is limited evidence that treatment outcome with different psychological therapies (including BT, CAT, CBT, IPT, family therapy, focal psychodynamic psychotherapy, and psychotherapy NOS) by the end of treatment and at follow-up (up to five years) is poor (in terms of weight gain/proportion of people recovered) in patients referred to tertiary referral centres (n = 258; Channon, 1989; Crisp, 1991; Dare, 2001; Hall, 1987; Treasure, 1995). I

---

[2] Here and elsewhere in the guideline, each study considered for review is referred to by a study ID (primary author and date of study publication, except where a study is *in press* or only submitted for publication, then a date is not used).

[3] The full list of all evidence statements generated from meta-analyses (and the associated forest plots) will be available on the CD-ROM that accompanies the guideline.

There is insufficient evidence to suggest that any particular psychological treatment (including CAT, CBT, IPT, family therapy, focal psychodynamic therapy) is superior to any other in the treatment of adult patients with anorexia nervosa either by the end of treatment or at follow-up (n = 297; Bachar, 1999; Channon, 1989; Crisp, 1991; Dare, 2001; McIntosh, submitted; Treasure, 1995). I

There is insufficient evidence to determine the efficacy of dietary counselling on its own as a treatment for anorexia nervosa (n = 65; Hall, 1987; Serfaty, 1999). I

There is insufficient evidence to determine any advantage for inpatient care over outpatient psychological treatments (individual therapy+family therapy+dietary counselling or group therapy+parents' group+dietary counselling) for patients who are not so severely ill as to need emergency treatment (n = 90; Crisp, 1991). I

In children and adolescents, there is insufficient evidence to determine whether conjoint or separate family therapy is more, or less, effective at the end of treatment or follow-up (Eisler, 2000; Robin, 1999). I

In children and adolescents, there is insufficient evidence to determine whether the addition of body awareness therapy to family therapy is superior to family therapy alone (Wallin, 2000).

Acceptability of outpatient psychological treatment given for the treatment of first episodes or later acute episodes

There is insufficient evidence to determine whether outpatient psychological treatments (including BT, CAT, CBT, family therapy, focal psychodynamic psychotherapy) are more, or less, acceptable to people with anorexia nervosa when compared to 'standard care' (n = 198; Channon, 1989; Crisp, 1991; Dare, 2001). I

There is insufficient evidence to suggest that any particular psychotherapy (including BT, CAT, CBT, family therapy, focal psychodynamic psychotherapy, IPT, psychotherapy NOS) is more, or less, acceptable to adults with anorexia nervosa (n = 297; Bachar, 1999; Channon, 1989; Crisp, 1991; Dare, 2001; McIntosh, submitted; Treasure, 1995). I

There is limited evidence to suggest that dietary counselling on its own is less acceptable to people with anorexia nervosa when compared to CBT (n = 35; Serfaty, 1999). I

There is limited evidence to suggest that inpatient treatment at a national tertiary eating disorder centre is less acceptable than tertiary outpatient psychological treatments provided at the same centre (n = 90; Crisp, 1991). I

In children and adolescents, there is insufficient evidence to determine whether conjoint or separate family therapy are more, or less, acceptable (n = 64; Eisler, 2000; Robin, 1999). I

In children and adolescents, there is insufficient evidence to determine whether the addition of body awareness therapy to family therapy is more, or less, acceptable compared to family therapy alone (n = 33; Wallin, 2000). I

6.2.4 Outpatient psychological treatments after weight restoration in hospital

Inpatient treatments aim to return body weight to a healthy level but even when this occurs patients remain very vulnerable to subsequent weight loss. Outpatient psychological treatments are offered to prevent this.

6.2.4.1 Psychological treatments reviewed

The following treatments were included:

- Cognitive behaviour therapy (CBT)

- Family therapy

- Dietary counselling

- Supportive therapy.

6.2.4.2 Studies considered

The review team conducted a new systematic search for RCTs of outpatient psychological treatments after weight restoration in hospital in people with anorexia nervosa. Three small trials were included (Geist, 2000; Pike, submitted; Russell, 1987), providing data on 138 participants ranging in age from adolescents to adults.

Full details of studies included and excluded from the guideline are given in Appendix 18.

6.2.4.3 Evidence statements[4]

The statements in this section relate to adults, except where explicitly stated.

Effect of treatment on symptoms (weight and/or proportion recovered or relapsed)

There is limited evidence that individual supportive psychotherapy is superior in terms of weight gain when compared to family therapy in a subgroup of adults with anorexia nervosa (with adult onset) at one year post-treatment follow-up (*n* = 21; Russell, 1987). I

There is limited evidence that for patients with an age of onset below 19 and with an illness duration of less than three years, family therapy focused explicitly on eating disorders is superior in terms of weight gain and the proportion classed as recovered when compared to individual supportive psychotherapy at one year post-treatment follow-up (*n* = 21; Russell, 1987). I

---

[4] The full list of all evidence statements generated from meta-analyses (and the associated forest plots) will be available on the CD-ROM that accompanies the guideline.

There is limited evidence suggesting that CBT is superior to dietary counselling in terms of proportion recovered and relapse rates, after weight restoration in hospital ($n = 33$; Pike, submitted). I

In children and adolescents, there is insufficient evidence to determine the efficacy of family group education versus conjoint family therapy following partial weight restoration in hospital ($n = 25$; Geist, 2000).

Acceptability of treatment

There is limited evidence suggesting that CBT is more acceptable to people with anorexia nervosa when compared to dietary counselling, after weight restoration in hospital ($n = 33$; Pike, submitted). I

In children and adolescents, there is insufficient evidence to determine the acceptability of family group education versus conjoint family therapy following partial weight restoration in hospital ($n = 25$; Geist, 2000).

6.2.5 Different types of psychological inpatient treatment regime

There has been some interest in the question of whether different types of inpatient regimes are more efficient than others in terms of achieving short-term weight restoration.

6.2.5.1 Inpatient psychological treatments reviewed

All inpatient treatments involving people with anorexia nervosa were considered in this section. These included specific forms of psychotherapy such as operant conditioning, and other behavioural regimes and psychodynamic psychotherapy, as well as (other) programmes focused on eating and weight gain.

6.2.5.2 Studies considered

The review team conducted a new systematic search for different types of psychological inpatient treatment regime in people with anorexia nervosa. Because of the difficulties associated with this type of treatment and the paucity of RCT data, lower levels of evidence were examined. Thus, two RCTs (Eckert, 1979; Weizman, 1985) and two non-randomised controlled studies were included (Herzog, 1996; Solanto, 1994), providing data on 374 participants ranging in age from adolescents to adults.

Full details of studies included and excluded from the guideline are given in Appendix 18.

Effect of treatment on symptoms (weight gain)

There is limited evidence (from one non-randomised study) to suggest that an inpatient programme with an explicit focus on changing eating disorder symptoms and weight is superior to a programme without this focus, in terms of producing short-term weight gain (*n* = 34; Herzog, 1996). IIa

There is very limited evidence from one small non-randomised study suggesting that increasing the four-day criterion weight gain from 0.4 to 0.5 kg in a behavioural contract produces more rapid weight gain (*n* = 53; Solanto, 1995). IIb

Acceptability of treatment

There is insufficient evidence to determine whether any one form of inpatient treatment is more, or less, acceptable to people with anorexia nervosa when compared with another form of inpatient care. I-IIb

6.2.6   Psychological treatments as adjuncts to inpatient treatment

Specialist inpatient treatment programmes for anorexia nervosa typically consist of multiple components, with the aim of providing comprehensive package of inpatient care. The relative importance and efficacy of these different components has so far received little research attention.

6.2.6.1   Psychological treatments reviewed

The following treatments, as adjuncts to inpatient treatment, were included:

- Behaviour therapy (systematic desensitisation)

- Relaxation training

- Social skills training.

6.2.6.2   Studies considered

The review team conducted a new systematic search for RCTs of psychological treatments as adjuncts to inpatient treatment in people with anorexia nervosa. Two small trials (Goldfarb, 1987; Pillay, 1981) were included, providing data on 41 participants ranging in age from adolescents to adults.

Full details of studies included and excluded from the guideline are given in Appendix 18.

---

[5] The full list of all evidence statements[5] generated from meta-analyses (and the associated forest plots) will be available on the CD-ROM that accompanies the guideline.

6.2.6.3 Evidence statements[6]

Effect of treatment on symptoms and acceptability

There is insufficient evidence to draw any conclusions from these studies as to the efficacy of behaviour therapy (systematic desensitisation), relaxation training or social skills training as an adjunct to inpatient treatment (*n* = 41; Goldfarb, 1987; Pillay, 1981). I

6.2.7 Additional considerations in the management of children and adolescents

There is a small but consistent evidence base, which indicates that family-based treatments are important in the treatment of adolescents with anorexia nervosa. Consensus as to what constitutes the best form of family intervention has not been achieved but two factors stand out as potentially important:

- Family interventions should have a focus on the eating disorder and how this impacts on family relationships, emphasising in the early stages of treatment the necessity for parents to take a central role in supporting their child's efforts to eat.

- Both separated (parents and patient meet separately with the therapist) and conjoint forms (parents and patient together with therapist) of family therapy may be beneficial.

Establishing a collaborative working relationship with families with a young person with anorexia nervosa presents a particular challenge that requires time and expertise to balance the competing needs of different family members. However, whilst there is an emphasis on family interventions the young person's individual rights and responsibilities should not be overlooked. Issues such as confidentiality and consent must be considered carefully and not simply overridden by clinicians or parents. For this reason, young people should be offered individual appointments with a therapist separate from those with their family members or carers. For children and adolescents it is also particularly important to ensure adequate physical monitoring and rapid commencement of treatment.

6.2.8 Clinical summary

Various forms of psychological treatment are associated with improvements in terms both of weight gain and recovery by the end of treatment compared to 'standard care' for certain populations. However, the long-term benefits may not be sustained. For patients not requiring emergency admission to hospital, outpatient psychological treatment may be as, or more, effective than admission. For those admitted to hospital, no particular psychological treatment regime, either as a central component of the treatment programme or as an adjunct has been shown to have beneficial effects.

---

[6] The full list of all evidence statements generated from meta-analyses (and the associated forest plots) will be available on the CD-ROM that accompanies the guideline.

There is limited evidence that family interventions focused explicitly on eating disorders may be of specific benefit to younger people, but there is insufficient evidence to determine whether conjoint (i.e. patient and parents meet together) or separated forms of family therapy (i.e. therapist meets patient and parents separately) are more effective.

6.2.9 Clinical practice recommendations

Common elements of the psychological treatment of anorexia nervosa

6.2.9.1 Therapies to be considered for the psychological treatment of anorexia nervosa include cognitive analytic therapy (CAT), cognitive behaviour therapy (CBT), interpersonal psychotherapy (IPT), focal psychodynamic therapy and family interventions focused explicitly on eating disorders. (C)

6.2.9.2 Patient and, where appropriate, carer preference, should be taken into account in deciding which psychological treatment is to be offered. (C)

6.2.9.3 The aims of psychological treatment should be to reduce risk, encourage weight gain and healthy eating, to reduce other symptoms related to an eating disorder, and to facilitate psychological and physical recovery. (C)

Outpatient psychological treatments in first episode and later episodes

6.2.9.4 Most people with anorexia nervosa should be managed on an outpatient basis with psychological treatment (with physical monitoring) provided by a health care professional competent to give it and to assess the physical risk of people with eating disorders. (C)*

6.2.9.5 Outpatient psychological treatment and physical monitoring for anorexia nervosa should normally be of at least six months' duration. (C)

6.2.9.6 For patients with anorexia nervosa, if during outpatient psychological treatment there is significant deterioration, or the completion of an adequate course of outpatient psychological treatment does not lead to any significant improvement, more intensive forms of treatment (for example, a move from individual therapy to combined individual and family work, day care or inpatient care) should be considered. (C)

6.2.9.7 Dietary counselling should not be provided as the sole treatment for anorexia nervosa. (C)

Psychological aspects of inpatient care

Psychological treatment is often a key element of an inpatient stay but evidence for what kind of treatment or approaches to treatment are effective is limited.

6.2.9.8 For inpatients with anorexia nervosa, a structured symptom-focused treatment regimen with the expectation of weight gain should be provided in order to achieve weight restoration. It is important to carefully monitor the patient's physical status during refeeding. (C)

6.2.9.9   Psychological treatment should be provided which has a focus both on eating behaviour and attitudes to weight and shape, and on wider psychosocial issues with the expectation of weight gain. (C)

6.2.9.10   Rigid inpatient behaviour modification programmes should not be used in the management of anorexia nervosa. (C)

Post-hospitalisation psychological treatment for adults with anorexia nervosa

For patients with anorexia nervosa following discharge from hospital it is usually necessary to extend the duration of psychological treatment over that normally provided to those who have not been hospitalised.

6.2.9.11   Following inpatient weight restoration, people with anorexia nervosa should be offered outpatient psychological treatment that focuses both on eating behaviour and attitudes to weight and shape, and on wider psychosocial issues, with regular monitoring of both physical and psychological risk. (C)

6.2.9.12   The length of outpatient psychological treatment and physical monitoring following inpatient weight restoration should typically be at least 12 months. (C)

Children and adolescents with anorexia nervosa

Special considerations are needed in the treatment of children and adolescents, of particular importance is the involvement of families and other carers. Support from education and peers may also play a role in recovery and clinicians will often need to liaise with schools over involvement in physical education and sitting examinations.

6.2.9.13   Family members including siblings, should normally be included in the treatment of children and adolescents with eating disorders. Interventions may include sharing of information, advice on behavioural management and facilitating communication. (C)*

6.2.9.14   Family interventions that directly address the eating disorder should be offered to children and adolescents with anorexia nervosa. (B)*

6.2.9.15   Children and adolescents with anorexia nervosa should be offered individual appointments with a health care professional separate from those with their family members or carers. (C)

6.2.9.16   The therapeutic involvement of siblings and other family members should be considered in all cases because of the effects of anorexia nervosa on other family members. (C)

6.2.9.17   In children and adolescents with anorexia nervosa the need for inpatient treatment and the need for urgent weight restoration should be balanced alongside the educational and social needs of the young person. (C)

6.3 Pharmacological interventions

6.3.1 Introduction

A diverse network of neurotransmitters and neurohormones are involved in the central and peripheral control of appetite and satiety. A variety of drugs that act on various receptors within these pathways have been examined in the treatment of anorexia nervosa.

6.3.2 Current practice

Antidepressant drugs are often used to treat the depressive symptoms in anorexia nervosa and their effects on weight gain have also been studied. Medications are also used to treat comorbid conditions such as major depressive disorder and obsessive-compulsive disorder. Antipsychotic drugs or minor tranquillisers or antihistamines are frequently used symptomatically to reduce the high levels of anxiety present with anorexia nervosa, but are not recommended for the promotion of weight gain.

However, an evidence base for current practice is lacking. There are few studies on which to base clinical decisions and the studies are of low statistical power. There is also doubt about generalising from the patient samples studied. Drugs are not as acceptable or as well tolerated as psychotherapy in this patient group (Treasure, 1998). Only short-term effects have been studied and the outcome measures used are often not comparable to those used in psychotherapy studies. Compromised nutritional status may also affect the mechanism of drug action and this is rarely considered in studies. For example, there is some evidence that antidepressants have lower efficacy in the context of low levels of oestrogen (Halbreich & Kahn, 2000). They may be also less effective if tryptophan levels are altered.

Because of the complications of starvation, vomiting, dehydration and over hydration in this clinical group, there may be problems in terms of pharmacokinetics (i.e. drug absorption and toxicity). Extremely malnourished patients and those with electrolyte abnormalities are at risk of cardiac complications. Drugs with cardiac side effects should be used with caution.

6.3.3 Pharmacological treatment

The aim of pharmacological treatment in people with anorexia nervosa is to produce weight gain and improve their quality of life or to alleviate some of the comorbidity such as depression, anxiety or obsessive-compulsive features. Three main classes of drugs have been considered in the treatment of anorexia nervosa, these are antidepressants, antihistamines and antipsychotics.

The following drugs were included:

- Antidepressants

    - Tricyclic antidepressants (amitriptyline, clomipramine)

    - SSRIs (fluoxetine, citalopram)

- Antihistamines (cyproheptadine)

- Antipsychotics (pimozide, sulipride).

Drugs that have had their licences withdrawn from the UK were not included in the guideline. Although there are studies assessing the use of lithium carbonate, these were not included, as it was felt inadvisable to use this drug given the potential risk of toxicity in these patients.

6.3.3.2   Studies considered

A new search was made for RCTs examining drugs used in the treatment of anorexia nervosa. One trial of both an antidepressant and an antihistamine (Halmi, 1986), five trials of antidepressants (Attia, 1998; Biederman, 1985; Fassino, 2002; Kaye, 2001; Lacey, 1980), one trial of an antihistamine (Goldberg, 1980), and three trials of antipsychotics (Ruggiero, 2001; Vandereycken, 1982 & 1984) met the eligibility criteria set by the GDG. Thus, ten RCTs involving 413 adult participants were included in this section.

Of the 11 trials, four trials involved a comparison of a tricyclic antidepressant (amitriptyline, clomipramine) with placebo (Biederman, 1985; Halmi, 1986; Kaye, 2001; Lacey, 1980), one compared a SSRI antidepressant (fluoxetine) with placebo (Attia, 1998), and one compared a SSRI antidepressant (citalopram) with a wait-list control (Fassino, 2002). Two trials involved a comparison of an antihistamine with placebo (Goldberg, 1980; Halmi, 1986). Two trials compared an antipsychotic with placebo (Vandereycken, 1982 & 1984), and one compared an antipsychotic with both another antipsychotic and with an antidepressant (Ruggiero, 2001).

Full details of studies included in the guideline and reasons for excluding studies are given in Appendix 18.

6.3.3.3   Evidence statements[7]

The data were analysed by combining all studies, irrespective of the class of antidepressant used. However, where the data are from a single drug, the class and name of drug are reported.

---

[7] The full list of all evidence statements generated from meta-analyses (and the associated forest plots) will be available on the CD-ROM that accompanies the guideline.

Effect of treatment on weight gain

There is evidence suggesting that it is unlikely there is a clinically significant difference between antidepressant drugs and placebo on weight gain by the end of multi-modal inpatient treatment (n = 146; Attia, 1998; Biederman, 1985; Halmi, 1986; Lacey, 1980). I

There is insufficient evidence to determine whether antipsychotics or antihistamines have any impact on weight compared with placebo during multi-modal inpatient treatment. I

There is insufficient evidence to determine whether there is any difference between antipsychotics and antidepressants with regard to weight gain. I

Effect of treatment on relapse/clinical deterioration

There is limited evidence suggesting that there is a clinically significant difference between an SSRI (fluoxetine) and placebo with fewer patients deteriorating clinically (which for the majority of patients was defined as a worsening or no improvement in symptoms) following inpatient weight restoration if given fluoxetine for one year (N = 1; n = 35; RR = 0.45; 95 per cent CI, 0.23 to 0.86). I

Acceptability of treatment

There is insufficient evidence to determine whether antidepressants, antipsychotics, or antihistamines are more, or less, acceptable to people with anorexia nervosa when compared to placebo or wait-list control. I

Tolerability of treatment

There is insufficient evidence to determine whether antidepressants, antipsychotics, or antihistamines produce a great risk of side effects in people with anorexia nervosa when compared to placebo. I

6.3.4 Additional considerations in the management of children and adolescents

It is uncertain whether any of the above findings can be generalised to children and adolescents. In general there are safety data available for sertraline and amisulpride used for other conditions in the under 18 group, but these drugs have not been studied in anorexia nervosa. There is no evidence specifically addressing the use of drugs in the child and adolescent age group.

6.3.5 Clinical summary

There is no evidence that drug treatment (antidepressants [tricyclics and SSRIs]), conventional antipsychotics and antihistamines) has additional benefit on weight gain in people undergoing multi-faceted inpatient treatment. There is limited preliminary evidence from one small trial that fluoxetine may reduce the likelihood of deterioration after inpatient weight restoration. It remains to be established whether or not new compounds (e.g. atypical antipsychotics) or new settings (e.g. day hospitals as a supplement to outpatient therapy) or new specifications (matching drug to clinical phenotype or endophenotype) will be of benefit. A further complication in interpreting these studies is that a number of the secondary features of anorexia nervosa that may respond to medication may also improve as the patient gains weight (e.g. depressed mood).

6.3.6 Clinical practice recommendations

6.3.6.1   Medication should not be used as the sole or primary treatment for anorexia nervosa. (C)

6.3.6.2   Caution should be exercised in the use of medication for comorbid features such as depressive or obsessive-compulsive features as they may resolve with weight gain alone. (C)

6.3.6.3   When medication is used to treat people with anorexia nervosa, the side effects of drug treatment (in particular, cardiac side effects), should be carefully considered because of the compromised cardiovascular function of many people with anorexia nervosa. (C)

6.3.6.4   Health care professionals should be aware of the risk of drugs that prolong the QTc interval on the ECG: for example, antipsychotics, tricyclic antidepressants, macrolide antibiotics, and some antihistamines. In patients with anorexia nervosa at risk of cardiac complications, the prescription of drugs with side effects that may compromise cardiac function should be avoided. (C)

6.3.6.5   If the prescription of medication that may compromise cardiac functioning is essential, ECG monitoring should be undertaken. (C)

6.3.6.6   All patients with a diagnosis of anorexia nervosa should have an alert placed in their prescribing record concerning the risk of side effects. (C)

6.4 Management of physical aspects

6.4.1 Introduction

Identification of those patients with short-term risk of serious harm or death is clearly important in clinical practice. Recommendations as to how to assess, what to monitor and when to intervene are, therefore, vital.

The vast majority of longer-term follow-up studies indicate that people with anorexia nervosa have an almost 10-fold risk of dying compared to healthy people the same age and sex. Standardised mortality rates range between 4.71 and 12.82 (Nielsen et al., 1998). Mortality in eating disorders is predominately related to malnutrition, methods of weight control and suicide. Among studies in which cause of death is documented, 54 per cent died of eating disorder complications, 27 per cent committed suicide and the remaining 19 per cent died of unknown or other causes (Nielsen, 2001).

6.4.2 Current practice

There is limited evidence as to how and where risk should be managed. Opinion and practice varies between (and within) countries, centres and clinicians. This is the case both in terms of threshold for hospital admission and the goals of the admission. For example, the APA guidelines (American Psychiatric Association, 2000) recommend admission to hospital when a BMI is less than 16 kg/m^2 or weight loss greater than 20 per cent. In both the US and Australia, patients are generally admitted for short-term medical stabilisation on a medical or paediatric ward. In the UK, patients at low weight are frequently managed in an outpatient setting in specialist eating disorder services. In these instances there is a higher threshold for inpatient treatment with admission often not occurring until the patient's BMI falls below 13 kg/m^2. However, managing these low weight patients in an outpatient setting can be hazardous and should rarely be done without specialist advice. In the majority of inpatient specialist services in the UK, the goal is full weight recovery and so admissions are longer term. Admission to either a medical/paediatric or general psychiatric unit may occur but this varies with availability of services.

6.4.3 Physical risk reduction and monitoring

Applying information about the best evidence to a specific patient's problem is not easy as the clinical picture is diverse physically, psychologically and socially. The patient's problems have to be clearly defined and placed within the context of a clinical risk assessment. This needs to include an assessment both of the acute risk and the longer-term prognosis.

Decisions on short-term risk involve a combined assessment of the physical risk and the person's psychological capacity to consent to treatment, taking into account the possible resources of motivation and psychosocial support. A diagram is provided (see Appendix 7) as a simple guide to medical practitioners and other members of the multidisciplinary team as a decision aid when evaluating this acute risk. Body mass index is a better marker than weight alone as a proxy measure of physical risk but a rigid cut off point is less good for the extremes of height as the relationship is non-linear. Children have smaller fat stores than mature women and so medical complications occur with less weight loss. Bulimic features or refusal to drink also increase the risk. In turn, these medical markers interact with a variety of clinical and psychosocial factors. High physical risk is often associated with an impairment of capacity for the consent to treatment.

Because of the paucity of data and the nature of the issue under review, the GDG chose to use an informal consensus process (see Chapter 3, Section 3.4.7. for details) to address questions related to risk reduction and monitoring. The review team conducted a systematic search for all available evidence relating to the issue. A number of studies met the GDG's eligibility criteria, including two systematic reviews of anorexia nervosa and mortality, and outcome at follow-up (Nielsen, 2001; Steinhassuen, 2002). Long-term follow-up studies on patients suffering from anorexia nervosa were also considered, and where possible predictors and causes of death were noted. This is an area in which there is limited research. Exact causes of death are rarely described. The majority of studies documented cause of death as being as a result of starvation in anorexia nervosa. In those studies where death certificates were examined, again the exact precipitant of death was not always established. There are few post-mortem results documented.

Physical factors associated with higher mortality include severity of weight loss, over-activity and vomiting, bulimia and purging (Nielsen, 2000; Steinhausen, 2002). A BMI less than 13 kg/m^2 in adults is of prognostic significance as it indicates a greater risk for mortality (Casper, 1996; Hebebrand et al., 1997). In the latter study, only seven out of the 14 patients with a BMI of 11 kg/m^2 at referral survived (Hebebrand, 1997). Data on malnourished females in famine indicate that with a BMI less than 11 kg/m^2, risk of mortality increases sharply (Collins, 1995). Prolonged QT intervals may predispose a person to life-threatening arrhythmias, and might be responsible for cases of sudden death. Furthermore, prolonged QT intervals in ECG were recorded seven days before sudden death (Isner, 1985). Abnormally low serum albumin levels and low weight are the best variables to predict a lethal course (Herzog et al., 1997).

In the studies documenting mortality in patients with anorexia nervosa, causes of death vary. Causes include dehydration, electrolyte (particularly hypokalaemia) and metabolic complications, infections (bronchopneumonia and sepsis) and cardiac complications (see Neumarker, 1997, for review). Comorbid alcoholism has also been shown to be associated with increased mortality (Keel et al., 2003). Rupture/perforation of the gastrointestinal tract has been less frequently described (Zipfel, 2000)

Few studies have reported exclusively on the mortality in adolescents. There is a suggestion that the mortality rate is lower. This may reflect the fact that chronicity and mortality increase with increasing age (Steinhausen, 2002). BMI measures in children and younger adolescents are an inadequate reflection of physical reserve. Weight centiles or percentage weight for height give a more accurate guide to the degree of weight loss. Rapid weight loss in children is potentially more dangerous than in adults, and children are known to dehydrate more quickly (Irwin, 1984). Clinical judgement and physical examination may be a better indicator than serum electrolyte levels as to the need for rehydration (Nicholls & Stanhope, 2000).

6.4.4 Clinical summary

Low weight (BMI less than 13 kg/m^2), dehydration and electrolyte abnormalities indicate an increased risk of mortality. Cardiac arrhythmias and low serum albumin and glucose are of particular concern.

6.4.5 Clinical practice recommendations

Managing weight gain

6.4.5.1   In most patients with anorexia nervosa an average weekly weight gain of 0.5 to 1 kg in inpatient settings and 0.5 kg in outpatient settings should be an aim of treatment. This requires about 3500 to 7000 extra calories a week. (C)

6.4.5.2   Regular physical monitoring and in some cases treatment with a multi-vitamin/multi-mineral supplement in oral form is recommended for people with anorexia nervosa during both inpatient and outpatient weight restoration. (C)

6.4.5.3   Health care professionals should advise people with eating disorders and osteoporosis or related bone disorders to refrain from physical activities that significantly increase the likelihood of falls. (C)

6.4.5.4   In children and adolescents with eating disorders, growth and development should be closely monitored. Where development is delayed or growth stunted despite adequate nutrition, paediatric advice should be sought. (C)

6.4.6 Long-term risk and its management

Apart from the concern of immediate physical risk in patients with anorexia nervosa, the long-term physical consequences are considerable. For the purposes of this section, the GDG chose to focus on the effects on the skeletal system, on reproduction and the associated hormonal abnormalities, including low oestradiol, low IGF-I, and high serum cortisol that may contribute to the bone loss. Gastrointestinal and dental complications are largely as a result of vomiting and laxative abuse. These are described in the chapter on bulimia nervosa. It should be noted however that many of these complications are exacerbated in patients with low weight and muscle weakness. Other consequences have also been described (e.g. cardiac, dermatological, haematological), but these will not be covered in this guideline.

The development of osteopenia and osteoporosis is a serious and long-term consequence of starvation. Oestrogen deficiency, malnutrition, low body mass and hyperactivity all play a part in this development. This section will consider evidence for the effect of weight gain and medication in the management of this complication. In children and adolescents, weight loss has particularly serious implications. Sixty per cent of bone accretion occurs during puberty (Golden, 1992). Gain in bone mass is most pronounced between 11 and 14 years of age and falls significantly after 16 years of age (Soyka et al., 2002). Therefore, it would be expected that the failure of bone mineral accrual in girls with anorexia nervosa would differ depending on the maturation age.

Failure of this accretion thus compounds bone loss in children and adolescents with anorexia nervosa. Growth retardation is a further complication in children and adolescents (Russell, 1985; Danziger, 1994) and failure to grow may indicate nutritional deficiencies. It is thought that with weight gain 'catch-up growth' can occur up until fusion of the epiphyses (Nicholls & Stanhope, 2000). Regular monitoring of height as well as weight is important in children and adolescents with anorexia nervosa. Recommended weight ranges have to be regularly adjusted to take into account changes in height and age. Hormonal treatments, although used, have not been evaluated in adolescents with anorexia nervosa. There is a risk that oestrogen administration may cause premature epiphyseal fusion and growth stunting (Nicholls & Stanhope, 2000).

With regard to the reproductive system, there are several areas of concern: infertility, persistent amenorrhoea and oligomenorrhoea, and polycystic ovaries. In adolescent anorexia nervosa there is a risk of pubertal delay and ultimately arrested pubertal development (Russell, 1985). The effect on fertility and pregnancy will be described below.

Dental erosion is the most common oral problem in patients with eating disorders who engage in self-induced vomiting. A discussion of the issues concerning dental complications can be found in the chapter on bulimia nervosa (Section 7.5.2).

Osteoporosis

People with anorexia nervosa have reduced bone mineral density (BMD) (Bachrach, Guido, Katzman, Litt & Marcus, 1990) which is associated with an increased fracture rate (Rigotti, Neer, Skates, Herzog & Nussbaum, 1991; Vestergaard *et al.*, 2002; Lucas, Melton, Crowson & O'Fallon, 1999; Soyka, Grinspoon, Levitsky, Herzog & Klibanski, 1999) and long-term disability such as pain, kyphosis and loss of height. Osteoporosis is manifest in some people after a year of illness and the severity gradually increases over time if the illness remains untreated. Fractures may occur after a few years of illness.

The factors that predict bone density in the majority of studies include: duration of amenorrhoea (Biller *et al.*, 1989; Seeman, Szmukler, Formica, Tsalamandris & Mestrovic, 1992), BMI, or some other variable that reflects body composition (Grinspoon *et al.*, 2000). Some studies find that age at menarche is also a predictor (Grinspoon *et al.*, 2000). Oestrogen use does not predict density in larger studies (Grinspoon *et al.*, 2000).

There have been several longitudinal studies that have examined changes in bone density over time. In the majority of cases the people are also engaged with treatment, commonly nutritional and psychological interventions. In some studies additional treatments such as fluoride and hormone replacement have been added. It is difficult to compare between studies as the presentation and type of data differs between studies, as does the case mix.

Adolescents. One of the largest studies in adolescents is that of Castro and colleagues (Castro *et al.*, 2001). They have an early intervention service with a young (mean age 14.4 years) and moderately severe (BMI 15 kg/m^2) group. They found that change over time depends on the severity of the osteoporosis at baseline and the degree of recovery made over the period of follow-up. The group with established osteopenia at baseline (i.e. z < −1.0) had an increase in bone density of over nine per cent at spine (5.7 per cent in the femur) over the follow-up interval (1.3 years).

Adults. In adults (mean age 22 years) with a severe illness (mean BMI 13.9 kg/m^2) followed over two years, when BMI increased to 17.1 kg/m^2 there was an overall two per cent increase in bone density which related to weight gain. The subgroup that had full recovery (weight gain and menstruation) had the largest increase in bone density (Iketani *et al.*, 1995).

An additional study (Zipfel *et al.*, 2001) in adults (21 years) with BMI 14 kg/m^2 found similar results.

Current Clinical Practice. The most effective treatment/preventative agent for osteoporosis in anorexia nervosa is not yet known. Adequate nutrition and weight are the most relevant factors but in some cases this is difficult to implement in the long term. Therefore, there has been interest in replacing some factors of relevance to bone turnover. These include oestrogen (in the form of hormone replacement therapy or the contraceptive pill) which inhibits bone resorption and Vitamin D, calcium, and insulin-like growth factors (Grinspoon, 1997 & 2002) and DHEA (Gordon, 2002).

Bisphosphonates and fluoride have also been tried (Maugars *et al.*, 1996). It is anticipated that further guidance on the management of osteoporosis will be available on the treatment and management of osteoporosis following the publication in 2005 of the NICE clinical practice guideline.

6.4.6.1   Treatments reviewed

The following treatments were included:

● De hydroepiandrosterone (DHEA)
● Insulin-like growth factor (IGF-I)
● Oestrogen supplementation.

6.4.6.2   Studies considered

The review team conducted a new systematic search for studies examining factors associated with the management of osteoporosis in people with anorexia nervosa. Five RCTs met the eligibility criteria set by the GDG (Gordon, 1999 & 2002; Grinspoon, 1996 & 2002; Klibanski, 1995), involving 207 participants.

Of the five studies included, one compared oestrogen supplementation with assessment only (Klibanski, 1995), one compared different doses of DHEA (Gordon, 1999), one compared DHEA with hormone replacement therapy (Gordon, 2002), one compared two different doses of IGF-I with placebo (Grinspoon, 1996), and one compared IGF-I, oestrogen supplementation, placebo and the combination of IGF-I and oestrogen (Grinspoon, 2002).

6.4.6.3   Evidence statements[8]

There is insufficient evidence to determine whether oestrogen supplementation improves bone density by the end of treatment. I

There is insufficient evidence to determine whether oral DHEA improves bone density compared to hormone replacement therapy by the end of treatment. I

There is limited evidence that both IGF-I alone and the combination of IGF-I and an oral contraceptive may improve bone density:

● There is limited evidence suggesting that there is a clinically significant difference between rhIGF-I and placebo with IGF being superior in terms of bone turnover/ density by the end of treatment (Grinspoon, 1996 & 2002). I

● There is limited evidence suggesting that there is a clinically significant difference between rhIGF-I+oral contraceptive and placebo with the combination being superior in terms of bone density by the end of treatment (Grinspoon, 2002). I

There is some evidence that the combination of rhIGF-I and an oral contraceptive is produces a better outcome than rhIGF-I alone.

---

[8] The full list of all evidence statements generated from meta-analyses (and the associated forest plots) will be available on the CD-ROM that accompanies the guideline.

There is insufficient evidence to determine whether oestrogen supplementation is more or less acceptable to people with anorexia nervosa when compared to no oestrogen supplementation. I

There is insufficient evidence to determine whether oral DHEA is more or less acceptable to people with anorexia nervosa when compared to hormone replacement therapy. I

Full recovery from anorexia nervosa with weight gain and return of menstruation leads to a marked increase in bone density (the rate depends on the initial level, but can be as much as five per cent or more a year). However in those that remain under weight with amenorrhoea bone loss continues. III

In adolescents with a good outcome and low initial bone density the increase in BMD is four-fold that of normal adolescents. III

6.4.7 Clinical summary

Bone loss is a serious problem in anorexia nervosa with serious long-term consequences. Weight restoration is associated in adolescents with important gains in bone density. Oral oestrogen and oral DHEA do not appear to have a positive impact on bone density and hormone replacement therapy is not recommended in children and adolescents as it may cause premature fusion of the bones. High impact exercise is associated with an increased risk of fracture in anorexia nervosa. rhIGF-I, alone or in combination with an oral contraceptive, is associated with improvements in bone metabolism and bone mineral density but intensive clinical monitoring is necessary and this treatment should only be given in specialist centres with appropriate skills and knowledge. The long-term effect is uncertain.

6.4.8 Clinical practice recommendations

6.4.8.1   Oestrogen administration should not be used to treat bone density problems in children and adolescents as this may lead to premature fusion of the epiphyses. (C)

6.4.9 Other physical interventions

Malnutrition is a core feature of anorexia nervosa. Refeeding is a necessary component of treatment but is not sufficient. The approach to refeeding varies between centres and countries. There is debate about the setting, means and rate of weight gain and limited evidence to support different views. In some centres the calorie deficit is made up with food, given as normal, albeit larger, meals or snacks. In other centres liquid foods can be used to supplement or replace some or all of the meals. An alternative, which is not used frequently within the UK, is nasogastric feeding. Rarely percutaneous endoscopic gastrostomy (PEG) or total parenteral nutrition (TPN) has been used. These interventions are only used when patients are not able to co-operate with oral refeeding and there is concern about physical risk. In these circumstances legal and ethical considerations need to be addressed.

A number of complications can occur during refeeding. This is a high-risk period for biochemical abnormalities. People at most risk are those with a BMI less than 12 kg/m^2, those who vomit, abuse laxatives and binge, and those with concurrent physical conditions. Physical monitoring is necessary during periods of refeeding. A range of electrolyte disturbances can occur during refeeding, which are sometimes referred to collectively as the 'refeeding syndrome'. Hypophosphataemia may develop rapidly during refeeding; if severe, it can cause cardiac and respiratory failure, delirium and fits. Ingestion of large quantities of carbohydrates, during rapid refeeding, may result in a precipitate drop in serum phosphate levels. Therefore, in the first few days of refeeding patients who have had very low or absent intakes for long periods, no attempt should be made to achieve net weight gain. Instead they should receive energy and protein provision at levels at or less than their estimated basal requirements with generous provision of balanced multi-vitamins and minerals especially thiamine, potassium, magnesium and phosphate.

Certain vitamin or mineral deficits have come under close scrutiny. For example, the similarity between some of the symptoms of zinc deficiency and the symptoms of anorexia nervosa has led to an interest in zinc replacement. A proportion of patients with anorexia nervosa may be deficient in thiamine, riboflavin, Vitamin C and Vitamin D. The clinical significance of many of these deficiencies is unclear but it is usual for there to be a general rather than a specific deficit and therefore a multi-vitamin/multi-mineral supplement in oral form (e.g. suitable preparations include Sanatogen Gold [non-NHS], Forceval 1–2 or Seravit capsules daily). Care should be taken to prevent the risk of vitamin A and D toxicity from excessive use of supplements.

There has been some research into the nutritional management of anorexia nervosa but all of the studies on nutritional approaches are quasi-experimental and small, and the studies on zinc are small.

There is controversy, but little evidence, about the appropriate time course used to achieve the goals of treatment. Some argue that it is important to restore normal weight as soon as possible, others argue for a slower increase in weight. The standard rate of weight gain in the UK is 0.5 to 1 kg per week. The majority of people with anorexia nervosa are treated as outpatients but for the small number who require admission most specialist eating disorder inpatient units aim to discharge people once weight is fully recovered. However, there is an alternative view that full weight recovery can be achieved by outpatient or day patient interventions following brief inpatient refeeding, and that discharge at an intermediate weight may provide an alternative.

There is also the argument that weight gain is only one outcome of interest. Another goal is to ensure that eating behaviour is normalised and maintained after discharge, that abnormal weight and shape cognitions are normalised and that there is improved quality of life in people with anorexia nervosa.

Physical therapies have been used in some European countries (e.g. Belgium and Norway), which have a long tradition of integrating physical therapies into psychotherapy. Physical rehabilitation programmes including riding, climbing, for example, have been used. This has not been the tradition in the UK. Indeed in many programmes in the UK exercise is restricted and bed rest is prescribed.

Feeding in the context of active resistance

This section relates to those occasions where the individual requires restraining to allow the refeeding to take place. Feeding in the context of active resistance raises ethical, legal and clinical issues for all involved. The reporting of it in the general media is often inaccurate and emphasises the emotive 'force feeding' and the suggested abuse of the individual's rights who is fed in this way. In the UK in the treatment of people with anorexia nervosa it is a very rare event and should only be done in a specialised treatment setting with access to the skills and experience required to manage it safely and effectively. It raises complex legal issues. It is interesting to note that all requests to the courts for permission to carry out this intervention in anorexia nervosa have been granted. It is undertaken using the Mental Health Act 1983, the Children Act 1989 and parental authority. Only a small proportion of patients who are admitted and treated compulsorily require this intervention. No studies have reported on the characteristics of those who are fed in this way, or have followed them up.

Methods of delivering this intervention vary across the country, as do the circumstances under which it is used. The risks associated with naso-gastric (NG) tube feeding, PEG, or spoon feeding, will be increased in the context of active physical resistance. Actions such as the pulling out the (NG) tube, interfering with or pulling out the PEG, and the physical condition of the patient increase the risk involved.

Clinical decisions as to when to start the intervention, how long to continue for, how often to repeat the intervention and when to stop are complex and difficult. There are further complications with children and adolescents where the urgency to intervene is increased because the low fat mass means that any weight loss is predominantly of lean tissue with higher medical consequences. As a result, children can become dangerously physically compromised. In addition, children and younger adolescents have a much greater tendency to restrict both fluid and food intake. The combination of these factors leads to a rapid breakdown of muscle tissue and dehydration, especially in pre-pubertal children.

6.4.9.1   Physical interventions reviewed

The following interventions were included:

- Nasogastric feeding

- TPN

- Zinc supplementation

- Massage

- Exercise.

6.4.9.2   Studies considered

The review team conducted a new systematic search for RCTs of physical interventions used in the treatment of anorexia nervosa. As there were few RCTs, the GDG elected to utilise lower levels of evidence where necessary. This included the APA guidelines and a recent expert review on the nutritional management of anorexia nervosa (EDSIG). Eight studies met the eligibility criteria set by the GDG (Arii, 1996; Birmingham, 1994; Hart, 2001; Katz, 1987; Lask, 1993; Pertschuk, 1981; Robb, 2002; Thien, 2000), involving 267 participants.

Of the eight studies, two involved nasogastric feeding (Arii, 1996; Robb, 2002), one TPN (Pertschuk, 1981), three zinc (Birmingham, 1994; Katz, 1987; Lask, 1993), one exercise (Thien, 2000), and one massage (Hart, 2001).

Full details of studies included in the guideline and reasons for excluding studies are given in Appendix 18.

6.4.9.3   Evidence statements[9]

Effect of treatment on weight gain

There is limited evidence suggesting that there is a clinically significant difference between nasogastric feeding and 'standard care' with nasogastric feeding being superior in terms of weight gain by the end of multi-modal inpatient treatment ($n = 116$; Arii, 1996; Robb, 2002). II

There is insufficient evidence to determine whether zinc supplementation has any impact on weight compared with placebo during multi-modal inpatient treatment. I

There is insufficient evidence to determine whether TPN has any impact on weight compared with placebo during multi-modal inpatient treatment. II

There is insufficient evidence to determine whether massage or exercise given in addition to 'standard care' have any impact on weight compared with 'standard care' alone by the end of treatment. I

Effect of treatment on symptoms of anorexia nervosa

There is limited evidence suggesting that there is a clinically significant difference between massage and 'standard care' with massage being superior on EDI scores by the end of treatment (N = 1; $n = 16$; SMD = 1.06; 95 per cent CI, 0.02 to 2.09). I

Acceptability of treatment

There is insufficient or no evidence to determine whether nasogastric feeding or TPN are more, or less, acceptable to people with anorexia nervosa when compared to placebo or 'standard care'. II

There is insufficient evidence to determine whether zinc supplementation is more, or less, acceptable to people with anorexia nervosa when compared to placebo or 'standard care'. I

---

[9] The full list of all evidence statements generated from meta-analyses (and the associated forest plots) will be available on the CD-ROM that accompanies the guideline.

There is insufficient evidence to determine whether massage or exercise are more, or less, acceptable to people with anorexia nervosa when compared with 'standard care'. I

Tolerability of treatment

There is evidence from a retrospective chart review that TPN may produce a greater risk of side effects than 'standard care':

● There is limited evidence suggesting that there is a clinically significant difference between TPN and 'standard care' with placebo being superior in terms of the number of people experiencing adverse events by the end of treatment ($n = 22$; Pertschuk, 1981). II

6.4.10 Clinical summary

Nasogastric feeding can confer some benefit in terms of increased rate of weight gain or actual weight gain, as part of a treatment programme. There was insufficient evidence that either TPN or zinc supplementation confer any benefit in terms of weight gain. TPN appears to be associated with more adverse events in one small study. Some limited benefit, on symptoms but not on weight gain, has also been identified from one small trial investigating massage.

6.4.11 Clinical practice recommendations

6.4.11.1   Total parenteral nutrition should not be used for people with anorexia nervosa, unless there is significant gastrointestinal dysfunction. (C)

6.4.12 Concurrent physical conditions

Diabetes

There does not appear to be an increased occurrence of anorexia nervosa in Type 1 diabetes, however the statistical power of the studies may be insufficient to rule this out (Nielsen, 2002). The mortality rate in 10 years of follow-up of population-based samples was found to be 2.2 (per 1000 person years) for Type 1 diabetes, 7.3 for anorexia nervosa and 34.6 for concurrent cases (the standardised mortality rates were 4.1 for Type 1 diabetes, 8.9 for anorexia nervosa, and 14.5 in concurrent cases) (Nielsen, 2002).

Close liaison and a shared knowledge base between the eating disorder and diabetes teams is essential in the management of anorexia nervosa with diabetes and they should have intensive regular physical monitoring as they are at high risk of complications and death.

Pregnancy

It is unusual for people with anorexia nervosa to become pregnant although a small proportion have fertility treatment to conceive or relapse into anorexia nervosa during the pregnancy. In a follow-up study of people with anorexia nervosa ($n = 140$) fertility was reduced to one-third of the expected, the rate of prematurity was twice that expected and perinatal mortality was increased six-fold (Brinch *et al.*, 1988). In a follow-up series of 66 women there was an increased miscarriage rate and more use of Caesarean sections and the offspring were more likely to be born prematurely and smaller (Bulik *et al.*, 1999). On the other hand Steiner found no difference in weight gain and foetal weight in their sample (Steiner, Smith, Rosenkranz & Litt, 1991). In a study in which pregnant women with anorexia nervosa were followed prospectively the infants grew slowly in utero especially in the last trimester (Treasure & Russell, 1988).

Women with anorexia nervosa are at greater risk for premature offspring and those that are small for gestational age. There are case series that suggest that some women with anorexia nervosa have difficulty feeding their children (Russell, Treasure & Eisler, 1998; Wezel-Meijler & Wit, 1989) and that the child's growth can be abnormal (Hodes *et al.*, 1997).

Management of laxative abuse

The management of laxative abuse is covered in the bulimia nervosa chapter (Section 7.5.2), as the management is essentially the same for both disorders.

6.4.13 Clinical practice recommendations

Managing risk

6.4.13.1   Health care professionals should monitor physical risk in patients with anorexia nervosa. If this leads to the identification of increased physical risk, the frequency and the monitoring and nature of the investigations should be adjusted accordingly. (C)

6.4.13.2   People with anorexia nervosa and their carers should be informed if the risk to their physical health is high. (C)

6.4.13.3   The involvement of a physician or paediatrician with expertise in the treatment of physically at-risk patients with anorexia nervosa should be considered for all individuals who are physically at risk. (C)

6.4.13.4   Pregnant women with either current or remitted anorexia nervosa may need more intensive prenatal care to ensure adequate prenatal nutrition and foetal development. (C)

Feeding against the will of the patient

6.4.13.5   Feeding against the will of the patient should be an intervention of last resort in the care and management of anorexia nervosa. (C)

6.4.13.6   Feeding against the will of a patient is a highly specialised procedure requiring expertise in the care and management of those with severe eating disorders and the physical complications associated with it. This should only be done in the context of the Mental Health Act 1983 or Children Act 1989. (C)

6.4.13.7   When making the decision to feed against the will of the patient the legal basis for any such action must be clear. (C)

6.5 Service interventions for anorexia nervosa

6.5.1 Introduction

The majority of people with eating disorders present first in primary care. However, it is probable that most patients presenting with anorexia nervosa are referred on to secondary care usually within mental health services, including both general mental health services and specialist eating disorder services. Specialist eating disorder services for anorexia nervosa are distributed patchily (Royal College of Psychiatrists, 2001). A substantial proportion of such tertiary provision, in particular inpatient care, is in the private sector and many NHS patients are treated in private hospitals.

6.5.2 Current practice

Most patients with anorexia nervosa receive treatment solely on an outpatient basis. However, a substantial minority receive inpatient treatment. The style and content of inpatient programmes for anorexia nervosa varies widely. Hospital admission may be aimed at ameliorating the effects of the illness on the patient's physical state or at achieving progress toward full recovery. The former sometimes involves admission to general medical settings. The latter is usually attempted within psychiatric hospitals. It is generally held that it is preferable for admission to be to settings where the staff are experienced in the treatment of the disorder. Furthermore, the setting needs to be appropriate to the age of the patient. Special day programmes are being developed as an alternative mode of intensive treatment for anorexia nervosa.

6.5.3 Effective service configurations

Although there is considerable variation in the pattern of service delivery there is a limited evidence base on which to develop effective patterns of service delivery. However, the principle that the right treatments should be offered to the right patients in the right setting if services are to be effective and cost-effective, should guide service development.

This review seeks to examine whether any particular level of service provision is associated with better outcomes in anorexia nervosa. In addressing this issue it may be useful to differentiate between two types of hospital admission.

First, inpatient treatment of anorexia nervosa may be aimed at the stabilisation and rectification of the patient's physical state. It is widely believed that such treatment can at times be life-saving. However, such management has not been the subject of systematic comparative research and is unlikely to be.

Second, inpatient treatment aimed at helping the patient to progress toward full recovery is widely practiced and is more amenable to study.

The literature contains many descriptions of special inpatient treatment regimes for anorexia nervosa, and some outcome data are available (e.g. Bowers & Anderson, 1994). However, comparison between centres is difficult because of the likelihood that the case mix varies widely across studies. There is less data available about outpatient or day patient approaches. (Particular outpatient therapies are described elsewhere.) There is very little on the comparison between outpatient and day or inpatient treatment or on the integration of different forms of care.

The St. George's study (Crisp, Norton, Gowers, Halek, Yeldham, Levett & Bhat, 1991) is alone in attempting a comparison within a randomised controlled trial of hospital admission and two forms of outpatient treatment. (There was also an assessment only condition but many participants went on to receive treatment elsewhere thereby confounding the comparison.)

The study lacked power and had other difficulties. However, it did demonstrate that many patients made progress with fairly modest outpatient treatment over one year (Gowers, Norton, Halek & Crisp 1994). Such outpatient treatment is widely practiced but poorly documented. In one study of a specialised secondary service nearly three-quarters of adults with anorexia nervosa were managed without hospital admission (Palmer, Gatward, Black & Park, 2000).

Specialised day patient treatment for anorexia nervosa has been described in this country and abroad and positive outcomes are documented at least in the short term (Birchall, Palmer, Waine, Gadsby & Gatward, 2002; Gerlinghof, Backmund & Franzen, 1998; Olmsted, McFarlane, Molleken & Kaplan, 2001; Robinson, 2003; Zipfel et al., 2002). However, it is uncertain whether the patients described might otherwise have been admitted as inpatients or managed as outpatients. There are no randomised comparisons. One study suggests that the addition of a day programme may reduce the use of inpatient beds (Birchall, Palmer, Waine, Gadsby & Gatward, 2002). It is unlikely that day care could ever abolish the need for inpatient treatment altogether. Indeed, the relative effectiveness and cost-effectiveness of the two forms of more intensive treatment have yet to be adequately studied.

It is widely believed that there may be benefits in the treatment of severe anorexia nervosa which has not responded to less intensive treatments within a specialised tertiary eating disorders service compared with less specialised secondary services. Both competence and confidence tend to develop in settings where such treatment is a regular and ongoing activity. However, there is a lack of studies that might provide evidence to support these views. One study of mortality in patients treated in two contrasting services suggested that there might be advantages associated with greater specialisation (Crisp, Callender, Halek & Hsu, 1992).

A single systematic review of inpatient versus outpatient treatment of anorexia nervosa was inconclusive because of lack of evidence (Meads, Gold & Burls, 2001).

6.5.4 Clinical summary

In a minority of patients, admission to hospital may at times be necessary to stabilise the physical state or even save the life of severely physically impaired patients. Inpatient treatment aimed at recovery usually leads to weight gain at least where admission has been to a unit where such treatment is a regular activity. Such treatment may have lasting effects although weight loss is common after discharge. There is no unequivocal evidence that inpatient treatment confers long-term advantage except as a short-term life-saving intervention in patients at high risk. However, inpatient treatment may well be a rational option for patients who have failed to respond to apparently adequate outpatient treatment. The place of day care as an alternative option in these circumstances has yet to be fully evaluated but seems promising.

6.5.5 Satisfaction with service setting/configuration and adherence to treatment

The area of patient and carer perceptions has been the focus of some research in the area of eating disorders. Much of this work has been focused on perceptions of inpatient treatment for anorexia nervosa or on mixed or poorly defined populations of people with eating disorders, therefore it should be treated with caution. This area of research is potentially informative when considering the relative merits of different service configurations although the major focus of such work has been on improving the acceptability of services, which may have benefits in terms of improved attendance rates and increased involvement with and effectiveness of programmes and treatments prescribed (Matoff & Matoff, 2001; Swain-Campbell et al., 2001). Taking account of user and carer perceptions when designing and delivering services may also facilitate help seeking over a prolonged period in people with recurrent mental health problems (Buston, 2002). This in turn may contribute to reduced morbidity.

Individuals with eating disorders, and anorexia nervosa in particular, are often described as being ambivalent about seeking treatment. Unlike most other psychiatric conditions, core features of eating disorders can be highly valued by the patient. In addition, the hospital environment can contribute to a sense of passivity and vulnerability, which can be linked to an increased sense of loss of control, one of the central characteristics of an eating disorder (Eivors et al., 2003). Such factors can contribute to a degree of reluctance to engage fully in interventions, resulting in relatively high levels of treatment refusal and premature drop-out, with related implications for long-term recovery and health care costs (Kahn & Pike, 2001; Swain-Campbell et al., 2001). Some centres report that up to 50 per cent of patients prematurely cease contact after assessment at an eating disorders service (Button et al., 1997; Vandereycken & Pierloot, 1993). Yager et al. (1989) draw attention to the fact that studies from many eating disorders centres suggest that drop-out rates for virtually all types of treatment are considerable, suggesting relatively high levels of patient dissatisfaction with services and treatments offered. Noordenbos et al. (1988) suggest that in people with a long-standing eating disorder, patients' dissatisfaction may be compounded by clinicians' beliefs about 'chronic' or 'untreatable' presentations.

People receiving inpatient treatment for anorexia nervosa have been found to be twice as likely to drop out of treatment compared to general psychiatric inpatients (Kahn & Pike, 2001). Reasons for drop out are likely to be varied and complex. One study found that drop out from adult inpatient treatment was modestly predicted by anorexia nervosa sub-type (being greater in the binge-purge sub-type) and length of illness (with associated higher number of previous hospitalisations) and not to severity of eating disorders symptomatology or associated psychopathology (Kahn & Pike, 2001). Another study concluded that very little of formal treatment is regarded by patients as essential to recovery in those who have been treated for and recovered from anorexia nervosa (Maine, 1985). Such findings suggested a complicated relationship between service setting, clinical outcome and patient experience that is difficult to tease out.

Models of service provision currently vary considerably. Newton (2001) reports that although various surveys have identified strengths and weaknesses in existing service provision, this information seems to have had little impact on service planning. Assessment of patient and carer satisfaction specifically in relation to service setting is rarely carried out. Similarly, patient adherence and drop out, specifically in relation to service setting is not usually investigated (Mahon, 2000). Information about patient and carer views tends to come from qualitative studies of service users, based on structured and semi-structured interviews (with data presented descriptively or, for example, using a type of thematic content analysis such as a grounded theory approach) or questionnaires. The latter are often used to measure characteristics of clinical presentation (rather than service setting), which are then correlated with, for example, satisfaction or drop out. In some cases forced choice responses about satisfaction or ratings of perceived helpfulness are used, but again these are rarely related specifically to service configurations. Research in the area of satisfaction surveys is particularly prone to bias.

This issue of satisfaction and adherence to treatment was considered across a number of different types of service setting (e.g. outpatient, inpatient, day patient, generalist, specialist, self-help; local, distant, etc.); and across different age groups (adults, adolescents, children).

The review team conducted a new systematic search for all relevant research. No studies were found that specifically investigated comparisons between types of service. Nevertheless, a number of studies provided useful data (Brinch, Isager & Tolstrup, 1988; Buston, 2002; Button *et al.*, 1997; Button & Warren, 2001; Carnell, 1998; Deeble & Bhat, 1991; Eivors *et al.*, 2003; Haigh & Treasure, 2003; Hsu, Crisp & Callender, 1992; Kahn & Pike, 2000; Kopec-Schrader *et al.*, 1993; Le Grange & Gelman, 1998; Mahon, 2000; Maine, 1985; Malson *et al.*, unpublished; Matoff & Matoff, 2001; Newton, 2001; Newton *et al.*, 1993a; Noordenbos *et al.*, 1988; Pettersen & Rosenvinge, 2002; Rosenvinge & Klusmeier, 2000; Sharkey-Orgnero, 1999; Stockwell *et al.*, 1987; Sturmey, 1992; Swain Campbell, Surgenor & Snell, 2001; Tozzi *et al.*, 2003; Vandereycken & Pierloot, 1983; Yager *et al.*, 1989). Seven further studies were consulted, but not used directly (Bowers & Andersen, 1994; Greenwood *et al.*, 1999; Lemberg & May, 1991; Neiderman *et al.*, 2000; Newton, Hartley & Sturmey, 1993b; Wilhelm & Clarke, 1998; Zipfel *et al.*, 2002).

The following findings emerged from the papers considered in this section:

- Greater treatment satisfaction is most commonly reported in relation to outpatient treatment (particularly regarding individual and group therapy) (Rosenvinge & Klusmeier, 2000; Newton *et al.*, 1993a).

- Lengthy waiting times for outpatient treatment have been identified as a major reason for being dissatisfied with health care, and problems and delays in accessing medical or other appropriate help are associated with lower levels of satisfaction (Rosenvinge & Klusmeier, 2000; Buston, 2002).

- Carers and parents of adolescents have identified a lack of and need for support, involvement and education about eating disorders for themselves (Kopec-Schrader *et al.*, 1993; Haigh & Treasure, 2003).

- Continuity of care with an individual professional has been found to be valued – this could be taken to support the notion of comprehensive services, which can be flexible in terms of intensity (Buston, 2002).

- People who perceive their therapists to be 'experts on eating disorders' have been found to be more satisfied with treatment. 'Expert' includes concepts of 'understanding' and having 'knowledge of eating disorders' with the former being rated as the more important therapist attribute (Rosenvinge & Klusmeier, 2000).

- Informal supportive social relationships outside the treatment setting and a supportive relationship with a partner have been identified as important in recovery in people with eating disorders (Maine, 1985; Pettersen & Rosenvinge, 2002; Tozzi et al., 2003).

- Surveys of self-help groups suggest that they are regarded by the majority of attendees as helpful, being positively associated with social involvement and supportive sharing. However, self-help groups can be experienced by some individuals as upsetting or promoting competitiveness in terms of weight loss and eating disorders behaviours (Deeble & Bhat, 1991).

- Some people who have received treatment for anorexia nervosa report a general negative perception of being treated as an illness or diagnosis rather than as a person (Brinch et al., 1988, Malson et al.). This may be associated with reduced likelihood of seeking psychiatric help later.

- Perceived negative staff attitudes, and an overemphasis on weight and weight restoration have been identified as unhelpful or harmful aspects of treatment by adults receiving inpatient treatment (Button & Warren, 2001). An overemphasis on weight gain has also been found to be associated with drop out from treatment (Newton et al., 1993a).

- The acceptability of inpatient treatment for anorexia nervosa in adolescence has been rated as low in regards to feeling pressured and watched, with authoritarian and restricting aspects of therapy causing anger and ambivalence (Brinch et al., 1988).

- Adolescents have reported a sense of lack of privacy and intrusiveness in the context of inpatient care (Buston, 2002).

- Parents of adolescents with anorexia nervosa have reported feeling blamed for their child's eating disorder by clinicians providing treatment (Sharkey-Orgnero, 1999).

6.5.5.1 Clinical summary

A wide range of views, experiences and levels of satisfaction is expressed, with responses ranging from totally satisfied to totally dissatisfied in relation to specific service settings. No consistent pattern emerges in relation to type of service setting, or age, with different people being satisfied or dissatisfied with different aspects of services or service settings. Treatment adherence, problem severity and eventual outcome are not always related to satisfaction and acceptability (Stockwell et al., 1987; Sturmey, 1992) and patients attribute a wide range of factors (independent of service setting) to recovery (Hsu et al., 1992; LeGrange & Gelman, 1998).

It is common that individuals remain ambivalent about treatment received, particularly those with anorexia nervosa (Brinch *et al.*, 1988, Carnell, 1998). Those who have anorexia nervosa in adolescence appear most likely to recall their treatment (whether inpatient or outpatient) in negative terms. This attitude tends to persist and does not appear to be related to treatment duration or intensity (Brinch *et al.*, 1988; Buston, 2002). The ambivalence characteristic of people with eating disorders in relation to treatment may be an important issue. This ambivalence stems in part from the functional aspects of the disorder itself, and must form part of the backdrop against which views about satisfaction are interpreted. In this respect it might be understandable that some suggest that unlike other psychiatric disorders, patient dissatisfaction will tend to be high in eating disorders (e.g. Swain Campbell *et al.*, 2001).

People (in Norway) asked to list recommendations to increase/improve health care services for people with eating disorders most frequently identified 'improving clinical competence and knowledge about eating disorders amongst GPs' (Rosenvinge & Klusmeier, 2000). The opportunity to talk and be understood seems to be more important than (type of) formalised psychotherapy or service setting in terms of user satisfaction (Button & Warren, 2001).

Finally, given that self-help groups do quite well on very or fairly helpful ratings, the fact that self-help group users tend to use other professional services, and the finding that supportive social relationships outside formal treatment settings are associated with recovery, it seems more could be possible in terms of integrated working between statutory and voluntary services/agencies.

6.5.6 Relationship between service setting and risk of death, suicide and self-harm

Anorexia nervosa is associated with an increased mortality (Nielsen, 2001). People at risk of death because of their extreme physical state are likely to be considered – appropriately – for admission to hospital. However, there is unlikely to be systematic evidence to support such practice. Furthermore, people suffering from anorexia nervosa may be at increased risk of self-harm and suicide (Favaro & Santonastaso, 2000). This is especially so with respect of the binge-purging sub-type of anorexia nervosa.

6.5.7 Compulsory admission and treatment

A decision to compulsorily treat people with eating disorders occurs infrequently but does raise debate amongst professionals working in the field, the individuals they treat and their families. People with anorexia nervosa often differ from others with mental health problems in that the central characteristics of the illness are perceived as functional and valued by the individual. The individual can be perceived as ambivalent about recovery and resistant to intervention. In (eating disorders) treatment an emphasis is placed on developing a collaborative therapeutic relationship with the individual. Under conditions of compulsion this may be more difficult. However individuals who have undergone such treatment report contrasting positive and negative views when asked to comment later.

Treatment in this context refers to inpatient treatment of anorexia nervosa in adults, children and adolescents. However in the case of children and adolescents compulsory treatment can take place on an outpatient basis under parental authority, under the Mental Health Act 1983 and more rarely, with specific Court Orders.

There are no reports of compulsory admission for the specific treatment of bulimia nervosa or binge eating disorder (BED) in the UK.

Compulsory admissions and treatment for adults are carried out using the Mental Health Act (MHA) 1983. The Mental Health Act Commission (Guidance note number 3) provides guidance on the use of the Act in anorexia nervosa. Practice with children and adolescents, varies throughout the country. The issues of the 'assessment of competence (in children/adolescents) and capacity (in adults)' are complex. Legislation used with this population includes the Mental Health Act 1983 and the Children Act 1989.

Individuals with anorexia nervosa may be ambivalent about their treatment and can experience treatment as compulsory whatever their legal status. Often there are no differences between treatment programmes for those admitted and treated compulsorily and those who are not. Patients with eating disorders are sometimes admitted compulsorily for treatment of comorbid conditions.

For the purpose of this guideline, compulsory admission and treatment will be defined as that carried out using the legal powers available under the Mental Health Act 1983 or the Children Act 1989 or the authority of the court.

A further aim of employing compulsion under the MHA 1983 is to offer the individual the protection that is provided for them in the Act. It is important to remember that compulsory treatment does not equate with 'feeding against the will of the person' or 'force feeding'. It is helpful to hold in mind the distinction between treatment carried out under the legislation with which the individual complies (for whatever reason) and that which the individual resists.

6.5.7.1   Studies considered

The review team conducted a new systematic search for all research relevant to the issue of compulsory admission and treatment. No RCTs or meta-analyses were found. However, a few case control and three cohort studies were included.

6.5.7.2   Evidence

There is a lack of research into the outcomes of compulsory admission for anorexia nervosa (Russell, 2001; Watson, 2000). The literature in this area relates mainly to those adults treated within specialist eating disorder settings or, individual case studies characterised by refusal of treatment in children and adolescents. There is a suggestion in the literature that those compulsorily treated have a poorer outcome but there is insufficient evidence to derive any conclusion from this (Ramsay et al., 1999).

The potential benefits of compulsory admission have been identified as weight gain (Ramsay et al., 1999), saving life (Honig & Bentovim, 1996), opportunities for further treatment and avoiding significant harm (Honig & Bentovim, 1996), improvement in mood and concentration and reduction in symptoms (Maloney & Farrell, 1980), and less starvation induced cognitive impairment (MacDonald, 2002).

The potential risks include: obstacles to the development of a therapeutic relationship (Orbach & Rathner, 1998; Lancely & Travers, 1993), negative physical and psychological effects (Dresser & Boisaubin, 1986), negative countertransference, stigma associated with the MHA 1983 affecting the persons future (Hebert *et al.*, 1991), damage to self-esteem, escalation of resistance (Rathner, 1998; Fichter, 1995).

The literature provides some guidance on when to employ compulsory treatment (Ramsay *et al.*, 1999). There is considerable guidance available to health care professionals and others involved in compulsory admissions which offers advice on the protection to all those involved and guidance on the use of ethical decision making (Manley *et al.*, 2002; Goldner, 1997, Honig & Jaffa, 2000) and the obtaining of consent particularly in the child and adolescent field. Practitioners should also be aware of the outcome of reported legal challenges to compulsory treatment in anorexia nervosa, including the use of forcible feeding if necessary which have tended to favour those applying for or defending the right to treat (Dolan, 1999). Proposed new legislation (the reform of the Mental Health Act 1983) may have a major impact on the issue of consent to treatment.

6.5.7.3   Clinical summary

Formal admission for the specific treatment of anorexia nervosa or for immediate life-saving is necessary in very rare circumstances, where substantial risk cannot be managed in any other way. Little is known about the outcomes of those who are compulsorily treated; they have a poorer outcome than those who are not compulsorily treated, but this may be due to the initial severity of illness on admission. Treatment under conditions of compulsion very rarely involves feeding in the context of active physical resistance. The successful management of anorexia nervosa in these circumstances requires special skill and expertise in the area of compulsory treatment of people with eating disorders.

Special considerations are required when using compulsory treatment with children and adolescents (in particular the assessment of competence to consent). The issues of consent and treatment refusal are complex in children and adolescents (see Department of Health guidelines – Reference Guide to Consent for Examination for Treatment, 2002) because of the need to assess competence and involve a third party (parents) in the discussion. When refusal of treatment repeatedly occurs expert legal advice should be sought to establish whether the use of mental health legislation (irrespective of the patient's age) or an application to the Court under the provision of the Children Act 1989 is the best way to proceed. As both physical and psychological development is compromised in patients with early onset anorexia nervosa, treatment should aim to balance the need for urgent weight restoration alongside the educational and social needs of the young person. It is not recommended to continue treatment relying indefinitely on parental consent. The legal basis under which treatment is being carried out should be clearly recorded for this patient group.

6.5.8 Clinical practice recommendations

6.5.8.1   Most people with anorexia nervosa should be treated on an outpatient basis. (C)

6.5.8.2   Inpatient treatment or day patient treatment should be considered for people with anorexia nervosa whose disorder has not improved with appropriate outpatient treatment, or for whom there is a significant risk of suicide or severe self-harm. (C)

6.5.8.3   Inpatient treatment should be considered for people with anorexia nervosa whose disorder is associated with high or moderate physical risk. (C)

6.5.8.4   Where inpatient management is required, this should be provided within a reasonable travelling distance to enable the involvement of relatives and carers in treatment, to maintain social and occupational links and to avoid difficulty in transition between primary and secondary care services. This is particularly important in the treatment of children and adolescents. (C)

6.5.8.5   People with anorexia nervosa requiring inpatient treatment should normally be admitted to a setting that can provide the skilled implementation of refeeding with careful physical monitoring (particularly in the first few days of refeeding) and in combination with psychosocial interventions. (C)*

6.5.8.6   Health care professionals without specialist experience in eating disorders, or in situations of uncertainty, should consider seeking advice from an appropriate specialist when contemplating a compulsory admission for a patient with anorexia nervosa regardless of the age of the patient. (C)

6.5.8.7   Health care professionals managing patients with anorexia nervosa, especially those with the binge-purging sub-type, should be aware of the increased risk of self-harm and suicide, particularly at times of transition between services or service settings. (C)

Additional considerations for children and adolescents

6.5.8.8   Health care professionals should ensure that children and adolescents with anorexia nervosa who have reached a healthy weight have the increased energy and necessary nutrients available in the diet to support growth and development. (C)

6.5.8.9   In the nutritional management of children and adolescents with anorexia nervosa, carers should be included in any dietary education or meal planning. (C)

6.5.8.10   Admission of children and adolescents with anorexia nervosa should be to age-appropriate facilities (with the potential for separate children and adolescent services), which have the capacity to provide appropriate educational and related activities. (C)

6.5.8.11   When a young person with anorexia nervosa refuses treatment that is deemed essential, consideration should be given to the use of the Mental Health Act 1983 or the right of those with parental responsibility to override the young person's refusal. (C)

6.5.8.12   Relying indefinitely on parental consent to treatment should be avoided. It is recommended that the legal basis under which treatment is being carried out should be recorded in the patient's case notes, and this is particularly important in the case of children and adolescents. (C)

6.5.8.13   For children and adolescents with anorexia nervosa, where issues of consent to treatment are highlighted, health care professionals should consider seeking a second opinion from an eating disorders specialist. (C)

6.5.8.14   If the patient with anorexia nervosa and those with parental responsibility refuse treatment, and treatment is deemed to be essential, legal advice should be sought in order to consider proceedings under the Children Act 1989. (C)

6.6 Predicting the outcome of treatment and recovery from anorexia nervosa

It is important to be able to predict how people with anorexia nervosa will respond to treatment. For example, those with a good prognosis may respond to less intensive treatment (i.e. outpatient treatment). Knowledge of the factors associated with outcome may also suggest modifications or alternative approaches for patients who do not respond to first line treatments.

Nielsen *et al.* (1998) reviewed the mortality rate from published outcome studies of anorexia nervosa and bulimia nervosa. In anorexia nervosa, the association of lower weight at presentation and elevated Standardised Mortality Rate (SMR) was highly significant. Age at presentation was also significant with the highest SMR for those presenting between 20 and 29 years of age. A recent review by Steinhausen (2002) considered 119 studies but did not consider issues relating to study or data quality. A number of other papers reviewed various comorbid conditions and their relationship to outcome in eating disorders (Holderness *et al.*, 1994; Herzog *et al.*, 1996; Rosenvinge *et al.*, 2000). A wide range of potential predictors of outcome have been studied, often those that are routinely or most easily collected at pre-treatment. Some predictors, such as readiness for change, which may be important, are rarely measured.

For the purposes of the guideline, a literature review was carried out using PsycLIT and MEDLINE to identify relevant studies published on or before January 2003. This augmented the search of clinical trials already performed as part of the review of the effectiveness of treatment interventions. A wide range of studies (cohort and treatment studies) of varying quality were identified. Studies of mixed eating disorder populations were excluded unless separate data for anorexia nervosa and bulimia nervosa were reported. Studies of all ages were included and all variables reported in the studies were included in the analysis. Most of the included studies are of inpatients, which limit the generalisability of the findings to less severe populations. Sample size ($N \geq 50$) was selected as the key inclusion criterion as it was not possible to derive robust measures of study quality. One exception was made to the key inclusion criteria; studies with a sample size of less than 50 were included where the follow-up period was four years or over. A total of 54 studies contributed to the final analysis with sample sizes ranging from 26 to 422. Many studies had repeated assessments at follow-up, the longest being 21 years (Lowe *et al.*, 2001).

The wide variability in method (e.g. different measures of a potential predictor, such as family dysfunction) did not permit a meta-analysis. There was insufficient data to justify analysing data separately for treatments, outcome measures or follow-up length. A detailed analysis of the number of participants leaving a study early, as an outcome measure, was beyond the scope of this review.

Outcome varied considerably across studies (e.g. weight, diagnostic status or Morgan-Russell categories). Some studies also focused on comorbid disorders as predictors of outcome. For consistency, all findings are expressed in relation to poor outcome.

Based on the number of studies showing a positive result relative to the number showing a negative result for each variable examined, a number of possible predictors emerged (for full details see Appendix 11). That is, in people with anorexia nervosa, a low BMI and a number of indices of physical deterioration prior to treatment are associated with a poorer outcome, as is the bulimic sub-type of anorexia nervosa (in particular vomiting). Previous treatment for anorexia nervosa is also associated with poorer outcome, but findings may be confounded by duration or severity of the disorder. Other pre-treatment predictors identified were personality or interpersonal problems, family disturbance, body image disturbance or dissatisfaction and low desired weight. These findings may indicate areas that need to be addressed within treatment. Age over 20 years at presentation is also associated with poorer outcome.

Post-treatment predictors of poor outcome include other psychiatric disorders, such as mood and personality disorders. This highlights the importance of comprehensive psychiatric and psychological interventions. Inadequate weight gain in treatment, low desired weight, and drive for thinness or continued dieting at post-treatment are also associated with poorer long-term outcome. This highlights the importance of addressing attitudes to food and weight within treatment. Poor social adjustment post-treatment is also associated with poorer long-term outcome indicating the potential needs of patients who do not recover.

6.6.1 Clinical practice recommendations

6.6.1.1   People with eating disorders should be assessed and receive treatment at the earliest opportunity. (C)

6.6.1.2   Early treatment is particularly important for those with or at risk of severe emaciation and such patients should be prioritised for treatment. (C)

7 Treatment and management of bulimia nervosa

7.1 Introduction

Bulimia nervosa was first described in 1979 in a paper titled 'Bulimia nervosa: an ominous variant of anorexia nervosa' (Russell, 1979). In this paper Russell described bulimia nervosa as 'intractable'. This view is no longer held. Within two years of Russell's paper a report was published describing a promising psychological treatment for the disorder, a specific form of CBT (Fairburn, 1981), and the following year there were two reports that antidepressant drugs also had a beneficial effect (Pope & Hudson, 1982; Walsh *et al.*, 1982). Since then, bulimia nervosa has been the subject of much research interest. There have been over 60 randomised controlled trials evaluating a range of treatments for bulimia nervosa and their findings are remarkably consistent. Evidence-based treatment is certainly possible.

In this chapter the research on psychological treatments is first reviewed. Then the drug studies are considered, followed by the trials evaluating psychological versus antidepressant drug treatment, and their combination. In addition, there are separate sections on the management of the physical aspects of bulimia nervosa and service level interventions. Finally, there is a section on predicting outcome to treatment and recovery from bulimia nervosa.

7.2 Psychological interventions

7.2.1 Introduction

The psychological treatment of bulimia nervosa has been the subject of much research interest. Within two years of the publication of Russell's seminal paper on bulimia nervosa (Russell, 1979), Fairburn (1981) described promising results with a specific form of cognitive behaviour therapy (CBT-BN) (Fairburn, 1981). The following year another promising psychological treatment was described, a form of exposure with response prevention (ERP) (Rosen & Leitenberg, 1982). By the mid-1980s randomised controlled trials evaluating these and other psychological treatments were beginning to be published (Lacey, 1983; Yates & Sambrailo, 1984; Ordman & Kirchenbaum, 1985; Fairburn *et al.*, 1986; Lee & Rush, 1986; Wilson *et al.*, 1986).

Since then research on the treatment of bulimia nervosa has continued apace. Certain trends are apparent. The studies have become larger, and therefore more statistically powerful (e.g. Agras *et al.*, 2000a), and more sophisticated in the questions that they have addressed (e.g. Fairburn *et al.*, 1993; Mitchell *et al.*, 2002). They have included studies of mediators of treatment effects (Wilson *et al.*, 2002) and moderators of treatment outcome (Agras *et al.*, 2000b). Generic research methods have improved too with the use of detailed treatment manuals (e.g. Fairburn, 1993, 1997) and procedures to ensure the treatments are well delivered (e.g. Agras *et al.*, 2000a). Standardised measures of outcome have been employed, the Eating Disorder Examination (EDE) (Cooper & Fairburn, 1987; Fairburn & Cooper, 1993) being widely viewed as the 'gold standard'. There has also been interest in not simply identifying effective treatments for bulimia nervosa but also in evaluating ways of disseminating them (e.g. Cooper *et al.*, 1996; Treasure *et al.*, 1996; Palmer *et al.*, 2003).

7.2.2 Current practice

There have been no UK-based studies of the treatments that are actually provided for patients with bulimia nervosa. Three studies in the US suggest that evidence-based treatments are not widely used (Crow *et al.*, 1999; Mussell *et al.*, 2000; Haas & Clopton, 2003). There is no reason to think that the situation is any different in the UK. There are likely to be wide variations in the nature of treatment provided, reflecting the resources available and the training and proclivity of the clinician involved. The findings of two UK-based studies suggest that most people with bulimia nervosa are not in treatment (Fairburn & Cooper, 1982; Fairburn *et al.*, 1996).

7.2.3 Psychological treatments versus wait-list or placebo control

7.2.3.1 Treatments reviewed

The following treatments were included:

● Cognitive behaviour therapy for bulimia nervosa (CBT–BN)

● CBT+exposure with response prevention (CBT+ERP)

● Focal supportive psychotherapy

● Guided self-help (GSH)

● Pure self-help (PSH)

● Simplified dialectical behaviour therapy (simplified DBT).

The Psychological Topic Group established definitions for each treatment (see Glossary). Two members of the Topic Group assessed each study for eligibility and classified each psychological treatment. Where disagreements arose, they were resolved by discussion.

7.2.3.2 Studies considered[10]

The review team used the existing Cochrane review 'Psychotherapy for bulimia nervosa and binging' (Hay & Bacaltchuk, 2003) as the starting point for this section.

---

[10] Here and elsewhere in the guideline, each study considered for use in the guideline is referred to by a study ID (primary author and date of study publication, except where a study is in press or only submitted for publication, then a date is not used).

Fourteen trials used in the existing Cochrane review were excluded because they did not meet the inclusion criteria set by the GDG (Bachar, 1999; Bossert, 1989; Bulik, 1998; Carter, 1998; Esplen, 1998; Laessle, 1987 & 1991; Loeb, 2000; Ordman, 1985; Peterson, 1998; Thackwray, 1993; Treasure, 1999; Wilfley, 1993; Wilson, 1986). A further six trials were excluded from this section, but included in the next section regarding different psychological treatments (Agras, 2000; Cooper, 1995; Fairburn, 1986 & 1991; Walsh, 1997; Wilson, 1991). The six remaining trials were included here (Agras, 1989; Freeman, 1988; Griffiths, 1994; Lee, 1986; Treasure, 1994; Wolf, 1992). In addition, one trial excluded from the Cochrane review (Mitchell, 1990) and six trials (Leitenberg, 1988; Mitchell, 2001a; Carter, 2003; Walsh, submitted; Sundgotborgen, 2002; Safer, 2001) found during the search for new evidence, were included. Thus, 13 RCTs comparing a psychological treatment with a wait-list control or placebo group, involving 1029 participants, were included.

Out of the included trials, 10 involved CBT-BN (Agras, 1989; Freeman, 1988; Griffiths, 1994; Lee, 1986; Leitenberg, 1988; Mitchell, 1990; Sundgotborgen, 2002; Treasure, 1994; Walsh, submitted; Wolf, 1992), three involved CBT+ERP (Agras, 1989; Leitenberg, 1988; Sundgotborgen, 2002), two involved focal supportive psychotherapy (Agras, 1989; Freeman, 1988), one used GSH (Walsh, submitted), three used PSH (Carter, 2003; Mitchell, 2001a; Treasure, 1994), and one involved simplified DBT (Safer, 2001).

Full details of the studies included in the guideline and the reasons for excluding studies are given in Appendix 18.

7.2.3.3   Evidence statements[11]

The level of evidence (I, IIb, IIb, III, IV) is given after each statement (see Section 3.4.6 for more information about the classification of evidence).

Effect of treatment on remission from binge eating/purging

There is strong evidence suggesting that there is a clinically significant difference between CBT–BN and wait-list control with CBT–BN being superior in terms of remission from binge eating (defined as cessation of binge eating) by the end of treatment (N = 3; n = 136; RR = 0.73; 95 per cent CI, 0.61 to 0.88; NNT = 4; 95 per cent CI, 3 to 9). I

There is limited evidence suggesting that there is a clinically significant difference between simplified DBT and wait-list control with simplified DBT being superior in terms of remission from binge eating/purging (defined as cessation of binge eating/purging) by the end of treatment (N = 1; n = 31; RR = 0.75; 95 per cent CI, 0.57 to 1.00; NNT = 4; 95 per cent CI, 3 to 100). I

---

[11] The full list of all evidence statements generated from meta-analyses (and the associated forest plots) will be available on the CD-ROM that accompanies the guideline.

There is limited evidence suggesting that it is unlikely that PSH improves remission from binge eating/purging by the end of treatment:

- There is evidence suggesting that it is unlikely there is a clinically significant difference between PSH and wait-list control in terms of remission from binge eating (defined as cessation of binge eating) by the end of treatment (N = 2; n = 139; RR = 0.96; 95 per cent CI, 0.85 to 1.09). I

- There is evidence suggesting that it is unlikely there is a clinically significant difference between PSH and wait-list control in terms of remission from purging (defined as cessation of purging) by the end of treatment (N = 2; n = 139; RR = 0.97; 95 per cent CI, 0.87 to 1.07). I

There is insufficient or no evidence to determine whether CBT+ERP, focal supportive psychotherapy, or GSH have any impact on remission rates.

Effect of treatment on frequency of binge eating and purging symptoms

There is strong evidence that CBT–BN reduces the frequency of binge eating and purging symptoms by the end of treatment:

- There is strong evidence suggesting that there is a clinically significant difference between CBT–BN and wait-list control with CBT-BN being superior on mean frequency of binge eating by the end of treatment (N = 5; n = 185; SMD = –0.75; 95 per cent CI, –1.05 to –0.44). I

- There is strong evidence suggesting that there is a clinically significant difference between CBT–BN and wait-list control with CBT–BN being superior on mean frequency of purging by the end of treatment (N = 6; n = 192; Random Effects SMD = -1.00; 95 per cent CI, –1.63 to –0.36). I

There is strong evidence suggesting that there is a clinically significant difference between CBT+ERP and wait-list control with CBT+ERP being superior on mean frequency of purging by the end of treatment (N = 2; n = 57; SMD = –0.83; 95 per cent CI, –1.37 to –0.28). I

There is strong evidence that focal supportive psychotherapy reduces the frequency of binge eating and purging symptoms by the end of treatment:

- There is strong evidence suggesting that there is a clinically significant difference between focal supportive psychotherapy and wait-list control with focal supportive psychotherapy being superior on mean frequency of binge eating by the end of treatment (N = 1; n = 50; SMD = –1.12; 95 per cent CI, –1.73 to –0.51). I

- There is strong evidence suggesting that there is a clinically significant difference between focal supportive psychotherapy and wait-list control with supportive psychotherapy being superior on mean frequency of purging by the end of treatment (N = 2; n = 84; SMD = –1.43; 95 per cent CI, –1.93 to –0.94). I

There is insufficient or no evidence to determine whether GSH, PSH, or simplified DBT have any impact on frequency of binge eating and purging symptoms.

Other effects of treatment

There is strong evidence suggesting that there is a clinically significant difference between CBT–BN and wait-list control with CBT–BN being superior with regard to the mean depression score by the end of treatment (N = 3; n = 87; Random Effects SMD = −1.19; 95 per cent CI, −1.99 to −0.39). I

There is strong evidence suggesting that there is a clinically significant difference between CBT+ERP and wait-list control with CBT+ERP being superior with regard to the mean depression score by the end of treatment (N = 1; n = 34 SMD = −1.20; 95 per cent CI, −1.94 to −0.46). I

There is insufficient or no evidence to determine whether focal supportive psychotherapy, GSH, PSH, or simplified DBT have any impact on depression. I

There is insufficient or no evidence to determine whether CBT-BN, CBT+ERP, focal supportive psychotherapy, GSH, PSH, or simplified DBT have any impact on interpersonal/ psychosocial functioning. I

Attrition from the study

There is evidence suggesting that it is unlikely there is a clinically significant difference between CBT–BN and wait-list control in terms of the number of people leaving the study early due to any reason by end of treatment (N = 9; n = 384; RR = 1.14; 95 per cent CI, 0.74 to 1.74). I

There is insufficient or no evidence to determine whether there is any difference between CBT+ERP, focal supportive psychotherapy, GSH, PSH, or simplified DBT and a wait-list control in terms of the number of people leaving the study early due to any reason by end of treatment.

7.2.4 Psychological treatments versus other psychological treatments

7.2.4.1   Treatments reviewed[12]

The following treatments were included:

● Behaviour therapy (BT)

● Cognitive behaviour therapy for bulimia nervosa (CBT–BN)

● CBT+exposure with response prevention (CBT+ERP).

---

[12] The full list of all evidence statements generated from meta-analyses (and the associated forest plots) will be available on the CD-ROM that accompanies the guideline.

- Focal supportive psychotherapy

- Group CBT

- Guided self-help (GSH)

- Individual CBT

- Interpersonal psychotherapy for bulimia nervosa (IPT-BN)

- Dietary counselling

- Psychodynamic psychotherapy.

7.2.4.2   Studies considered

The review team used the existing Cochrane review 'Psychotherapy for bulimia nervosa and binging' (Hay & Bacaltchuk, 2003) as the starting point for this section.

Fourteen trials used in the existing Cochrane review were excluded because they did not meet the inclusion criteria set by the GDG (Bachar, 1999; Bossert, 1989; Bulik, 1998; Carter, 1998; Esplen, 1998; Laessle, 1987 & 1991; Loeb, 2000; Ordman, 1985; Peterson, 1998; Thackwray, 1993; Treasure, 1999; Wilfley, 1993; Wilson, 1986). A further two trials were excluded from this section, but included in the earlier section of psychological treatments versus wait-list control or placebo (Griffiths, 1994; Lee, 1986). The 10 remaining trials were included in the present section (Agras, 1989 & 2000; Cooper, 1995; Fairburn, 1986 & 1991; Freeman, 1988; Treasure, 1994; Walsh, 1997; Wilson, 1991; Wolf, 1992). In addition, eight trials (Bailer, in press; Chen, 2003; Garner, 1993; Hsu, 2001; Jansen, 2002; Kirkley, 1985; Leitenberg, 1988; Sungotborgen, 2002) found during the search for new evidence, were included. Thus, 18 RCTs comparing two different psychological treatments, involving 1343 participants, were included in this section.

Out of the included trials, three involved a comparison of CBT–BN with BT (Fairburn, 1991; Freeman, 1988; Wolf, 1992), with follow-up periods ranging from three to 12 months. Four trials involved a comparison of CBT with CBT+ERP (Bulik, 1998; Cooper, 1995; Leitenberg, 1988; Wilson, 1991) with all using 12 months' follow-up, except Leitenberg, 1988 (six-months' follow-up). Two trials involved a comparison of CBT–BN with IPT–BN (Agras, 2000; Fairburn, 1991) using a follow-up period of eight and 12 months, respectively. One trial involved a comparison of CBT–BN with psychodynamic psychotherapy (Garner, 1993), but presented no follow-up data. Four trials had a comparison of CBT–BN with focal supportive psychotherapy (Agras, 1989; Fairburn, 1986; Freeman, 1988; Kirkley, 1985) using follow-up periods ranging between three and 12 months. One trial compared CBT–BN with dietary counselling (Sungotborgen, 2002) using a follow-up of 18 months, and one trial compared CBT–BN with GSH (Bailer, in press) using a follow-up of 12 months. Another trial compared CBT–BN with PSH (Treasure, 1994) with no follow-up.

In addition, one trial compared CBT+ERP with focal supportive psychotherapy (Agras, 1989) and two compared CBT+ERP with dietary counselling (Hsu, 2001; Jansen, 2002), all without follow-up data. One trial compared BT with IPT–BN (Fairburn, 1991) using a follow-up period of 12 months, and one compared BT with focal supportive psychotherapy (Freeman, 1988). Finally, one compared individual CBT with group CBT (Chen, 2003) with six-months' follow-up.

Full details of the studies included in the guideline and the reasons for excluding studies are given in Appendix 18.

7.2.4.3   Evidence statements[13]

Effect of treatment on remission from binge eating and purging

There is evidence from two trials that CBT–BN when compared to IPT–BN improves remission from binge eating and purging by the end of treatment, but is no longer superior at post-treatment follow-up:

- There is strong evidence suggesting that there is a clinically significant difference between CBT–BN and IPT–BN with CBT–BN being superior in terms of remission from binge eating (defined as cessation of binge eating) by the end of treatment (N = 2; n = 270; RR = 0.77; 95 per cent CI, 0.67 to 0.87; NNT = 5; 95 per cent CI, 4 to 20). I

- There is strong evidence suggesting that there is a clinically significant difference between CBT–BN and IPT–BN with CBT–BN being superior in terms of remission from purging (defined as cessation of purging) by the end of treatment (N = 1; n = 220; RR = 0.76; 95 per cent CI, 0.67 to 0.86; NNT = 5; 95 per cent CI, 4 to 8). I

- There is evidence suggesting that it is unlikely there is a clinically significant difference between CBT–BN and IPT–BN in terms of remission from binge eating (defined as cessation of binge eating/purging) at follow-up (N = 2; n = 270; RR = 0.93; 95 per cent CI, 0.82 to 1.06). I

There is insufficient or no evidence to determine whether there is any difference between CBT-BN and BT on remission rates. I

Effect of treatment on frequency of binge eating and purging

There is limited evidence suggesting that there is a clinically significant difference between CBT–BN and CBT+ERP with CBT-BN being superior in terms of mean frequency of binge eating at follow-up (N = 1; n = 25; SMD = -0.90; 95% CI, –1.73 to –0.07). I

There is limited/strong evidence that CBT-BN when compared with dietary counselling is superior at reducing the frequency of purging by both the end of treatment and post-treatment follow-up:

---

[13] The full list of all evidence statements generated from meta-analyses (and the associated forest plots) will be available on the CD-ROM that accompanies the guideline.

- There is limited evidence suggesting that there is a clinically significant difference between CBT-BN and dietary counselling with CBT-BN being superior on mean frequency of purging by the end of treatment (N = 1; n = 31; SMD = –0.95; 95 per cent CI, –1.70 to –0.20). I

- There is strong evidence suggesting that there is a clinically significant difference between CBT–BN and dietary counselling with CBT–BN being superior on mean frequency of purging at follow-up (N = 1; n = 31; SMD = –1.34; 95 per cent CI, –2.13 to –0.55). I

It is unlikely that CBT-BN is superior to BT at reducing the frequency of binge eating and purging by the end of treatment:

- There is evidence suggesting that it is unlikely there is a clinically significant difference between CBT–BN and BT on mean frequency of binge eating by the end of treatment (N = 3; n = 131; SMD = –0.11; 95 per cent CI, –0.45 to 0.24). I

- There is evidence suggesting that it is unlikely there is a clinically significant difference between CBT–BN and BT on mean frequency of purging by the end of treatment (N = 3; n = 131; SMD = 0.08; 95 per cent CI, –0.27 to 0.42). I

It is unlikely that CBT–BN is superior to IPT–BN at reducing the frequency of binge eating by both the end of treatment or post-treatment follow-up:

- There is evidence suggesting that it is unlikely there is a clinically significant difference between CBT–BN and IPT–BN on mean frequency of binge eating by the end of treatment (N = 2; n = 262; SMD = –0.24; 95 per cent CI, –0.48 to 0.01). I

- There is evidence suggesting that it is unlikely there is a clinically significant difference between CBT–BN and IPT–BN in terms of mean frequency of binge eating at follow-up (N = 2; n = 257; SMD = –0.04; 95 per cent CI, –0.29 to 0.20). I

It is unlikely that CBT–BN is superior to focal supportive psychotherapy at reducing the frequency of binge eating and purging by the end of treatment:

- There is evidence suggesting that it is unlikely there is a clinically significant difference between CBT–BN and focal supportive psychotherapy on mean frequency of binge eating by the end of treatment (N = 3; n = 111; SMD = 0.00; 95 per cent CI, –0.37 to 0.38). I

- There is evidence suggesting that it is unlikely there is a clinically significant difference between CBT–BN and focal supportive psychotherapy on mean frequency of purging by the end of treatment (N = 4; n = 144; SMD = –0.13; 95 per cent CI, -0.46 to 0.20). I

It is unlikely that CBT-BN is superior to PSH at reducing the frequency of binge eating by the end of treatment:

- There is evidence suggesting that it is unlikely there is a clinically significant difference between CBT–BN and PSH on mean frequency of binge eating by the end of treatment (N = 1; n = 80; SMD = 0.03; 95 per cent CI, –0.43 to 0.49). I

There is limited evidence from one trial that GSH when compared to CBT–BN is superior at reducing the frequency of binge eating and purging by the end of treatment:

● There is limited evidence suggesting that there is a clinically significant difference between CBT–BN and GSH with GSH being superior on mean frequency of binge eating by the end of treatment (N = 1; n = 56; SMD = 1.20; 95 per cent CI, 0.63 to 1.78). I

● There is limited evidence suggesting that there is a clinically significant difference between CBT–BN and GSH with GSH being superior on mean frequency of purging by the end of treatment (N = 1; n = 56; SMD = 0.55; 95 per cent CI, 0.01 to 1.08). I

Other effects of treatment

There is insufficient or no evidence to determine whether CBT–BN differs from BT in its effects on depression, general psychiatric symptoms, or psychosocial/interpersonal functioning by the end of treatment or post-treatment follow-up. I

There is insufficient or no evidence to determine whether CBT–BN differs from CBT+ERP in its effects on depression, general psychiatric symptoms, or psychosocial/interpersonal functioning by the end of treatment or post-treatment follow-up. I

There is insufficient or no evidence to determine whether CBT–BN differs from IPT–BN in its effects on depression or psychosocial/interpersonal functioning by the end of treatment or post-treatment follow-up. I

There is insufficient or no evidence to determine whether CBT-BN differs from psychodynamic psychotherapy in its effects on psychosocial/interpersonal functioning by the end of treatment or post-treatment follow-up, or on general psychiatric symptoms at follow-up. I

There is insufficient evidence to determine whether CBT–BN differs from focal supportive psychotherapy in its effects on general psychiatric symptoms or psychosocial/interpersonal functioning by the end of treatment or post-treatment follow-up. I

There is no evidence to determine whether CBT–BN differs from dietary counselling in its effects on depression, general psychiatric symptoms or psychosocial/interpersonal functioning by the end of treatment or post-treatment follow-up. I

There is insufficient or no evidence to determine whether CBT–BN differs from GSH or PSH in its effects on depression, general psychiatric symptoms or psychosocial/interpersonal functioning by the end of treatment or post-treatment follow-up. I

There is insufficient or no evidence to determine whether CBT+ERP differs from focal supportive psychotherapy or dietary counselling in its effects on depression, general psychiatric symptoms or psychosocial/interpersonal functioning by the end of treatment or post-treatment follow-up. I

There is insufficient or no evidence to determine whether BT differs from IPT–BN or focal supportive psychotherapy in its effects on depression, general psychiatric symptoms or psychosocial/interpersonal functioning by the end of treatment or post-treatment follow-up. I

Acceptability of treatment

There is insufficient evidence to determine whether CBT–BN is more, or less, acceptable to people with bulimia nervosa when compared with BT, CBT+ERP, IPT–BN, psychodynamic psychotherapy, focal supportive psychotherapy, dietary counselling, GSH or PSH. I

There is insufficient evidence to determine whether CBT+ERP is more, or less, acceptable to people with bulimia nervosa when compared with focal supportive psychotherapy or dietary counselling. I

There is insufficient evidence to determine whether BT is more, or less, acceptable to people with bulimia nervosa when compared with IPT–BN or focal supportive psychotherapy. I

7.2.5 Additional considerations in the management of children and adolescents

Bulimia nervosa is rarely, if ever, seen in children. It does occur in adolescents although in clinical practice most patients are young adults. There has been no research on the treatment of adolescents with bulimia nervosa. This omission needs to be rectified. In line with much current clinical practice, the GDG took the view that, subject to adaptation to their age, circumstances and level of development, adolescent patients with bulimia nervosa should receive the same type of treatment as adults with the disorder. In the treatment of adolescents with CBT-BN consideration should also be given to the appropriate involvement of the family.

7.2.6 Clinical summary

Four main conclusions may be drawn from these analyses and the studies upon which they are based. First, until recently, most of the studies of the psychological treatment of bulimia nervosa have been small in size and, therefore, lacking in statistical power. They have therefore been vulnerable to Type II error. Thus, the great majority of the many statistically non-significant findings cannot be interpreted. Second, the weight of evidence as measured in terms of the strength and consistency of the findings and the number of relevant studies indicates that CBT–BN (delivered on a one-to-one basis) is the most effective treatment for bulimia nervosa. Third, CBT+ERP is also effective in the short term. However, its use has fallen from favour because it is difficult to implement and disliked by patients (Bulik *et al.*, 1998) and time-consuming. Lastly, IPT–BN appears to be as effective as CBT-BN at eight to 12-month post-treatment follow-up (i.e. one year after starting treatment). Prior to this, CBT–BN is more effective than IPT–BN.

7.2.7 Clinical practice recommendations

7.2.7.1   As a possible first step, patients with bulimia nervosa should be encouraged to follow an evidence-based self-help programme. (B)

7.2.7.2   Health care professionals should consider providing direct encouragement and support to patients undertaking an evidence-based self-help programme as this may improve outcomes. This may be sufficient treatment for a limited subset of patients. (B)

7.2.7.3   Cognitive behaviour therapy for bulimia nervosa (CBT–BN), a specifically adapted form of CBT, should be offered to most adults with bulimia nervosa. The course of CBT-BN should normally be of 16 to 20 sessions over four to five months. (A)*

7.2.7.4   Adolescents with bulimia nervosa may be treated with CBT–BN adapted as needed to suit their age, circumstances, level of development and including the family as appropriate. (C)*

7.2.7.5   When people with bulimia nervosa have not responded to or do not want CBT, other psychological treatments should be considered. (B)

7.2.7.6   Interpersonal psychotherapy should be considered as an alternative to CBT, but patients should be informed it takes eight to 12 months to achieve results comparable to CBT. (B)

7.3 Pharmacological interventions

7.3.1 Introduction

A diverse network of neurotransmitters/neurohormones are involved in the central and peripheral control of appetite and satiety. A wide array of drugs that act on various receptors within these pathways have been examined in the treatment of bulimia nervosa.

7.3.2 Current practice

Antidepressants are often employed as a first line treatment as they are easily used in primary care.

Drugs are not as acceptable or as well tolerated as psychological treatments in this patient group. Only short-term effects have been studied and the outcome measures used are often not comparable to those used in studies of psychological treatments.

People with bulimia nervosa have an increased risk of self-harm and so risks of overdose need to be considered. Drugs that require dietary restrictions, such as monoamine-oxidase inhibitors (MAOIs) may be less appropriate in this group. They may also be using a wide variety of non-prescription medication the effects of which are unknown and may interact adversely with prescription medication. Particular consideration needs to be given to the possibility of pregnancy and breast-feeding. Very few drugs are recommended for children and adolescents aged less than 18. There are safety data available for other conditions for sertraline and amisulpride in the under 18 group but the use of these medications has not been studied in adults with bulimia nervosa.

7.3.3 Antidepressant drug treatment

In clinical practice, it has often been found that any drug effect is poorly sustained and it is often necessary to switch medication in an effort to sustain a remission of symptoms. The effective dose of fluoxetine is 60 mg, and as such is higher than the standard dose for depression. No other drug studies have compared different doses.

7.3.3.1   Drugs reviewed

The following drugs were included:

- Antidepressants

    - MAOIs (moclobemide, phenelzine)

    - SSRIs (fluoxetine)

    - Tricyclic antidepressants (desipramine, imipramine)

    - Other antidepressants (bupropion, trazodone, mianserin)

- Opioid antagonist (naltrexone)

- Antiemetics.

Drugs that have had their licences withdrawn from the UK were not included in the guideline. Although there are studies assessing the use of lithium carbonate, these were not included, as it was felt inadvisable to use this drug given the potential risk of toxicity in people with bulimia nervosa.

7.3.3.2   Studies considered

The review team used the existing Cochrane review 'Antidepressants versus placebo for people with bulimia nervosa' (Bacaltchuk & Hay, 2003) as the starting point for the present analysis.

Five trials used in the existing Cochrane review were excluded because they did not meet the inclusion criteria set by the GDG (Agras, 1987; Kennedy, 1988 & 1993; Mitchell, 1984; Rothschild, 1994). The 11 remaining trials were included in this section (Fluoxetinebulim, 1992; Goldstein, 1995; Horne, 1988; Kanerva, 1994; McCann, 1990; Mitchell, 1990; Popo, 1983 & 1989; Sabine, 1983; Walsh, 1987 & 1991). In addition, four trials of antidepressants (Carruba, 2001; Mitchell, 2001a; Ramano, 2002; Walsh, submitted), two trials of naltrexone (Huseman, 1990; Mitchell, 1989a) and two of ondansetron (Faris, 1989 & 2000) were found during the search for new evidence. Thus, 19 RCTs involving 1851 participants were included.

Of the 19 trials, 15 compared antidepressants with placebo. Of these, four compared tricyclic antidepressants with placebo (McCann, 1990; Mitchell, 1990; Pope, 1983; Walsh, 1991), five compared SSRIs with placebo (Fluoxetinebulim, 1992; Goldstein, 1995; Kanerva, 1994; Mitchell, 2001a; Walsh, submitted), two compared MAOIs with placebo (Walsh, 1987; Carruba, 2001), and three compared other antidepressants with placebo (Horne, 1988; Pope, 1989, Sabine, 1983). The trials ranged in duration from 26 to 365 days, with a median of 56 days.

Full details of the studies included in the guideline and the reasons for excluding studies are given in Appendix 18.

7.3.3.3   Evidence statements[14]

The data were analysed in two ways. First, by combining the results across all classes of antidepressants (referred to below as 'antidepressants'). Secondly, by combining the results across each class separately (i.e. MAOIs, SSRIs, and tricyclics).

Effect of treatment on remission from binge eating/purging

There is limited evidence suggesting that there is a clinically significant difference between antidepressants and placebo, with antidepressants being superior in terms of remission from binge eating/purging (defined as cessation of binge eating/purging) by the end of treatment (N = 6; n = 697; RR = 0.88; 95 per cent CI, 0.83 to 0.94; NNT = 9; 95 per cent CI, 6 to 15). I

There is limited evidence suggesting that there is a clinically significant difference between the MAOIs and placebo with MAOIs being superior in terms of remission from binge eating (defined as cessation of binge eating) by the end of treatment (N = 1; n = 62; RR = 0.77; 95 per cent CI, 0.62 to 0.95; NNT = 5; 95 per cent CI, 3 to 17). I

There is insufficient evidence to determine whether SSRIs or tricyclics are preferable in improving remission rates by the end of treatment. I

Effect of treatment on frequency of binge eating and purging

There is strong evidence suggesting that there is a clinically significant difference between antidepressants and placebo with antidepressants being superior in terms of clinical improvement (defined as at least a 50 per cent reduction in the frequency of binge eating) by the end of treatment (N = 6; n = 855; RR = 0.68; 95 per cent CI, 0.60 to 0.78; NNT = 5; 95 per cent CI, 4 to 8). I

---

[14] The full list of all evidence statements generated from meta-analyses (and the associated forest plots) will be available on the CD-ROM that accompanies the guideline.

However, using a continuous measure of binge eating or purging, there is insufficient evidence to determine whether antidepressants reduce the frequency of binge eating and purging by the end of treatment. |

There is strong evidence from three trials that SSRIs when compared to placebo produce clinical improvement in binge eating and purging by the end of treatment:

- There is strong evidence suggesting that there is a clinically significant difference between the SSRIs and placebo with SSRIs being superior in terms of clinical improvement (defined as at least a 50 per cent reduction in frequency of binge eating) by the end of treatment (N = 3; n = 706; RR = 0.73; 95 per cent CI, 0.62 to 0.84; NNT = 6; 95 per cent CI, 5 to 12). |

- There is strong evidence suggesting that there is a clinically significant difference between SSRIs and placebo with SSRIs being superior in terms of clinical improvement (defined as at least a 50 per cent reduction in the frequency of purging) by the end of treatment (N = 2; n = 656; RR = 0.66; 95 per cent CI, 0.57 to 0.76; NNT = 5; 95 per cent CI, 4 to 7). |

There is strong evidence suggesting that there is a clinically significant difference between tricyclics and placebo with tricyclics being superior in terms of clinical improvement (defined as at least a 50 per cent reduction in the frequency of binge eating) by the end of treatment (N = 1; n = 22; RR = 0.30; 95 per cent CI, 0.11 to 0.80; NNT = 2; 95 per cent CI, 2 to 4). |

There is strong evidence suggesting that there is a clinically significant difference between tricyclics and placebo with tricyclics being superior on mean frequency of binge eating by the end of treatment (N = 3; n = 120; SMD = -0.82; 95 per cent CI, −1.20 to −0.45). |

There is insufficient evidence to determine whether appetite suppressants or antiemetics reduce the frequency of binge eating or purging when compared to placebo by the end of treatment. |

Other effects of treatment

There is limited evidence suggesting that there is a clinically significant difference between antidepressants and placebo, with antidepressants being superior in terms of mean depression scores by the end of treatment (N = 6; n = 293; SMD = −0.28; 95 per cent CI, −0.51 to −0.05). |

There is limited evidence suggesting that there is a clinically significant difference between tricyclics and placebo with tricyclics being superior in terms of mean depression scores by the end of treatment (N = 3; n = 120; SMD = −0.47; 95 per cent CI, −0.83 to −0.10). |

There is insufficient evidence to determine whether MAOIs or SSRIs reduce the symptoms of depression by the end of treatment. |

Acceptability of treatment

There is limited evidence from five trials favouring SSRIs over placebo in terms of treatment acceptability:

- There is limited evidence suggesting that there is a clinically significant difference between the SSRIs and placebo with SSRIs being superior in terms of the number of people leaving the study early due to any reason by end of treatment (N = 5; *n* = 803; RR = 0.79; 95 per cent CI, 0.67 to 0.95). I

There is strong evidence from four trials that tricyclics are less acceptable to people with bulimia nervosa than placebo by the end of treatment:

- There is strong evidence suggesting that there is a clinically significant difference between tricyclics and placebo with placebo being superior in terms of the number of people leaving the study early due to any reason by end of treatment (N = 4; *n* = 217; RR = 2.03; 95 per cent CI, 1.18 to 3.49; NNH = 7; 95 per cent CI, 4 to 20). I

There is insufficient evidence to determine whether appetite suppressants or antiemetics are more, or less, acceptable to people with bulimia nervosa than placebo. I

Tolerability of treatment

There is limited evidence suggesting that there is a clinically significant difference between antidepressants and placebo, with placebo being superior in terms of the number of people leaving the study early due to adverse events by end of treatment (N = 9; *n* = 1078; RR = 1.90; 95 per cent CI, 1.20 to 2.99; NNH = 20; 95 per cent CI, 13 to 50). I

There is insufficient evidence to determine whether a specific class of antidepressant is more, or less, tolerated in people with bulimia nervosa. I

7.3.4 Additional considerations in the management of children and adolescents

Antidepressant drugs may be used for the treatment of bulimia nervosa in adolescents but they are not licensed for this age group and there is no evidence base for this practice. They should not be considered as a first line treatment in adolescent bulimia nervosa.

7.3.5 Clinical summary

There are a limited number of studies and inevitably this must lead to rather tentative conclusions. Antidepressants, in particular fluoxetine, can produce benefits in overall symptomatology but the evidence is not as strong for specific behaviours such as binge eating and purging. Antidepressants, specifically SSRIs, appear to be reasonably tolerated. The major problem in interpreting the outcome of these trials is their short duration and lack of follow-up data for most trials and the consequent absence of any evidence for long-term effectiveness.

7.3.6 Clinical practice recommendations

7.3.6.1   As an alternative or additional first step to using an evidence-based self-help programme, adults with bulimia nervosa may be offered a trial of an antidepressant drug. (B)*

7.3.6.2   Patients should be informed that antidepressant drugs can reduce the frequency of binge eating and purging, but the long-term effects are unknown. Any beneficial effects will be rapidly apparent. (B)

7.3.6.3   Selective serotonin reuptake inhibitors (SSRIs) (specifically fluoxetine) are the drugs of first choice for the treatment of bulimia nervosa in terms of acceptability, tolerability and reduction of symptoms. (C)

7.3.6.4   For people with bulimia nervosa, the effective dose of fluoxetine is higher than for depression (60 mg daily). (C)

7.3.6.5   No drugs, other than antidepressants, are recommended for the treatment of bulimia nervosa. (B)

7.4 Antidepressant drugs compared to psychological interventions and their combination

7.4.1 Introduction

Psychological and pharmacological treatments for bulimia nervosa have not only been evaluated on their own but they have also been compared. In addition, they have been studied in combination to see whether any advantages come from using them together. The only drugs to be studied in this way have been antidepressant drugs. These studies are now reviewed starting with the direct comparative studies and then the evaluations of the two treatments combined.

7.4.2 Current practice

There are no data available on the combined use of antidepressant drugs and psychological treatment in the management of bulimia nervosa in routine clinical practice.

7.4.3 Psychological treatments versus antidepressant drugs

7.4.3.1.   Treatments reviewed

The following psychological treatments were included:

- CBT

- Focal supportive psychotherapy

- PSH.

The following antidepressant drugs were included:

- SSRIs (fluoxetine)

- Tricyclic antidepressants (desipramine, imipramine).

The review team used the existing Cochrane review 'Antidepressants versus psychological treatments and their combination for bulimia nervosa' (Bacaltchuk, Hay & Trefiglio, 2003) as the starting point for the present analysis.

All five trials comparing a psychological treatment with an antidepressant, used in the existing Cochrane review, were included in the present section (Agras, 1992; Goldbloom, 1997; Mitchell, 1990; Leitenberg, 1994; Walsh, 1997). In addition, three trials (Mitchell, 2001A; Jacobi 2002; Walsh, submitted) found during the search for new evidence, were included. Thus, eight RCTs involving 694 participants were included.

Out of the included trials, five compared CBT with an antidepressant (Agras, 1992; Goldbloom, 1997; Jacobi, 2002; Leitenberg, 1994; Walsh, 1997), and two compared PSH with an antidepressant (Mitchell, 2001a; Walsh, submitted). In addition, Walsh, 1997, compared focal supportive psychotherapy with an antidepressant.

Full details of the studies included in the guideline and the reasons for excluding studies are given in Appendix 18.

7.4.3.3.   Evidence statements[15]

The data were analysed by comparing each psychological treatment to any antidepressant, irrespective of drug class.

Effect of treatment on remission from binge eating/purging

There is limited evidence from five trials favouring CBT over antidepressants with regard to remission from binge eating and purging (defined as cessation of binge eating/ purging) by the end of treatment:

---

[15] The full list of all evidence statements generated from meta-analyses (and the associated forest plots) will be available on the CD-ROM that accompanies the guideline.

- There is limited evidence suggesting that there is a clinically significant difference between CBT and antidepressants with CBT being superior in terms of remission from binge eating by the end of treatment (N = 5; n = 270; RR = 0.78; 95 per cent CI, 0.67 to 0.92; NNT = 6; 95 per cent CI, 4 to 15). I

- There is limited evidence suggesting that there is a clinically significant difference between CBT and antidepressants with CBT being superior in terms of remission from purging by the end of treatment (N = 5; n = 196; RR = 0.78; 95 per cent CI, 0.66 to 0.92; NNT = 6; 95 per cent CI, 4 to 15). I

There is insufficient evidence to determine whether CBT differs from antidepressants with respect to remission from binge eating or purging at post-treatment follow-up. I

There is insufficient or no evidence to determine whether PSH or focal supportive psychotherapy differ from antidepressants with respect to remission from binge eating or purging by the end of treatment or post-treatment follow-up. I

Effect of treatment on frequency of binge eating and purging

Overall, it is unlikely that there is any difference between CBT and antidepressants with respect to the frequency of binge eating or purging by the end of treatment:

- There is insufficient evidence to determine if there is a clinically significant difference between CBT and antidepressants on mean frequency of binge eating by the end of treatment (N = 4; n = 149; SMD = −0.19; 95 per cent CI, −0.52 to 0.14). I

- There is evidence suggesting that it is unlikely there is a clinically significant difference between CBT and antidepressants on mean frequency of purging by the end of treatment (N = 5; n = 158; SMD = −0.14; 95 per cent CI, −0.46 to 0.19). I

There is insufficient evidence to determine whether CBT differs from antidepressants with respect to the frequency of binge eating or purging at post-treatment follow-up. I

There is insufficient or no evidence to determine whether PSH or focal supportive psychotherapy differ from antidepressants with respect to the frequency of binge eating or purging by the end of treatment or post-treatment follow-up. I

Other effects of treatment

There is insufficient or no evidence to determine whether CBT, PSH or focal supportive psychotherapy differ from antidepressants on depression or general psychiatric symptoms by the end of treatment or post-treatment follow-up. I

Acceptability of treatment

There is insufficient evidence to determine whether CBT is more, or less, acceptable to people with bulimia nervosa when compared with antidepressants. I

However, closer inspection of the data indicated significant heterogeneity in the data set. A sensitivity analysis was conducted by removing one study (Jacobi, 2002) from the analysis as this study appeared to be an outlier. The authors of this study speculated that their findings might differ from previous studies due to cultural differences in the health care systems (i.e. the study was conducted in Germany, whereas the other studies were North American). The sensitivity analysis indicated that:

- There is strong evidence suggesting that there is a clinically significant difference favouring CBT–BN over antidepressants in terms of the number of people leaving the study early due to any reason by end of treatment (N = 3; n = 149; RR = 0.48; 95 per cent CI, 0.28 to 0.83). I

There is insufficient or no evidence to determine whether PSH or focal supportive psychotherapy are more, or less, acceptable to people with bulimia nervosa when compared with antidepressants. I

Tolerability of treatment

There is insufficient or no evidence to determine whether antidepressants have more, or less, side effects in people with bulimia nervosa when compared with CBT, PSH or focal supportive psychotherapy. I

7.4.4 Psychological treatments versus the combination of psychological treatment and antidepressants

7.4.4.1   Treatments reviewed

The following psychological treatments were included:

- CBT

- Focal supportive psychotherapy

- Dietary counselling

- PSH.

The following antidepressant drugs were included:

- SSRIs (fluoxetine)

- Tricyclic antidepressants (desipramine, imipramine).

7.4.4.2   Studies considered

The review team used the existing Cochrane review 'Antidepressants versus psychological treatments and their combination for bulimia nervosa' (Bacaltchuk, Hay & Trefiglio, 2003) as the starting point for the present analysis.

All seven trials comparing a psychological treatment to the combination of a psychological treatment and an antidepressant, used in the existing Cochrane review, were included in this section (Agras, 1992; Beumont, 1997; Fichter, 1991; Goldbloom, 1997; Leitenberg, 1994; Mitchell, 1990; Walsh, 1997). In addition, three trials (Mitchell, 2001a; Jacobi, 2002; Walsh, submitted) found during the search for new evidence, were included here. Thus, 10 RCTs involving 801 participants were included.

Out of the included trials, seven used CBT as the psychological treatment (Agras, 1992; Fichter, 1991; Goldbloom, 1997; Jacobi, 2002; Leitenberg, 1994; Mitchell, 1990; Walsh, 1997), two used PSH (Mitchell, 2001a; Walsh, submitted) and one used dietary counselling (Beumont, 1997). In addition, Walsh (1997) included a focal supportive psychotherapy group.

Full details of the studies included in the guideline and the reasons for excluding studies are given in Appendix 18.

7.4.4.3   Evidence statements[16]

The data were analysed by comparing each psychological treatment to the combination of the psychological treatment and any antidepressant, irrespective of drug class.

Effect of treatment on remission from binge eating/purging

There is insufficient evidence to determine whether CBT differs from the combination of CBT and antidepressants with respect to remission from binge eating or purging by either the end of treatment or post-treatment follow-up. I

There is insufficient evidence to determine whether PSH or focal supportive psychotherapy differs from the combination of PSH or focal supportive psychotherapy and antidepressants with respect to remission from binge eating or purging by either the end of treatment or post-treatment follow-up. I

There is insufficient evidence to determine whether dietary counselling differs from the combination of dietary counselling and antidepressants with respect to remission from binge eating or purging by the end of treatment. However, at follow-up there is evidence from one study favouring the combination:

● There is limited evidence to suggest that there is a clinically significant difference between dietary counselling and a combination of dietary counselling and an antidepressant with dietary counselling being superior in terms of remission from binge eating/purging at follow up (N = 1; n = 67; RR = 0.70; 95 per cent CI, 0.50 to 0.97; NNT = 4; 95 per cent CI, 3 to 25). I

---

[16] The full list of all evidence statements generated from meta-analyses (and the associated forest plots) will be available on the CD-ROM that accompanies the guideline.

Effect of treatment on the frequency of binge eating and purging

There is evidence from five trials that the combination of CBT and antidepressants is equivalent to CBT alone with respect to the reduction of binge eating or purging by the end of treatment:

- There is limited evidence suggesting that there is a statistically significant difference between CBT and a combination of CBT and an antidepressant but the difference is unlikely to be clinically significant in terms of the mean frequency of binge eating by the end of treatment (N = 5; n = 185; SMD = 0.38; 95 per cent CI, 0.09 to 0.68). I

- There is evidence suggesting that it is unlikely there is a clinically significant difference between CBT and a combination of CBT and an antidepressant on mean frequency of purging by the end of treatment (N = 5; n = 157; SMD = 0.16; 95 per cent CI, −0.16 to 0.48). I

There is insufficient evidence to determine whether CBT differs from the combination of CBT and antidepressants with respect to the frequency of binge eating or purging at post-treatment follow-up. I

There is insufficient or no evidence to determine whether PSH or focal supportive psychotherapy differ from the combination of these psychological treatments and antidepressants with respect to the frequency of binge eating or purging by either the end of treatment or post-treatment follow-up. I

There is insufficient evidence to determine whether dietary counselling differs from the combination of dietary counselling and antidepressants with respect to the frequency of binge eating or purging by either the end of treatment or post-treatment follow-up. I

Other effects of treatment

There is insufficient or no evidence to determine whether CBT differs from the combination of CBT and antidepressants on depression or general psychiatric symptoms by either the end of treatment or post-treatment follow up. I

There is insufficient or no evidence to determine whether PSH, focal supportive psychotherapy or dietary counselling differ from the combination of these psychological treatments and antidepressants with respect to depression or general psychiatric symptoms by either the end of treatment or post-treatment follow-up. I

Acceptability of treatment

There is insufficient evidence to determine whether CBT is more, or less, acceptable to people with bulimia nervosa when compared with the combination of CBT and antidepressants. I

There is insufficient evidence to determine whether PSH or focal supportive psychotherapy are more, or less, acceptable to people with bulimia nervosa when compared with the combination of these psychological treatments and antidepressants. I

There is insufficient evidence to determine whether dietary counselling is more, or less, acceptable to people with bulimia nervosa when compared with the combination of dietary counselling and antidepressants. I

7.4.5 Antidepressant drugs versus the combination of antidepressant drugs and psychological treatment

7.4.5.1   Treatments reviewed

The following antidepressant drugs were included:

● SSRIs (fluoxetine)

● Tricyclic antidepressants (desipramine, imipramine).

The following psychological treatments were included:

● CBT

● Focal supportive psychotherapy

● Dietary counselling

● PSH.

7.4.5.2   Studies considered

The review team used the existing Cochrane review 'Antidepressants versus psychological treatments and their combination for bulimia nervosa' (Bacaltchuk, Hay & Trefiglio, 2003) as the starting point for the present analysis.

All five trials comparing an antidepressant to a combination of an antidepressant and a psychological treatment, used in the existing Cochrane review, were included in this section (Agras, 1992; Goldbloom, 1997; Leitenberg, 1994; Mitchell, 1990; Walsh, 1997). In addition, three trials (Mitchell, 2001a; Jacobi 2002; Walsh, submitted) found during the search for new evidence, were included here. Thus, eight RCTs involving 694 participants were included.

Of the included trials, six used CBT as the psychological treatment (Agras, 1992; Goldbloom, 1997; Jacobi, 2002; Leitenberg, 1994; Mitchell, 1990; Walsh, 1997) and two used self-help (Mitchell, 2001a; Walsh, submitted). In addition, Walsh (1997) used a focal supportive psychotherapy group.

Full details of the studies included in the guideline and the reasons for excluding studies are given in Appendix 18.

The data were analysed by comparing any antidepressant to any antidepressant combined with a specific psychological treatment.

Effect of treatment on remission from binge eating/purging

There is insufficient evidence to determine whether antidepressants differ from the combination of CBT and antidepressants with respect to remission from binge eating or purging by either the end of treatment or post-treatment follow-up. I

There is insufficient evidence to determine whether antidepressants differ from the combination of PSH or focal supportive psychotherapy and antidepressants with respect to remission from binge eating or purging by either the end of treatment or post-treatment follow-up. I

Effect of treatment on the frequency of binge eating and purging

There is evidence from five trials favouring the combination of CBT and antidepressants over antidepressants alone in terms of the frequency of binge eating and purging by the end of treatment:

●   There is strong evidence suggesting that there is a clinically significant difference between antidepressants and a combination of CBT and an antidepressant with the combination being superior on mean frequency of binge eating by the end of treatment (N = 4; n = 133; SMD = 0.55; 95 per cent CI, 0.21 to 0.90). I

●   There is limited evidence suggesting that there is a clinically significant difference between antidepressants and a combination of CBT and an antidepressant with the combination being superior on mean frequency of purging by the end of treatment (N = 5; n = 141; SMD = 0.49; 95 per cent CI, 0.15 to 0.83). I

There is insufficient evidence to determine whether antidepressants differ from the combination of CBT and antidepressants with respect to the frequency of binge eating or purging at post-treatment follow-up. I

There is insufficient or no evidence to determine whether antidepressants differ from the combination of PSH or focal supportive psychotherapy and antidepressants with respect to the frequency of binge eating or purging by either the end of treatment or post-treatment follow-up. I

Other effects of treatment

There is insufficient or no evidence to determine whether antidepressants differ from the combination of CBT and antidepressants on depression or general psychiatric symptoms by either the end of treatment or post-treatment follow-up. I

---

[17] The full list of all evidence statements generated from meta-analyses (and the associated forest plots) will be available on the CD-ROM that accompanies the guideline.

There is insufficient or no evidence to determine whether antidepressants differ from the combination of PSH or focal supportive psychotherapy and antidepressants on depression or general psychiatric symptoms by either the end of treatment or post-treatment follow-up. I

Acceptability of treatment

There is insufficient evidence to determine whether antidepressants are more, or less, acceptable to people with bulimia nervosa when compared with the combination of CBT and antidepressants. I

There is insufficient or no evidence to determine whether antidepressants are more, or less, acceptable to people with bulimia nervosa when compared with the combination of PSH or focal supportive psychotherapy and antidepressants. I

Tolerability of treatment

There is insufficient evidence to determine whether antidepressants have more, or less, side effects in people with bulimia nervosa when compared with the combination of CBT and antidepressants. I

There is insufficient or no evidence to determine whether antidepressants have more, or less, side effects in people with bulimia nervosa when compared with the combination of PSH or focal supportive psychotherapy and antidepressants. I

7.4.6 Clinical summary

Four points emerge from these analyses and the studies upon which they are based. First, there have been few comparisons of psychological and pharmacological treatments, and their combination, with the result that any practice recommendations must be tentative. Second, few studies have included post-treatment follow-up periods, a problem with almost all the studies that have used drugs. Third, the comparisons of CBT-BN with antidepressant drugs indicate that CBT-BN is the more potent treatment. Finally, the combination of CBT with antidepressant drugs is superior to antidepressant drugs on their own.

7.5 Management of the physical aspects of bulimia nervosa

7.5.1 Introduction

For the majority of people with bulimia nervosa, serious medical complications are rare. Severe problems can arise when there is comorbidity with diabetes. In addition, some of the compensatory behaviours can be toxic (herbal preparations, high dose analgesics, diuretics and Ipecac). The longer-term physical risks include damage to teeth from vomiting and overuse of carbonated drinks, damage to the gut from laxative abuse and potentially fatal electrolyte (K+) imbalance.

The crude mortality rate (CMR) of bulimia nervosa was 0.4 per cent (11 deaths in 2692 patients), when two meta-analyses were combined (Keel & Mitchell, 1997; Nielsen, 2001). No information is available as to the distribution of causes of death.

In one meta-analysis (Nielsen, 2001), the overall aggregate SMR of bulimia nervosa in studies with five to 11 years of follow-up was 7.4 (95 per cent CI, 2.9 to 14.9).

In addition to the general nutritional deficiency that may be present in bulimia nervosa, there may be specific nutritional problems related to meal content and patterning and purging.

The physical management of bulimia nervosa, therefore, falls (with the exceptions described below) into normal medical practice with the provisos set out in the introduction and primary care section concerned with detection and appropriate investigations. Good history taking and skilled empathic interviewing are necessary to elicit the full range of compensatory behaviours as these are often secretive, shameful and can be illegal.

The physical risk assessment screen used for anorexia nervosa may also be considered for bulimia nervosa.

7.5.2 Physical complications of binge eating/purging

The physical consequences of bulimia nervosa result largely from the compensatory behaviours of vomiting, laxative and diuretic abuse. For the purposes of this section the following complications were considered: fluid and electrolyte disturbances, damage to the gastrointestinal tract and dental complications. Evidence for the management of these difficulties is limited to descriptive reviews, other guidelines and knowledge of common medical practice.

Fluid and electrolyte disturbances

Fluid and electrolyte disturbances occur in bulimia nervosa and relate to the severity of symptoms and the general nutritional status. Common abnormalities include:

- Dehydration

- Hypokalaemia

- Hypochloraemia

- Alkalosis.

Dehydration can cause volume depletion and consequently low blood pressure and a rapid pulse. Patients can complain of dizziness because of orthostatic hypotension and weakness. In extreme cases renal function can be compromised. Secondary hypoaldosteronism can lead to rebound, fluid retention and peripheral oedema when laxatives and diuretics are withdrawn (Mitchell, 1988).

Low potassium causes weakness in all muscle and most worryingly cardiac arrhythmias, which may lead to death in severe cases. Renal function can also be affected. Metabolic alkalosis may augment potassium depletion. Diuretic abuse, particularly thiazide and loop diuretics, can produce marked potassium and sodium depletion.

Low sodium and magnesium levels occur less commonly but both have potentially serious consequences. If severe the former may cause central nervous system disturbances, whilst the latter results in muscle weakness, cardiac arrhythmias and mood changes. Low magnesium is also associated with other abnormalities such as hypocalcaemia and hypokalaemia. Clinicians should consider the presence of low magnesium levels in the face of refractory hypokalaemia.

In general, these abnormalities settle with cessation of purging behaviours. If needed, oral rather than IV supplementation (with substances such as rehydrate in severe cases) is advised. Advice from a physician and/or paediatrician may be necessary if there is severe metabolic disturbance (Connan, Lightman & Treasure, 2000). Very rarely patients may require hospital admission to manage severe purging behaviour.

Gastrointestinal damage

Loss of the gag reflex and gastro-oesophageal reflux has been found in patients with bulimia nervosa. Frequent and severe vomiting can cause more serious complications of oesophageal tears, perforation, and oesophagitis. These may require surgical intervention.

Laxative abuse

The prevalence of daily laxative abuse in patients with bulimia nervosa has been reported as up to 20 per cent (Mitchell *et al.*, 1985) and 75 per cent of patients report using laxatives at some point (Fairburn & Cooper, 1984). Patients usually take laxatives with the mistaken assumption that there is a consequent reduction in calorie absorption. The fluid loss that results from laxative action on the colon can provide a feeling of emptiness and weight loss. However laxatives have been shown to be an ineffective method of reducing calorie absorption (Bo-Linn *et al.*, 1983). The majority of patients use stimulant rather than bulk laxatives. The former have been shown to cause degeneration of the colonic nerve supply (Oster, 1980).

Laxative abuse carries the acute complication of electrolyte and fluid disturbances and can be particularly dangerous in low weight individuals. Abrupt cessation of laxatives in those who are taking them regularly can result in reflex fluid and sodium retention, and consequent weight gain, and oedema. This can increase patient anxiety and reluctance to curtail the use of laxatives. To avoid this effect a gradual reduction in laxative use is advised.

Long-term excessive laxative use can decrease the motility of the colon. This results in constipation and more worryingly an atonic cathartic colon. Recommended treatment of the constipation is regular food intake, bulk laxatives, adequate fluids and exercise (Robinson, 2000). Some patients may find these measures uncomfortable. Rarely surgical intervention may be required.

Dental complications

Dental erosion is the most common oral problem in patients with eating disorders who engage in self-induced vomiting. Erosion of the enamel of the tooth surface is caused by exposure to gastric acid. Teeth may become discoloured and change shape. Tooth sensitivity (pain on eating hot or cold meals) has also been reported. The chaotic eating pattern may also lead to high levels of dental caries (decay).

Detailed clinical guidelines on the diagnosis and prevention of dental erosion are available (http://www.rcseng.ac.uk/dental/fds/clinical_guidelines). These guidelines stress that recognition and management of the underlying aetiology (i.e. the eating disorder) is essential. It is noted that referral by dental practitioners to the general practitioner for treatment may be required and that 'initiation of medical help is a sensitive undertaking'. Dental practitioners are advised to monitor the erosion, to offer advice and provide treatment to prevent further erosion and improve appearance. Restorative treatment may prove difficult in the face of ongoing vomiting.

For clinicians involved with the management of the eating disorder, it is important to advise patients on the dental consequences and refer to a dental practitioner. Although any treatment of the eating disorder will aim to limit vomiting, patients should be given the following advice:

● Brushing teeth after vomiting should be avoided as it may increase tooth damage

● Mouth rinsing after vomiting with water and sodium bicarbonate (or other non-acid mouth wash) will neutralise the acid environment

● Visit the dentist regularly

● Fluoride mouth rinses and toothpastes may be helpful for desensitisation.

A high intake of acidic foods may increase dental erosion. These foods include fruit, fruit juice, carbonated drinks, pickled products, yoghurt and some alcoholic drinks. Dental practitioners guidelines recommend detailed dietary advice, which these patients may find difficult to follow. This advice includes:

● Limiting acidic foods and drinks to mealtimes

● Finishing meals with alkaline foods (e.g. milk or cheese)

● Avoiding acid foods and drinks last thing at night

● Avoiding habits such as prolonged sipping, holding acidic beverages in the mouth and 'frothing' prior to swallowing

● Avoiding toothbrushing after acidic substances

- Chewing sugar-free gum after meals to stimulate salivary flow (although this may cause increased gastric secretions).

Whilst this guidance will contribute to a reduction in dental erosion, it may not always be possible to follow it, particularly in the early stages of the treatment plan. For example, the consumption of some acidic foods (yoghurt and fruit) may be a necessary stage in stabilising a chaotic eating pattern, while encouraging other strategies to limit acid in the mouth.

Other physical consequences

Fasting and binge eating foods high in refined carbohydrates, especially if this is followed by vomiting, can lead to high levels of insulin release with large fluctuations in blood sugar levels (Johnson, Jarrell, Chupurdia & Williamson, 1994). This may disrupt the appetite control mechanisms and the utilisation and deposition of energy

Serotonin is implicated in appetite regulation (there may be a particular role in carbohydrate balance) (Leibowitz & Alexander, 1998)), disruptions in serotonin levels may be affected by the impact of insulin on its precursor, tryptophan, the levels of which can be adversely affected by dieting, particularly in women. In turn acute tryptophan depletion may lead to an increase in calorie intake and irritability in bulimia nervosa (Weltzin, Fernstrom, Fernstrom, Neuberger & Kaye, 1995) and may be related to decreased mood, increased rating in body image concern and subjective loss of control of eating in people who have recovered from bulimia nervosa (Smith, Fairburn & Cowen, 1999). People with bulimia nervosa appear to have dysregulation in the release of factors involved in the peripheral response to food such as cholecystokinin (Geracioti & Liddle, 1988) and ghrelin (Tanaka *et al.*, 2002). There is some suggestion of dysregulation in the systems that are involved in longer-term energy balance such as leptin (Brewerton, Lesem, Kennedy & Garvey, 2000; Monteleone *et al.*, 2000; Jimerson, 2002), which may persist after recovery (Jimerson, 2002).

In summary, people with bulimia nervosa may have abnormal levels of tryptophan and central serotonin along with a potential disruption in both the acute and the longer-term mechanisms controlling hunger and satiety.

7.5.3 Clinical practice recommendations

7.5.3.1   Patients with bulimia nervosa who are vomiting frequently or taking large quantities of laxatives (and especially if they are also underweight) should have their fluid and electrolyte balance assessed. (C)

7.5.3.2   When electrolyte disturbance is detected, it is usually sufficient to focus on eliminating the behaviour responsible. In the small proportion of cases where supplementation is required to restore the patient's electrolyte balance, oral rather than intravenous administration is recommended, unless there are problems with gastrointestinal absorption. (C)

7.5.3.3   Where laxative abuse is present, patients should be advised to gradually reduce laxative use and informed that laxative use does not significantly reduce calorie absorption. (C)

7.5.3.4   Patients who are vomiting should have regular dental reviews. (C)

7.5.3.5   Patients who are vomiting should be given appropriate advice on dental hygiene, which should include avoiding brushing after vomiting, rinsing with a non-acid mouthwash after vomiting, and reducing an acid oral environment (for example, limiting acidic foods). (C)

7.5.4 Somatic interventions

One of the risk domains for bulimia nervosa relates to dieting and weight control. People with bulimia nervosa frequently have a personal or family history of obesity. One of the important maintaining factors is the perceived need (or wish) to control weight. There has been recent interest in the use of somatic interventions including exercise and massage. In the case of some exercise, this relates to the evidence that it may be of benefit in improving mood (Babyak *et al.*, 2000). It is also frequently used in the treatment of obesity. However, current practice is not underpinned by a strong evidence base. For this section two interventions were considered:

● Exercise

● Massage.

7.5.4.1   Studies considered

The review team conducted a new systematic search for RCTs that assessed the efficacy of exercise or massage for people with bulimia nervosa.

Two trials met the eligibility criteria set out by the GDG. One compared exercise with a non bulimia nervosa focused form of CBT (Sundgotborgen, 2002), and one trial compared massage in addition to 'standard care' with 'standard care' alone (Field, 1998a). Thus, two trials involving 88 participants were included in this section.

Full details of the studies included in the guideline and the reasons for excluding studies are given in Appendix 18.

7.5.4.2   Evidence statements[18]

Exercise

Effect of treatment on the frequency of binge eating and purging

There is limited evidence suggesting that there is a clinically significant difference between exercise and a non bulimia nervosa focused form of CBT with exercise being superior in terms of mean frequency of binge eating by 18 months' post-treatment follow-up (N = 1; n = 26; SMD = –0.83; 95 per cent CI, –1.64 to –0.02). I

---

[18] The full list of all evidence statements generated from meta-analyses (and the associated forest plots) will be available on the CD-ROM that accompanies the guideline.

There is insufficient evidence to determine whether exercise differs from CBT with respect to the frequency of purging by follow-up. I

Acceptability of treatment

There is insufficient evidence to determine whether exercise is more, or less, acceptable to people with bulimia nervosa than CBT. I

Massage

Other effects of treatment

There is limited evidence to suggest that the addition of massage to 'standard care' is superior to 'standard care' alone in terms of mean scores on the Eating Disorders Inventory by the end of treatment (*n* = 24; Field, 1998a). I

Acceptability of treatment

There is insufficient evidence to determine whether massage is more, or less, acceptable to people with bulimia nervosa than 'standard care'. I

7.5.5 Clinical summary

The use of somatic treatments (exercise and massage) is not frequent in the UK. There is limited evidence from one small RCT suggesting that moderate exercise may reduce the frequency of binge eating when compared to a non bulimia nervosa focused form of CBT. In addition, massage may produce some benefit over and above 'standard care'. However, there are currently no RCTs comparing exercise or massage with psychological interventions shown to be effective for the treatment of people with bulimia nervosa. Until a more substantial evidence base is established it is unlikely that either will form part of the routine practice of eating disorder services in the UK.

7.5.6 Concurrent physical conditions

A number of physical conditions present particular problems when they present comorbidly with bulimia nervosa. The problems presented by these conditions are set out below, followed by a summary on approaches to the management of the problems as they present.

Diabetes

Diabetes is over-represented in people with bulimia nervosa. There is a three-fold increase in the odds ratio for bulimia nervosa (OR = 2.9; 95 per cent CI, 1.0 to 8.4) and a significant two-fold increase in odds ratio for both EDNOS and sub-threshold eating disorders in people with Type 1 diabetes (Nielsen, 2002). It has been suggested that Type 1 diabetes may precede the eating disorder (Neilson *et al.*, 2002). Omission or intentional under-dosing of insulin so called 'insulin-purging' is increased (OR = 12.6; 95 per cent CI, 7.8 to 21.1). This leads to poor control of blood sugar and an increased risk of physical complications. Increased retinopathy is also found where eating disorders co-exist with Type 1 Diabetes (OR = 4.8; 95 per cent CI, 3.0 to 7.8).

In the largest (N = 91) longitudinal study (four years) of a cohort of people with eating disorders and Type 1 diabetes, disturbed eating persisted in 60 per cent of cases and was associated with a three-fold increase in retinopathy (Rydall, Rodin, Olmsted, Devenyi & Daneman, 1997). In a cohort of young diabetics (N = 43 males, N = 33 females) followed over 10 years, those with behavioural problems in adolescence had a worse outcome (Bryden, Peveler, Stein, Neil, Mayou & Dunger, 2001).

The presence of Type 1 diabetes presents challenges not only for physical management but also for psychological treatment. One of the goals of CBT for bulimia nervosa is to relax control over eating and this can conflict with the nutritional advice given to diabetics (Peveler, Davies, Mayou, Fairburn & Mann, 1993). On the other hand it is most important that these patients are helped to overcome their eating disorder given the associated physical complications. There are guidelines for adapting CBT–BN for these patients (Peveler & Fairburn, 1992).

One empirical study, an RCT, compared psycho-education with 'standard care' for people with bulimia nervosa and Type 1 diabetes (Olmsted, 2002). In this study, 212 women attending a paediatric diabetes clinic were screened for signs of eating disturbance. One-hundred-and-thirty passed the screening and were invited to participate in the intervention phase of the study. Eighty-five participants were randomised to psychoeducation or 'standard care'. Assessments were conducted before and after treatment and at six-month follow-up.

An intention-to-treat group by time multivariate analyses of variance (MANOVA) indicated significant reductions following psychoeducation on the Restraint and Eating Concern subscales of the Eating Disorder Examination (EDE) and on the Drive for Thinness and Body Dissatisfaction subscales of the Eating Disorder Inventory (EDI), but no improvement in frequency of purging by insulin omission (mean 1.4 insulin omission days at baseline and 1.3 at six-months' follow-up) or haemoglobin A1c levels (mean at baseline 9.2 and at six-months' follow-up 9.3). Psychoeducation was associated with reductions in eating disturbance, but not with improved metabolic control.

7.5.7 Clinical summary

The conclusions to be drawn from the review are that females with Type 1 diabetes have an increased risk of bulimia nervosa and EDNOS and that poor adherence to insulin treatment is frequent in eating disordered Type 1 diabetes individuals. This comorbidity complicates psychological interventions. Psychoeducation may have some limited benefit on eating disorder symptoms but not on diabetic control. In the management of people with bulimia nervosa and Type 1 diabetes, close liaison and a shared knowledge base between the eating disorder and diabetes teams is essential.

7.5.8 Clinical practice recommendations

7.5.8.1   Treatment of both subthreshold and clinical cases of an eating disorder in people with diabetes is essential because of the greatly increased physical risk in this group. (C)

7.5.8.2   Patients with Type 1 diabetes and an eating disorder should have intensive regular physical monitoring as they are at high risk of retinopathy and other complications. (C)

Pregnancy and the postnatal period

The peak age of prevalence of eating disorders is in the childbearing years. Women with bulimia nervosa are at risk of unplanned pregnancies due to mistaken beliefs about fertility in the presence of oligomenorrhoea (Morgan, Lacey & Sedgwick, 1999), and also because many women take an oral contraceptive pill which they inadvertently vomit. In the majority of cases bulimic symptoms will improve during pregnancy and for a period of time after the birth. Lemberg and Phillips (1989) found that the fear of losing control over weight gain was one of the most common worries during pregnancy. Most women had not mentioned their eating disorder to their obstetricians.

In a small case series a higher than expected number of complications were reported (Lacey & Smith, 1987). It is not certain whether such complications can be ascribed to the core symptoms/behaviours of bulimia nervosa or whether they are caused by comorbidity such as alcohol and drug abuse found among these patients (Key, Mason & Bolton, 2001; Abraham, 1998). Women with bulimia nervosa are at risk of delivering low birth weight infants, and have higher rates of Caesarean sections and perinatal problems (Franko et al., 2001). A two-fold increase in miscarriage rate was reported for a bulimic population (Abraham, 1998; Willis & Rand, 1988). In Waugh and Bulik's study (1999) the children of mothers with eating disorders had a significantly lower birth weight and length.

Eating disorder symptomatology has been found to increase in the post-partum in the majority of studies on small clinical samples of women with eating disorders (Lacey & Smith, 1987; Lemberg & Phillips, 1989; Morgan, Lacey & Sedgwick, 1999; Stein & Fairburn, 1996). Mothers had difficulties in maintaining breast-feeding and in making positive comments about food and eating at mealtimes, they were less likely to cook or eat with their children (Waugh & Bulik, 1999). The infants of mothers with eating disorders have a lower mean weight than controls. The infants' weight was associated with conflict during mealtimes and mothers' concerns about their own weight (Stein, Woolley, Cooper & Fairburn, 1994). Moreover, in a small prospective study on women with eating disorders, mothers used a less regular feeding schedule for their infants and used food more for non-nutritive purposes (Agras, Hammer & McNicholas, 1999). They also had higher concerns about their daughters' weight from the age of two onwards. Lacey & Smith (1987) reported that 15 per cent of mothers in their series reported attempting to 'slim down' their babies.

Also mothers report increase problematic interactions, for example, increased irritability and inability to cope with the child's demands while binge eating. Children of mothers with eating disorders showed more negative affect, mainly sadness and crying (Agras et al., 1999). In addition to emotional problems, language and speech problems have been reported shown (Franzen & Gerlinghoff, 1997). Also there have been reports of inappropriate involvement of children in their parent's illness, with 'parenting' on the part of the child and role-reversal (Brandes & Lackstrom, 1993; Woodside, Shekter-Wolfson, Garfinkel & Olmsted, 1995).

7.5.9 Clinical summary

Although for many women with bulimia nervosa pregnancy can pass uneventfully, for some pregnancy and the post-partum period can present considerable challenges. For this at-risk group four points should be considered. First, women with bulimia nervosa may have more complications during pregnancy and the children who are smaller at birth. Secondly, they may also have problematic interactions feeding their infants and children and use food for instrumental rather nutritive reasons. Thirdly, they tend to be more concerned about their child's weight and shape. Finally, they may have more problematic interactions with their children.

7.5.10 Clinical practice recommendations

7.5.10.1   Pregnant women with eating disorders require careful monitoring throughout the pregnancy and in the post-partum period. (C)

7.6 Service level interventions

7.6.1 Introduction

In the UK, most people presenting with bulimia nervosa do so in primary care and over the last 20 years the numbers doing so have increased markedly (Turnbull, Ward, Treasure, Jick & Derby, 1996). Some patients may receive adequate help there. For many people interventions may consist of the prescription of antidepressant drugs or the reading of books or using similar self-help materials with or without professional guidance. The number referred onto secondary care services, whether general mental health services or specialist eating disorder services is not known. However, the filters on the pathway to more specialised secondary and tertiary care are complex. As indicated in the introduction, the availability of appropriate expertise is variable and may be the greatest single determinant of the kind of help an individual with bulimia nervosa receives. Whether an individual receives appropriate and effective services depends upon many factors including the existence and availability of such services. Within secondary services, bulimia nervosa is almost always treated on an outpatient basis. Inpatient treatment is usually reserved for the management of severe psychiatric comorbidity and physical complications. Special inpatient programmes for the treatment of bulimia nervosa are unusual in the UK, although they are more common in the rest of Europe.

7.6.2 Effective service configurations

The treatment of bulimia nervosa may involve a range of interventions from self-help in primary care through to, in occasional cases, inpatient treatment. Treatments vary in type and in the service level – outpatient, day patient or inpatient – at which they are delivered. The idea of 'stepped care' has been widely advocated (Fairburn & Peveler, 1990; Dalle Grave, Ricca & Todesco, 2001). This idea proposes that patients should be offered simpler and less expensive interventions first and that more complex and expensive interventions should be reserved for those who have not benefited.

The related ideas of sequencing and integration of different types of treatment has also been advocated (Garner & Needleman, 1997).

Unfortunately there have been no systematic comparisons of outcome in different service levels. The few comparisons are not randomised and are difficult to interpret. (Williamson, Prather, Bennett, Davis, Watkins & Grenier, 1989). The great majority of reports are of outpatient treatments. All of the current evidence-based therapies for bulimia nervosa are designed to be delivered in an outpatient setting.

The place of inpatient treatment for bulimia nervosa is not supported by research evidence. Special inpatient and day patient treatment regimes have been described (Zipfel *et al.*, 2002). However, in these cases the role of admission would seem to be advocated mainly in relation to extreme severity, comorbidity or suicidal risk. There are some reports on special treatment programmes for severe bulimia nervosa complicated by self-harm, substance abuse and similar behaviours in patients who often also fulfil criteria for borderline personality disorder (Lacey, 1997). Such programmes have not been adequately evaluated and most such patients can be managed on an outpatient basis.

7.6.3 Satisfaction with services

The area of patient and carer perceptions has been the focus of some research in the area of eating disorders. Much of this work has been focused on perceptions of inpatient treatment for anorexia nervosa or on mixed or poorly defined populations of people with eating disorders, therefore it should be treated with caution in the specific context of bulimia nervosa. The reader is referred to the chapter on anorexia nervosa for a fuller review of the evidence base for satisfaction with services.

7.6.4 Death, suicide and self-harm, and the relationship to service setting

Bulimia nervosa is associated with a significant risk of deliberate self-harm behaviour (Anderson, McIntosh, Joyce & Bulik, 2002; Favaro & Santonastaso, 1997). The results of studies of overall mortality suggest a possible increase in bulimia nervosa although the extent is not clear (Nielsen, 2001). However, it is certainly the case that patients may die prematurely as a result of the disorder or its complications. People with bulimia nervosa may be offered treatment in outpatient, day patient or inpatient settings with the aim of ameliorating the risk of death through complication or suicide, or to contain self-harm.

7.6.5 Clinical practice recommendations

7.6.5.1   The great majority of patients with bulimia nervosa should be treated in an outpatient setting. (C)

7.6.5.2   For patients with bulimia nervosa who are at risk of suicide or severe self-harm, admission as an inpatient or a day patient or the provision of more intensive outpatient care, should be considered. (C)

7.6.5.3   Psychiatric admission for people with bulimia nervosa should normally be undertaken in a setting with experience of managing this disorder. (C)

7.7 Predicting the outcome of treatment and recovery from bulimia nervosa

Predicting response to treatment in bulimia nervosa is difficult and currently poorly understood. A particular complication is that comorbidity in bulimia nervosa is common and it is often unclear whether patients presenting with such problems should have a standard treatment or how such treatment should be modified, enhanced or complemented. Even with the best treatments currently available, up to 50 per cent of all bulimia nervosa patients may not respond adequately. In principle, it is desirable not to allocate patients to initial interventions that are unlikely to be of benefit as this may demoralise patients and be wasteful of resources. It is, therefore, important to identify which factors may influence outcome.

Two papers provide narrative reviews of predictors of outcome for bulimia nervosa. Keel and Mitchell (1997) reviewed data on 60 studies, which assessed outcome at least six months after presentation. They concluded that there were few consistent factors although 'personality traits such as impulsivity may contribute to poor outcome'. Vaz (1998) reviewed data on 'individual, environmental and therapeutic' factors. In the reviews so far conducted, a distinction has not always been made between studies employing a mixed eating disorder population and those of a single diagnosis. A number of papers review various concurrent psychopathology and its relationship to outcome in eating disorder populations (Holderness *et al.*, 1994; Herzog *et al.*, 1996; Rosenvinge *et al.*, 2000). Bell (2002) reviewed the evidence specifically for bulimia nervosa and concluded that there is no consistent relationship between psychiatric comorbidity and outcome for bulimia nervosa, but the presence of co-existing impulse control problems or cluster B personality disorder is probably associated with poorer outcome.

A wide range of potential predictors of outcome have been studied, often those which are routinely or most easily collected at pre-treatment. Some predictors, such as readiness for change, which may be important, are rarely measured. The impact of a potential predictor will vary at different points in the course of a disorder and few studies address this (Garner *et al.*, 1990; Fahy & Russell, 1993; and those of the Oxford group are exceptions). A number of different factors may influence speed of response to treatment, outcome at end of treatment, outcome at follow-up, relapse and chronicity. Most studies assess relationships between pre-treatment measures and outcome at end of treatment; some report on outcome at follow-up. Factors which predict end-of-treatment outcome may not predict outcome at follow-up.

For the purposes of the guideline, a literature review was carried out using PsycLIT and MEDLINE, which augmented the search of clinical trials already performed as part of the review of the effectiveness of treatments. A wide range of studies (cohort and treatment studies) of varying quality were considered. Studies of mixed eating disorder populations were excluded unless separate data for anorexia nervosa and bulimia nervosa were reported. Sample size ($n \geq 50$) was selected as the key inclusion criterion as it was not possible to derive robust measures of study quality, and both positive and negative findings were included. All variables reported in the studies were included in the analysis. One exception was made to the key inclusion criteria; studies with positive findings and a sample size of less than 50 were included if the follow-up was one year or over. A total of 60 studies contributed to the final analysis with sample sizes ranging from 17 to 647. All but two studies (Fairburn *et al.*, 2003; Stice & Agras, 1998) were of outcome in response to specific treatments.

The wide variability in method did not permit a meta-analysis. A detailed analysis by intervention was also beyond the scope of this review, though the data suggest a difference between interventions with respect to the frequency of pre-treatment binge eating and purging. A detailed analysis of the number of participants leaving a study early, as an outcome measure, or an analysis by follow-up was also beyond the scope of the review.

Outcome measures varied considerably across studies (abstinence, diagnostic status, changes or percentage reduction in the frequency of binge eating/purging). Some studies also examined comorbid disorders as measures of outcome. For consistency all findings are expressed in relation to poor outcome. A wide range of statistical techniques was used in the studies under review but an assessment of their quality and appropriateness was not undertaken.

Based on the number of studies showing a positive result relative to the number showing a negative result for each variable examined, a number of possible predictors emerged (for full details see Appendix 11). There is less robust evidence for predictors of outcome in bulimia nervosa than anorexia nervosa, but those with lower motivation for change prior to treatment had poorer outcomes. This was also the case for concurrent substance misuse and a history of obesity. Higher levels of binge eating and purging prior to treatment were associated with poorer outcome in abbreviated treatments. Continuing bulimic behaviours at the end of treatment is also associated with poorer long-term outcome. It is possible that treatment that is terminated before abstinence is achieved may compromise long-term recovery, but in the absence of firm evidence this remains speculative. There is some evidence to suggest that patients with concurrent borderline features do less well but this needs further research.

Those who respond poorly to treatment have a wide range of problems at the end of treatment including poor social adjustment, lack of a stable relationship, and depressive features. Disordered eating attitudes, body dissatisfaction and drive for thinness at the end of treatment and their associated behaviours (i.e., dietary restriction and vomiting) were associated with poorer outcome in the longer term. Outcome for these patients may be improved by addressing these issues within treatment.

7.7.1 Clinical practice recommendation

7.7.1.1   Health care professionals should be aware that patients with bulimia nervosa who have poor impulse control, notably substance misuse, may be less likely to respond to a standard programme of treatment. As a consequence treatment should be adapted to the problems presented. (C)

8 Treatment and management of atypical eating disorders (eating disorders not otherwise specified) including binge eating disorder

8.1 Introduction

In the absence of research evidence to guide the management of atypical eating disorders (Fairburn & Harrison, 2003) (also termed Eating Disorders Not Otherwise Specified, EDNOS; APA, 1994), other than binge eating disorder (BED), it is recommended that clinicians treat these patients following the principles advocated for treating the eating disorder that their eating problem most closely resembles.

In addition to the evidence base for anorexia nervosa and bulimia nervosa covered in other chapters of this guideline, BED has a growing evidence base relating to CBT, IPT and self-help approaches. There is also emerging research on antidepressants and appetite suppressants. To date, the research has focused primarily on the treatment of cases with comorbid obesity. It is not known whether equivalent findings would be obtained with patients who do not have obesity. Similar treatment approaches may well be helpful in adolescent cases though this has not been researched. There is no evidence about service setting for the treatment of BED.

8.2 Psychological interventions

8.2.1 Introduction

Psychological treatments for atypical eating disorders have been little studied, although patients with these disorders comprise a very significant proportion of those who present for treatment in the NHS (Fairburn & Harrison, 2003). The past 10 years has seen a growing interest in the treatment of BED with the development of specialised forms of CBT and IPT along with simplified forms of DBT. Behavioural weight management programmes have also been evaluated as a form of treatment for BED when it co-occurs with obesity.

8.2.2 Current practice

As indicated above, although patients with atypical eating disorders comprise a significant percentage of patients with eating disorders in specialist service settings, little is known about their current management. It is clearly a priority that treatment of these patients receives research attention.

8.2.3 Psychological treatments compared with wait-list controls

8.2.3.1 Treatments reviewed

The treatments included in this section are for BED only, usually in the presence of obesity.

The following treatments were included:

- Behavioural weight control (BWC)

- Cognitive behaviour therapy for binge eating disorder (CBT-BED)

- Interpersonal psychotherapy for binge eating disorder (IPT-BED)

- Simplified dialectical behaviour therapy (simplified DBT).

The Psychological Topic Group established definitions for each treatment (see Glossary). Two members of the Topic Group assessed each study for eligibility and classified each psychological treatment. Where disagreements arose, they were resolved by discussion.

8.2.3.2 Studies considered[19]

The review team conducted a new review of psychological treatments compared to wait-list control for BED. Seven trials met the eligibility criteria set by the Psychological Topic Group (Agras, 1995; Eldredge, 1997; Gorin, 2001; Reeves, 2001; Telch, 1990 & 2001; Wilfley, 1993). Of these, four used CBT–BED as the active treatment (Agras, 1995; Eldredge, 1997; Gorin, 2001; Telch, 1990), one used BWC (Reeves, 2001), one used simplified DBT (Telch, 2001), and one used IPT–BED (Wilfley, 1993). Thus, seven RCTs comparing a psychological treatment with a wait-list control group, involving 432 participants, were included in this section.

Full details of studies included in this review and reasons for excluding studies are given in Appendix 18.

8.2.3.3 Evidence statements[20]

The level of evidence (I, IIa, IIb, III, IV) is given after each statement (see Section 3.4.6 for more information about the classification of evidence).

---

[19] Here and elsewhere in the guideline, each study considered for review is referred to by a study ID (primary author and date of study publication, except where a study is in press or only submitted for publication, then a date is not used).

[20] The full list of all evidence statements generated from meta-analyses (and the associated forest plots) will be available on the CD-ROM that accompanies the guideline.

Effect of treatment on remission from binge eating

There is strong evidence suggesting that there is a clinically significant difference between CBT–BED and wait-list control with CBT–BED being superior in terms of remission (defined as cessation of binge eating) by the end of treatment (N = 4; n = 226; Random Effects RR = 0.64; 95 per cent CI, 0.49 to 0.84; NNT = 3; 95 per cent CI, 2 to 7). I

There is strong evidence suggesting that there is a clinically significant difference between simplified DBT and wait-list control with simplified DBT being superior in terms of remission (defined as cessation of binge eating) by the end of treatment (N = 1; n = 44; RR = 0.30; 95 per cent CI, 0.15 to 0.60; NNT = 2; 95 per cent CI, 1 to 3). I

There is strong evidence suggesting that there is a clinically significant difference between IPT–BED and wait-list control with IPT–BED being superior in terms of remission (defined as cessation of binge eating) by the end of treatment (N = 1; n = 38; RR = 0.56; 95 per cent CI, 0.37 to 0.84; NNT = 3; 95 per cent CI, 2 to 5). I

Effect of treatment on frequency of binge eating

There is strong evidence suggesting that there is a clinically significant difference between CBT–BED and wait-list control with CBT–BED being superior on mean frequency of binge eating by the end of treatment (N = 4; n = 214; Random Effects SMD = –1.30; 95 per cent CI, –2.13 to –0.48). I

There is insufficient evidence to determine whether simplified DBT has any impact on the frequency of binge eating by the end of treatment. I

There is strong evidence suggesting that there is a clinically significant difference between IPT–BED and wait-list control with IPT–BED being superior on mean frequency of binge eating by the end of treatment (N = 1; n = 38; SMD = –1.44; 95 per cent CI, –2.16 to –0.72). I

There is limited evidence suggesting that there is a clinically significant difference between BWC and wait-list control with BWC being superior on mean frequency of binge eating by the end of treatment (N = 1; n = 82; SMD = –0.45; 95 per cent CI, –0.89 to –0.01). I

Effect of treatment on weight

There is evidence suggesting that it is unlikely there is a clinically significant difference between CBT–BED and wait-list control in terms of mean body weight (BMI where possible) by the end of treatment (N = 3; n = 176; SMD = –0.02; 95 per cent CI, –0.33 to 0.30). I

There is insufficient evidence to determine whether BWC has any impact on body weight by the end of treatment. I

Other effects of treatment

There is evidence suggesting that it is unlikely there is a clinically significant difference between CBT–BED and wait-list control in terms of mean depression scores by the end of treatment (N = 4; n = 214; SMD = –0.18; 95 per cent CI, –0.46 to 0.10). I

There is limited evidence suggesting that there is a clinically significant difference between IPT-BED and wait-list control with IPT-BED being superior on mean depression scores by the end of treatment (N = 1; n = 38; SMD = –0.80; 95 per cent CI, –1.46 to –0.13). I

There is insufficient or no evidence to determine whether CBT-BED, simplified DBT or IPT–BED have any impact on general psychiatric state or interpersonal/social functioning by the end of treatment. I

Attrition from the study

There is limited evidence suggesting that there is a clinically significant difference favouring the wait-list control group over CBT–BED in terms of the number of people leaving the study early due to any reason by end of treatment (N = 4; n = 222; RR = 1.86; 95 per cent CI, 1.10 to 3.15; NNH = 7; 95 per cent CI, 4 to 34). I

There is insufficient evidence to determine whether there is any difference between simplified DBT, IPT–BED or BWC and wait-list control in terms of the number of people leaving the study early due to any reason by the end of treatment. I

8.2.4 Psychological treatments compared with other psychological treatments

The treatments included in this section are for BED only, usually in the presence of obesity.

8.2.4.1   Psychological treatments reviewed

The following treatments were included:

- Behavioural weight control (BWC)

- Cognitive behaviour therapy for binge eating disorder (CBT-BED)

- Guided self-help (GSH)

- Interpersonal psychotherapy for binge eating disorder (IPT-BED)

- Pure self-help (PSH).

The review team conducted a new review of psychological treatments compared to other psychological treatments for BED. Four RCTs met the eligibility criteria set by the Psychological Topic Group (Carter, 1998; Loeb, 2000; Nauta, 2000; Wilfley, 1993 & 2002). Of these, one compared CBT–BED with BWC (Nauta, 2000) using a follow-up period of six months, and two compared CBT–BED with IPT–BED (Wilfley, 1993 & 2002), with only the latter study using a follow-up of 12 months. A further two trials compared GSH with PSH (Carter, 1998; Loeb, 2000), with the former study using a six-month follow-up. Both studies used the book *Overcoming Binge Eating* (Fairburn, 1995).

Thus, four trials, involving a total of 404 participants, were included in this review.

Full details of studies included in this review and reasons for excluding studies are given in Appendix 18.

8.2.4.3   Evidence statements[21]

Effect of treatment on remission from binge eating

There is insufficient evidence to determine whether or not there is any difference between CBT-BED and IPT-BED or BWC in terms of remission (defined as cessation of binge eating) by either the end of treatment or post-treatment follow-up. I

There is strong evidence suggesting that there is a clinically significant difference between CBT-BED and BWC with CBT-BED being superior in terms of remission (defined as cessation of binge eating) at follow-up (N = 1; n = 37; RR = 0.25; 95 per cent CI, 0.08 to 0.79; NNT = 3; 95 per cent CI, 2 to 8). I

There is insufficient evidence to determine whether GSH differs from PSH on remission of binge eating by end of treatment. I

Effect of treatment on frequency of binge eating

It is unlikely that CBT–BED and IPT–BED differ with regard to their effect on mean frequency of binge eating by either the end of treatment or follow-up:

●   There is evidence suggesting that it is unlikely there is a clinically significant difference between CBT-BED and IPT-BED on mean frequency of binge eating by the end of treatment (N = 2; n = 194; SMD = –0.07; 95 per cent CI, –0.35 to 0.22). I

●   There is evidence suggesting that it is unlikely there is a clinically significant difference between CBT-BED and IPT-BED on mean frequency of binge eating at follow-up (N = 1; n = 138; SMD = 0.14; 95 per cent CI, –0.19 to 0.48). I

---

[21] The full list of all evidence statements generated from meta-analyses (and the associated forest plots) will be available on the CD-ROM that accompanies the guideline.

There is insufficient evidence to determine whether CBT-BED differs from BWC on mean frequency of binge eating by post-treatment follow-up. I

There is limited evidence suggesting that there is a clinically significant difference between GSH and PSH with GSH being superior on mean frequency of binge eating by the end of treatment (N = 2; *n* = 109; SMD = −0.48; 95 per cent CI, −0.86 to −0.09). I

There is insufficient evidence to determine whether GSH differs from PSH on mean frequency of binge eating by post-treatment follow-up. I

Effect of treatment on weight

There is evidence suggesting that it is unlikely there is a clinically significant difference between CBT-BED and IPT-BED on mean weight (BMI where possible) by the end of treatment (N = 1; *n* = 158; SMD = 0.06; 95 per cent CI, −0.26 to 0.37). I

There is insufficient evidence to determine whether CBT-BED differs from IPT-BED or BWC on mean weight by post-treatment follow-up. I

There is evidence suggesting that it is unlikely there is a clinically significant difference between GSH and PSH on mean weight (BMI where possible) by the end of treatment (N = 2; *n* = 109; SMD = 0.08; 95 per cent CI, −0.30 to 0.46). I

There is insufficient evidence to determine whether GSH differs from PSH on mean weight by post-treatment follow-up. I

Other effects of treatment

There is insufficient evidence to determine whether CBT-BED differs from IPT-BED or BWC in terms of depression by the end of treatment. I

There is evidence suggesting that it is unlikely there is a clinically significant difference between CBT-BED and IPT-BED on mean depression scores at follow-up (N = 1; *n* = 138; SMD = 0.10; 95 per cent CI, −0.24 to 0.43). I

There is insufficient evidence to determine whether CBT-BED differs from BWC in terms of depression by post-treatment follow-up. I

There is evidence suggesting that it is unlikely there is a clinically significant difference between CBT-BED and IPT-BED on mean general psychiatric symptom scores by the end of treatment (N = 1; *n* = 158; SMD = 0.06; 95 per cent CI, −0.25 to 0.37). I

There is evidence suggesting that it is unlikely there is a clinically significant difference between CBT-BED and IPT-BED on mean psychosocial/interpersonal functioning scores by the end of treatment (N = 2; *n* = 194; SMD = 0.06; 95 per cent CI, −0.22 to 0.35). I

There is insufficient evidence to determine whether CBT–BED differs from IPT–BED in terms of mean psychosocial/interpersonal functioning scores by post-treatment follow-up. I

There is evidence suggesting that it is unlikely there is a clinically significant difference between CBT-BED and IPT-BED on mean general psychiatric scores at follow-up (N = 1; *n* = 138; SMD = 0.13; 95 per cent CI, −0.20 to 0.47). I

There is insufficient evidence to determine whether GSH differs from PSH in terms of mean general psychiatric scores by either the end of treatment or post-treatment follow-up. I

Acceptability of treatment

There is insufficient evidence to determine whether CBT-BED is more, or less, acceptable to people with BED than IPT-BED or BWC. I

There is insufficient evidence to determine whether GSH is more, or less, acceptable to people with BED than PSH. I

8.2.5 Additional considerations in the management of children and adolescents

Nothing is known about the treatment of atypical eating disorders in adolescents. Binge eating disorder does occur in some children and adolescents, especially among those with obesity (e.g. Decaluwe *et al.*, 2003). The prevalence of BED in this age group is not known. There have been no studies of their treatment. This omission needs to be rectified. In the meantime, it is the view of the GDG that child and adolescent patients with BED should receive the same type of treatment as adults but adapted to suit their age, circumstances and level of development and with appropriate family involvement.

8.2.6 Clinical summary

There has been no research specifically directed at the treatment of atypical eating disorders other than BED. The view of the GDG is that clinicians should manage the large number of these cases according to the guidelines for anorexia nervosa or bulimia nervosa depending on the clinical presentation and age of the patient.

With regard to BED, given the apparently good response, at least in the short term, to a range of different psychological interventions including self-help and given the lower level of acute physical and psychiatric risk compared to anorexia and bulimia nervosa, treatment for BED may often be deliverable in primary care through the use of evidence-based self-help manuals. Children and adolescents with binge eating problems should receive the same type of treatment as adults but adapted to suit their age, circumstances and level of development, with appropriate family involvement.

8.2.7 Clinical practice recommendations

8.2.7.1   In the absence of evidence to guide the management of atypical eating disorders (also known as eating disorders not otherwise specified) other than binge eating disorder, it is recommended that the clinician considers following the guidance on the treatment of the eating problem that most closely resembles the individual patient's eating disorder. (C)*

8.2.7.2   As a possible first step, patients with binge eating disorder should be encouraged to follow an evidence-based self-help programme. (B)

8.2.7.3   Healthcare professionals should consider providing direct encouragement and support to patients undertaking an evidence-based self-help programme as this may improve outcomes. This may be sufficient treatment for a limited subset of patients. (B)

8.2.7.4   Cognitive behaviour therapy for binge eating disorder (CBT–BED), a specifically adapted form of CBT, should be offered to adults with binge eating disorder. (A)*

8.2.7.5   Other psychological treatments (interpersonal psychotherapy for binge eating disorder and modified dialectical behaviour therapy) may be offered to adults with persistent binge eating disorder. (B)

8.2.7.6   Patients should be informed that all psychological treatments for binge eating disorder have a limited effect on body weight. (A)

8.2.7.7   When providing psychological treatments for patients with binge eating disorder, consideration should be given to the provision of concurrent or consecutive interventions focusing on the management of any comorbid obesity. (C)

8.2.7.8   Suitably adapted psychological treatments should be offered to adolescents with persistent binge eating disorder. (C)

8.3 Pharmacological interventions

8.3.1 Introduction

Antidepressants, antiepileptics and appetite suppressants have been suggested as possible treatments for BED. The evidence base for such practice is very limited.

8.3.2 Current practice

Little is known about the use of medication in the treatment of BED or other atypical eating disorders in the NHS.

8.3.3 Pharmacological treatment

All the studies reviewed below are on BED.

The following drugs were included:

- Antidepressants

- Antiepileptics.

Drugs that have had their licences withdrawn from the UK were not included in the guideline.

The review team conducted a new review of RCTs involving pharmacological treatment in people with BED. Five trials met the eligibility criteria (Arnold, 2002; Hudson, 1998; Laederachhofman, 1999; McElroy, 2000; McElroy, in press). Three trials compared a SSRI antidepressant (fluoxetine, fluvoxamine, sertraline) with placebo (Arnold, 2002; Hudson, 1998; McElroy, 2000), one trial compared a tricyclic antidepressant (imipramine) with placebo (Laederachhofman, 1999), and one trial (McElroy, in press) compared an antiepileptic (topiramate) with placebo. Thus, five RCTs comparing a pharmacological treatment with placebo, involving 271 participants, were included for review.

Full details of studies included in this review and reasons for excluding studies are given in Appendix 18.

Effect of treatment on remission

There is limited evidence suggesting that there is a clinically significant difference between antidepressants (SSRIs) and placebo with antidepressants being superior in terms of remission (defined as cessation of binge eating) by the end of treatment (N = 3; n = 179; RR = 0.77; 95 per cent CI, 0.63 to 0.93; NNT = 6; 95 per cent CI, 4 to 17). I

There is limited evidence suggesting that there is a clinically significant difference between topiramate and placebo with topiramate being superior in terms of remission (defined as cessation of binge eating) by the end of treatment (N = 1; n = 61; RR = 0.56; 95 per cent CI, 0.34 to 0.92; NNT = 4; 95 per cent CI, 2 to 15). I

---

[22] The full list of all evidence statements generated from meta-analyses (and the associated forest plots) will be available on the CD-ROM that accompanies the guideline.

Effect of treatment on symptoms

There is limited evidence suggesting that there is a clinically significant difference between antidepressants and placebo with antidepressants being superior on mean frequency of binge eating by the end of treatment (N = 3; *n* = 91; SMD = -0.61; 95 per cent CI, −1.04 to −0.18). I

Effect of treatment on weight

There is insufficient evidence to determine whether antidepressants have any impact on weight when compared with placebo at the end of treatment. I

Other effects of treatment

There is strong evidence suggesting that there is a clinically significant difference between antidepressants and placebo with antidepressants being superior on mean depression scores by the end of treatment (N = 2; *n* = 65; SMD = −0.78; 95 per cent CI, −1.30 to −0.27). I

Acceptability of treatment

There is insufficient evidence to determine whether antidepressants or antiepileptics are more, or less, acceptable to people with BED. I

Tolerability of treatment

There is insufficient evidence to determine whether antidepressants or antiepileptics produce side effects in people with BED. I

8.3.4 Clinical summary

There have been no studies of the use of drugs to treat atypical eating disorders other than BED. In BED there is limited evidence that by the end of treatment antidepressants can bring about improved remission from binge eating, reduced frequency of binge eating and improved mood. One small trial has demonstrated a positive impact of an antiepileptic (topiramate) on remission. No long-term follow-up data exists for any drug.

8.3.5 Clinical practice recommendations

8.3.5.1   As an alternative or additional first step to using an evidence-based self-help programme, consideration should be given to offering a trial of a SSRI antidepressant drug to patients with binge eating disorder. (B)

8.3.5.2   Patients with binge eating disorders should be informed that SSRIs can reduce binge eating, but the long-term effects are unknown. Antidepressant drugs may be sufficient treatment for a limited subset of patients. (B)

8.4 Management of physical aspects

The predominant long-term risks for patients with BED are with the physical consequences of any comorbid obesity. As current treatment programmes for BED appear to have minimal or no impact on weight, appropriate physical monitoring, advice and management strategies for obesity should be adopted. The physical consequences and management of obesity is beyond the scope of this guideline.

Binge eating disorder is the predominant eating disorder to occur in Type 2 diabetes and this usually occurs in the context of obesity. In nearly 90 per cent of cases the eating disorder preceded the onset of the diabetes (Herpertz *et al.*, 1998).

The management of physical complications accompanying atypical eating disorders other than BED (e.g. severe underweight, electrolyte disturbance) should follow the guidance specified for anorexia nervosa and bulimia nervosa.

8.5 Service level interventions

Little is known about the optimal management of people with atypical eating disorders (including BED) in the NHS. Sometimes the strict use of referral criteria specifying full syndrome eating disorders may mean that they are excluded from specialised services. Most patients with atypical eating disorders referred to secondary care are treated as outpatients unless the management of comorbid states required admission to hospital. The GDG considered any evidence that certain levels of service provision – outpatient, day patient or inpatient – were associated with better outcomes in atypical eating disorders. No additional data relating specifically to atypical eating disorders (including BED) were identified. Therefore, it was agreed that the recommendations concerning the general approach for bulimia nervosa and anorexia nervosa be also applied to the atypical eating disorders. This should be borne in mind when considering the recommendations for this group of patients.

9 Health economics evidence

Data on the economic burden of eating disorders and cost-effectiveness evidence of the different treatment options for eating disorders were collected and assessed as part of the development of the guideline in order to help decision making.

9.1 Systematic literature review

A systematic review of the health economic evidence in the field of eating disorders was conducted. The aim of the review was three-fold:

1. To identify all publications with information about the economic burden of eating disorders;

2. To identify previously conducted economic evaluations of any psychological, pharmacological or service level interventions for the treatment of eating disorders, or any interventions for the management of the physical aspects of eating disorders; and

3. To find studies with relevant resource use and cost data, or quality-of-life evidence generalisable to the UK context to facilitate possible cost-effectiveness modelling.

9.1.1 Search strategy

Bibliographic electronic databases and health economic databases were searched for studies using the combination of a specially developed health economics search filter and a general filter for eating disorders. A combination of subject headings and free text searches were used where possible. The search strategies and the databases searched are presented in Appendix 12.

The search for further evidence included papers from reference lists of eligible studies and relevant reviews. Experts in the field of eating disorders and mental health economics were also contacted to identify additional relevant published and unpublished studies. Studies included in the clinical evidence review and stakeholders' submissions were also screened for economic evidence.

9.1.2 Review process

The database searches identified 770 possibly eligible references. A further five studies were identified by hand searching and recommendations from experts. Titles/abstracts of all references were checked to identify papers of potential relevance. The full texts of all potentially eligible studies (or where relevance/eligibility was not clear from the abstract)

(62 papers) were obtained and tested against a set of standard inclusion criteria by the health economist.

Papers eligible for inclusion were subsequently assessed for internal validity. The quality assessment of economic evaluations was based on the 32-point checklist used by the British Medical Journal to assist referees in appraisal of economic analyses (Drummond & Jefferson, 1996), or on a shortened 18-point version in the case of costing studies (Appendix 13).

9.1.3 Selection criteria

Cost-of-illness/economic burden studies

- There was no restriction placed on language or publication status of the papers.

- Studies published from 1980 until September 2002 were included. This date restriction was imposed in order to obtain data relevant to current health care settings and costs.

- Only studies from OECD countries were included as the aim of the review was to identify economic burden information relevant to the current UK context.

- Selection criteria based on types of clinical conditions and patients were identical to the clinical literature review section.

- The study provided sufficient details regarding methods and results to enable judgement of the quality of the study and the use of the study's data and results.

Economic evaluations

- The studies used an analytical method of cost-minimisation analysis, cost-effectiveness analysis, cost-utility analysis or cost-benefit analysis.

- Clinical evidence was sourced from meta-analyses, randomised controlled trials, quasi-experimental trials or a cohort studies.

- There was no restriction placed on language or publication status of the papers.

- Studies published from 1980 until September 2002 were included. This date restriction was imposed in order to obtain data relevant to current health care settings and costs.

- Only studies from OECD countries were included as the aim of the review was to identify cost-effectiveness information relevant to the current UK context.

- Selection criteria based on types of clinical conditions, patients, treatments and settings were identical to the clinical literature review section.

- The studies provided sufficient details regarding methods and results to enable judgement of the quality of the study and the use of the study's data and results.

- All types of costing studies were considered for inclusion, regardless of study design. However, this was subject to the study providing sufficient details on methods and results to enable judgement of the quality of the study.

- There was no restriction placed on language or publication status of the papers.

- Studies published from 1980 until September 2002 were included. This date restriction was imposed in order to obtain data relevant to current health care settings and costs.

- Only studies from the UK were included as the aim of the review was to identify cost information relevant to the current UK context.

- Selection criteria based on types of clinical conditions, patients, treatments and settings were identical to the clinical literature review section.

Health related quality-of-life studies

- All formal quality-of-life studies reporting utilities and involving people with eating disorders were considered for inclusion.

- There was no restriction placed on language or publication status of the papers.

- Studies published from 1980 until September 2002 were included.

- Selection criteria based on types of clinical conditions, patients, treatments and settings were identical to the clinical literature review section.

9.1.4 Data extraction

Data were abstracted by a single abstractor using the economic data extraction form (Appendix 14). Masked assessment, whereby data extractors are blind to the details of journal, authors, etc., was not undertaken because there is no evidence to support the claim that this minimises bias (Cochrane, 2001).

9.1.5 Evidence synthesis

Cost-of-illness/economic burden studies

Altogether 12 publications were deemed eligible for the economic burden review (Brown, 1997; Crow, 2003; Garvin, 2002; Hoek, 1991; Hoek, 2003; Howlett, 1995; Krauth, 2002; Lemouchoux, 2001; Office of Health Economics, 1994; Striegel-Moore, 2000; Turnbull, 1996; Vos, 2001). Results of these studies were summarised in the form of a narrative review about the socioeconomic burden of eating disorders in Section 2.6.

The GDG also had the initial attempt to establish the usual care pathway and health service use of people with eating disorders in the UK. However, the group later agreed that such task would require significant further primary research and so it is outside the scope of the guideline development process.

Economic evaluations

One economic evaluation was selected for data abstraction.

Koran *et al.* (1995) conducted an exploratory post hoc study that compared the cost-effectiveness of five different treatment strategies for 71 women with bulimia nervosa based on the randomised controlled trial by Agras *et al.* (1992, 1994). The five strategies were: 18 sessions of CBT (CB), 16 weeks and 24 weeks of desipramine (Med16, Med24) and CBT combined with desipramine for those durations (Combo16, Combo24). They calculated the average median treatment costs per successfully treated patient on an intention-to-treat basis. At 32 weeks these cost estimates were $3948, $2338, $2972, $6613 and $4141, respectively. The same estimates at one year were: $3230, $3117, $1982, $6613 and $4832. The authors did not carry out sensitivity analysis. Overall, these estimates are average cost-effectiveness ratios, and so cannot be used for the assessment of incremental efficiency.

Costing studies

Two costing studies relevant to the UK setting were included in the economic evidence review, although the quality of both studies was poor and they did not provide sufficient methodological details to be able to judge the robustness of their estimates.

A review by Meads *et al.* (2001) investigated the costs of outpatient and inpatient care for the treatment of anorexia nervosa in 1998 prices. They collected unpublished data and carried out a telephone survey of District Health Authorities in the West Midlands. The review showed that the mean cost per inpatient episode varied between £18,924 and £32,636. The mean number of outpatient sessions per patient per year varied between five and 13 with a cost range of £60 to £90 per outpatient episode. Based on these data the authors estimated that the cost of outpatient treatment is approximately one-tenth of the cost of inpatient treatment in the UK.

Birchall *et al.* (2002) costed an intensive day programme for the treatment of severe anorexia nervosa in Leicestershire. They compared the number of hospital days for their cohort of anorexia nervosa patients in the three years prior to the opening of the day programme (1994–1997) with another cohort in the three years following (1997–2000). They estimated the average cost of an inpatient day for eating disorder treatment at £216.73 and a day programme day at £111.07. The average number of inpatient days per patient greatly reduced after the introduction of the day programme from 217 to 90, but the number of day programme days significantly increased from 0 to 153. The average total cost of hospital use per patient was £3919 and £2434.20 before and after the day care programme was available, respectively.

Three further costing studies not relevant for the UK setting were also identified by the review (Kachele, 1999; Mitchell, 1998; Williamson, 2001).

One study was identified that measured the quality-of-life of patients with eating disorders using the Nottingham Health Profile (NHP). Both patients with anorexia nervosa and bulimia nervosa showed significantly more impairment than average female student controls in the health domains of the NHP. In addition to health difficulties, the patient groups also reported functional difficulties in daily living. However, the study did not provide the necessary data to inform a cost-utility analysis (Keilen *et al.*, 1994).

9.2 Cost-effectiveness modelling

9.2.1 Background

The GDG in collaboration with the health economist discussed a few possible areas within the scope of the guideline with major cost impacts in an attempt to conduct primary economic evaluations alongside the guideline development process. Based on the preliminary analysis of the clinical evidence these areas were the following:

- Comparative cost-effectiveness of CBT versus IPT for the treatment of bulimia nervosa

- Comparative cost-effectiveness of individual CBT versus group CBT

- Comparative cost-effectiveness of psychotherapy versus antidepressant therapy for the treatment of bulimia nervosa

- Comparative cost-effectiveness of psychotherapy versus combination of psychotherapy and antidepressant therapy for the treatment of bulimia nervosa

- Comparative cost-effectiveness of antidepressant therapy versus combination of psychotherapy and antidepressant therapy for the treatment of bulimia nervosa

- Comparative cost-effectiveness of inpatient versus day patient management of anorexia nervosa

- Comparative cost-effectiveness of stepped care model versus conventional model for the management of eating disorders.

However, where there is little clinical evidence of comparative clinical efficacy/ effectiveness of different treatment options, it is difficult to model the difference in cost-effectiveness between the alternatives.

The GDG identified one area where enough clinical data were available to develop a decision analytic model and provide robust cost-effectiveness information for the decision making process. This was the comparative cost-effectiveness of antidepressant therapy, cognitive behaviour therapy (CBT) and the combination of the two for the treatment of bulimia nervosa.

9.2.2 Treatment strategies and model structure

As part of the health economic evidence presented for the guideline, a formal decision analytic model was constructed in order to explore the incremental cost-effectiveness of antidepressant therapy, individual cognitive behaviour therapy (CBT) and the combination of the two for the treatment of bulimia nervosa in the UK. Originally three strategies for the management of bulimia nervosa were modelled:

● Strategy A: antidepressant treatment given for 16 weeks

● Strategy B: 20 sessions of CBT

● Strategy C: combination of 16 weeks antidepressant treatment and 20 sessions of CBT.

However, the clinical evidence reviewed in the guideline development process showed no overall superiority of combination therapy on treatment outcomes over CBT, and there was insufficient evidence to determine whether antidepressants differ from combination therapy with respect to the primary outcome by the end of treatment or post-treatment follow-up (see Section 7.4). The clinical evidence together with the higher treatment cost of the combination therapy compared to the costs of either antidepressant therapy alone or CBT alone resulted in the dominance of the two single therapies over the combination therapy. Hence, strategy C was excluded from the final cost-effectiveness analysis.

Costs and outcomes of the alternative strategies were compared post-treatment. Although the original attempt was to compare the cost-effectiveness at 12-month follow-up, it was later amended according to the clinical evidence to four months, since there was insufficient evidence regarding the effects of antidepressant medication by post-treatment follow-up to draw firm conclusions about the relative outcome by the different treatment options (see Section 7.4).

The structure of the decision tree is presented in Appendix 15.

9.2.3 Treatment outcomes

Since no health related quality-of-life data of people with bulimia nervosa were available, economic evaluation in the form of a cost-utility analysis was not possible. In the clinical evidence review, more than one outcome measure was used; of these, remission/no remission from binge eating was chosen as the most appropriate primary outcome measure for the cost-effectiveness analysis.

Clinical parameter estimates were collected as part of the clinical evidence review. Mean values from the guideline meta-analyses were used as baseline estimates in the model, and 95 per cent confidence intervals or minimum/maximum values from the clinical evidence reviews were used as the minimum/maximum estimates in the sensitivity analyses. Estimates of the absolute effectiveness of CBT were calculated from the relative risk data and the absolute effectiveness of antidepressant therapy to be as consequent as possible with the clinical evidence. No discounting of benefits was applied since the time horizon of the analysis did not exceed one year. Full details of the clinical outcome parameters used in this analysis are given in Appendix 16 and the corresponding clinical evidence review section of this guideline (Section 7.4).

9.2.4 Resource use and unit costs

Costing of the different treatment strategies was carried out as part of the guideline development process since no formal UK costing study of the different bulimia nervosa treatment strategies could be identified in the literature review.

The costs were identified from the UK National Health Service's perspective using UK specific costs. All cost data are for year 2002–2003. No discounting was applied since the time horizon of the analysis did not exceed one year.

Input data for the base case and the sensitivity analysis of the model were obtained from a broad range of sources. Resource utilisation and unit cost data were collected as part of the literature review, from other published sources, or from the GDG acting as an expert panel. All baseline estimates, the ranges used in the sensitivity analyses and the sources of the information are listed in Appendix 16.

For calculating drug costs, the generic price of the drug from the British National Formulary 45 was used. However, the scenario of prescribing Prozac, the proprietary version of fluoxetine, instead of the generic equivalent, was also explored in the sensitivity analysis.

Unit cost estimates for staff fees were taken from Netten *et al.* (2002). The staff unit cost estimates used in this analysis are without qualification costs, but include salary costs, salary oncosts, overheads, capital overheads and ongoing training costs.

Estimated resource utilisation was then combined with the unit cost information to give the average cost associated with each treatment strategy. Treatment costs were also adjusted by the cost savings incurred by people leaving the treatment early.

No estimates were available for the total health service costs or for the health service use of an average patient with bulimia nervosa from the literature. This calculation was also outside of the scope of the guideline, hence no such formal estimate was available for the cost-effectiveness analysis.

9.2.5 Assumptions of the model

- A cohort of 1000 patients in each arm

- Each patient in the model has a well-established diagnosis of bulimia nervosa

- The treatment outcomes used are based on intention-to-treat analyses

- CBT is provided by a suitably qualified and trained psychologist. (Clinical psychologists were chosen as a representative example of therapists providing bulimia nervosa specific CBT for the model)

- The protocol of CBT used in the analysis is based on the clinical manual of bulimia nervosa specific CBT (Fairburn *et al.*, 1993) and personal communication with Professor Christopher Fairburn.

- The typical antidepressant treatment of bulimia nervosa is fluoxetine in 60 mg/day dose (BNF, 2003)

- Since there was insufficient evidence that antidepressant therapy given for longer than 16 weeks is more effective than given only for 16 weeks, 16 weeks was chosen as the base case for the length of antidepressant therapy. However, the scenario of 24 weeks was also explored

- Antidepressant therapy can be prescribed in primary care by a general practitioner or in secondary care on an outpatient basis by a psychiatrist, and the clinical effectiveness of antidepressant does not depend on the qualification of the prescribing doctor

- The minimum amount of fluoxetine prescribed at one time is its monthly dose

- Those patients who leave the treatment early do not incur full treatment cost, only a proportion of it corresponding to the mean drop out time.

9.2.6 Result of the cost-effectiveness analysis

The patient groups to which the results apply are identical to those described in the clinical evidence section.

9.2.6.1 Treatment outcomes

The systematically reviewed clinical evidence shows that the number of patients remitting is significantly higher for CBT than for antidepressant treatment. The end of treatment absolute risk of no remission by antidepressants was found to be 0.807 and the relative risk of no remission by antidepressant treatment versus CBT was 1.28 (see Paragraph 7.4). Although there was insufficient evidence to draw firm conclusions about the comparable longer-term treatment outcomes of CBT and antidepressant therapy, it is anticipated that the relapse rate with CBT is lower than that with antidepressants (Agras, 2001).

9.2.6.2 CBT costs

On average, one course of bulimia nervosa specific CBT costs £967.00 when provided by a suitably qualified and trained clinical psychologist.

The unit cost and resource utilization data used for this calculation are listed in Appendix 16.

9.2.6.3 Antidepressant treatment costs

Due to the different service-level possibilities for prescribing antidepressant treatment for people with bulimia nervosa, multiple scenarios were considered to calculate the cost of fluoxetine therapy:

- The estimated average cost of generic fluoxetine treatment prescribed by a general practitioner is £118.48.

- Fluoxetine prescribed by a psychiatrist in secondary care on an outpatient basis is estimated to be a less costly alternative of antidepressant therapy for people with bulimia nervosa, average total treatment cost of £94.66, than primary care provision when prescribed by a specialist registrar level physician. However, it is estimated to be more costly option, average total treatment cost of £238.66, when consultant level physician fees are used for the calculation.

No estimates exist for the health care costs due to the complications of antidepressant therapy in bulimia nervosa, and so they could not be included in the calculation.

9.2.6.4 Cost of no remission from bulimia nervosa

Bulimia nervosa is a chronic psychiatric disorder, a high percentage of the people do not achieve remission at all or relapse in a few months post-treatment. Although no formal estimate exists about the magnitude of the additional health service use of people with bulimia nervosa, it is well known that people unsuccessfully treated continue to impose considerable extra costs for the health care sector (due to the need for extra eating disorder treatments, and additional medical and dental expenses due to symptomatic behaviour and comorbidities). Patients with bulimia nervosa also incur substantial extra costs for the broader society due to lost productivity and have greatly decreased quality-of-life as shown by Keilen et al. (1994). Hence it is anticipated that CBT, which has a significantly higher remission rate compared to antidepressant treatment for people with bulimia nervosa, also averts important additional health care costs.

9.2.6.5 Incremental cost-effectiveness of CBT versus antidepressant therapy

Since CBT was estimated to be both more effective and more costly, the difference in costs and effects were compared between CBT and antidepressant therapy. However, it needs to be emphasised that these estimates do not include the potential cost savings of CBT by averting additional and longer term health service use in the NHS. As a consequence, the net health service cost of CBT and the incremental cost-effectiveness ratio of CBT versus antidepressants are likely to be significantly overestimated in the analysis.

The incremental cost of CBT per successfully treated bulimia nervosa case is estimated to be the following:

- £4807.24 when generic fluoxetine is prescribed by a general practitioner.

- £4942.23/£4126.41 when generic fluoxetine is prescribed by a psychiatrist in secondary care on an outpatient basis.

Comparison of the costs and effects of CBT and antidepressant therapy (AD) for two cohorts of 1000 people with bulimia nervosa are summarised in Table 1 (overleaf).

Table 1: Costs and effects of CBT versus antidepressant therapy for people with bulimia nervosa

	CBT	AD	Incremental effectiveness	Incremental cost (£)	Incremental cost per successfully treated bulimia nervosa case (CBT vs. AD)
Number of people with bulimia nervosa starting treatment	1000	1000			
Number of patients achieving remission	370	193	177		
Total treatment cost (GP prescription)	£967,000	£118,483		£848,517	£4807.24
Total treatment cost (specialist registrar prescription)	£967,000	£94,656		£872,344	£4942.23
Total treatment cost (consultant psychiatrist prescription)	£967,000	£238,656		£728,344	£4126.41

9.2.7 Sensitivity analyses

9.2.7.1 One-way sensitivity analysis

There is considerable uncertainty about the parameter estimates used in the model and the policy implications of point estimates are uncertain. To explore the effect of this uncertainty a one-way sensitivity analysis was carried out, whereby individual parameters were varied while maintaining all remaining parameters at their base value. The ranges of parameters used in the sensitivity analyses together with the ranges of the calculated incremental cost-effectiveness ratios are listed in Table 2 (overleaf). The one-way sensitivity analysis shows that the most significant component of the uncertainty around the comparative cost-effectiveness of the two treatment strategies is the relative risk of no remission between antidepressant therapy and CBT. All other factors such as number of prescribing visits, length of prescribing visits, qualification of the prescribing physician, length of CBT sessions or the absolute risk of no remission by antidepressant therapy play only minor roles in the variation of the estimate.

9.2.7.2 Worst-case/best-case scenario sensitivity analysis

Worst-case/best-case scenarios were also investigated using the least favourable/most favourable parameter values for CBT and the most favourable/least favourable parameter values for antidepressant therapy, respectively. These showed that the extreme values of the incremental cost per successfully treated bulimia nervosa case are £19,209.12 and −£249.47.

9.2.7.3 Probabilistic sensitivity analysis

To demonstrate the joint uncertainty around the parameters used in the cost-effectiveness model, a probabilistic sensitivity analysis was conducted. The theoretical basis of probabilistic sensitivity analysis is described in detail by Briggs and Gray (1999). The methodology applied in this analysis is based on the study by Briggs *et al.* (2002). Using the baseline estimates and the minimum/maximum values of the different variables, special distributions were assigned to all parameters included in the sensitivity analysis and then the incremental cost-effectiveness ratio was simulated 1000 times.

The result of the probabilistic analysis is illustrated in the form of a cost-effectiveness acceptability curve in Figure 1. This gives an estimate of the proportion of the simulated incremental cost-effectiveness ratios that lie below a given threshold. (The threshold value is the maximum value a decision maker is willing to pay for a unit of effect, in this case for an additional successfully treated bulimia nervosa case.) Equally, it shows the probability that CBT is cost-effective when compared to antidepressant treatment for bulimia nervosa in the UK.

Table 2: One-way sensitivity analysis

Qualification of prescribing physician	Parameter	Base value	Alternative value/range used	Alternative value/range of cost per successfully treated bulimia nervosa case
General practitioner	Antidepressant cost/month	£22.83 (generic fluoxetine)	£47.61 (Prozac)	£4357.99
	Length of antidepressant therapy	16 weeks	24 weeks	£4471.61
	Number of antidepressant therapy visits	4	3–8	£4752.02 – £4517.70
	Length of antidepressant therapy visits	9.36 minutes	4–15 minutes	£4954.62 – £4652.16
	Length of CBT sessions	50 minutes	40–60 minutes	£3711.54 – £5902.94
	Relative risk of no remission by antidepressants vs. CBT	1.28	1.09–1.5	£12,735.84 – £3154.75
	Absolute risk of no remission by antidepressants	0.807	0.667–0.913	£5818.42 – £4248.37

Continued alongside

Qualification of prescribing physician	Parameter	Base value	Alternative value/range used	Alternative value/range of cost per successfully treated bulimia nervosa case
Specialist	Antidepressant cost	£22.83 (generic fluoxetine)	£47.61 (Prozac)	£4492.98
	Length of antidepressant therapy	16 weeks	24 weeks	£4674.10
	Cost of specialist per hour contact	£27 (specialist registrar)	£207 (consultant psychiatrist)	£4126.41
	Number of antidepressant therapy visits	4	3–8	£4861.70 – £4804.56
	Length of antidepressant therapy visits	15 minutes	10–20 minutes	£4983.02 – £4901.44
	Length of CBT sessions	50 minutes	40–60 minutes	£3846.53 – £6037.93
	Relative risk of no remission by antidepressants vs. CBT	1.28	1.09–1.5	£13,093.48 – £3243.34
	Absolute risk of no remission by antidepressants	0.807	0.667–0.913	£5981.80 – £4367.67

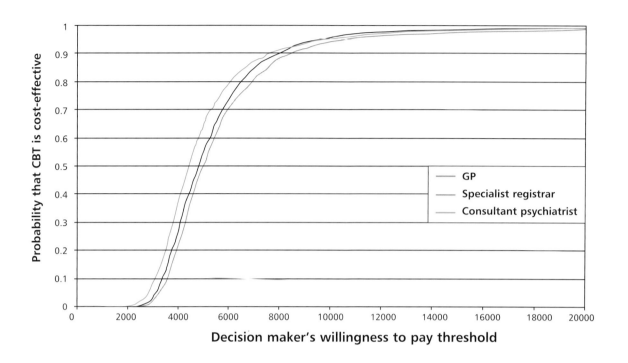

Figure 1. Cost-effectiveness acceptability curves of CBT versus antidepressant therapy for the treatment of bulimia nervosa depending on the qualification of the prescribing physician.

9.2.8 Discussion of the health economic evidence

The systematic literature review identified only one economic evaluation within the scope of the guideline and two costing studies relevant to the UK setting, but no health related quality-of-life study with the necessary data for a cost-utility analysis. Based on the available literature, no firm conclusions could be made about the comparative cost-effectiveness of the different competing therapeutic options either for the treatment of anorexia nervosa, bulimia nervosa or EDNOS.

The question of the comparative cost-effectiveness of antidepressants and CBT for people with bulimia nervosa was identified within the scope of the guideline as having a major economic consequence and enough clinical evidence to conduct a primary cost-effectiveness analysis. Present analysis shows that CBT is both more effective and more costly than antidepressant therapy. The point estimate of its incremental cost per successfully treated bulimia nervosa case varies between £4807.24, £4942.23 and £4126.41 depending on whether the antidepressant is prescribed in primary care or in secondary care by a more junior doctor or by a consultant psychiatrist, respectively. However, it is anticipated that these values are overestimations of the real incremental cost-effectiveness of CBT since its potential savings in additional health care costs were not included in the analysis due to the lack of available resource use data.

Uncertainty around these estimates was explored by sensitivity analyses, including probabilistic analysis. Under present circumstances this shows that if decision makers are not willing to pay more for additional benefit, CBT is unlikely to be cost-effective. On the other hand, if decision makers are willing to pay £4000–£5000 more for an additional successfully treated bulimia nervosa case, the probability of CBT being cost-effective is 50 per cent. The likelihood of CBT being cost-effective would increase to approximately

95 per cent if the decision maker's willingness to pay threshold for the same benefit is £10,000. However, it is assumed that if broader health service costs could be included in the analysis, the cost-effectiveness curve would shift to the left and the probability of CBT being cost-effective would increase at each threshold values. Depending on the size of the additional averted health care costs by CBT, CBT could be even cost saving for the health service sector and clearly superior to antidepressant therapy.

Based on the reviewed evidence, combination therapy of CBT and antidepressants for the treatment of bulimia nervosa is highly unlikely to be cost-effective for the NHS.

Significant uncertainty around these results still exists (e.g. the true cost of side effects of antidepressant therapy are unknown, nor have attempts been made to quantify possible costs averted due to successful treatment). When further research is carried out, it will be necessary to re-estimate the cost-effectiveness of each alternative incorporating such influences. However, all these influences are likely to favour bulimia nervosa specific CBT and so current estimates may be considered conservative.

No other cost-effectiveness analyses could be carried out as part of the guideline development process due to the lack of sufficient clinical evidence or available resource use data.

When such data will become available, other areas within the scope of this guideline identified as having possible major cost implications for the NHS should be explored (see Paragraph 9.2.1). In particular, the efficiency of a stepped care model for eating disorders is an important area considering the usual waiting time for and the great training requirements of psychotherapies. It is also recommended to investigate the comparative cost-effectiveness of IPT versus bulimia nervosa specific CBT for the treatment of bulimia nervosa in the UK with regard to the non-disease specific nature of IPT.

9.2.9 Implementation costs of the guideline

There are insufficient data about the health service utilization patterns of patients with eating disorders and about the currently available health care resources for the treatment and management of eating disorders; hence at present it is impossible to calculate the estimated cost impact of the implementation of this guideline for the NHS.

However, it is anticipated that the recommended shift towards CBT in the management of bulimia nervosa would impose a great need for health care professionals trained in bulimia nervosa specific CBT. The NHS cost of bulimia nervosa specific CBT training per person was calculated using the resource use information provided by the GDG. The estimate is based on the teaching programme of the Department of Psychiatry, University of Oxford, UK including a two-day workshop, 20 four-hour long meetings and the additional time required by the trainer for a group of five trainees. Clinical psychologists were chosen as a representative example of trainees for bulimia nervosa specific CBT for the calculation. The total training cost per trainee was estimated to be £4326 in year 2002–2003 assuming that currently enough resources are available in the NHS to train health care professionals in bulimia nervosa specific CBT. Consequently, this estimate does not include any qualification costs. Further, possible travel costs and the cost of time spent on travelling related to the training could not be included in the analysis due to the lack of such data.

10 Criteria for auditing the management of eating disorders

10.1 Objectives for the audit

One or more audits can be carried out in different care settings to ensure that:

- Individuals with an eating disorder are involved in their care

- Treatment options, including psychological interventions, are appropriately offered for individuals with an eating disorder.

10.2 Individuals to be included in an audit

A single audit could include all individuals with an eating disorder. Alternatively, individual audits could be undertaken on specific groups of individuals such as:

- People with a specific eating disorder, e.g. bulimia nervosa

- Sample of patients from particular populations in primary care.

10.3 Measures that could be used as a basis for an audit

See table alongside.

Criterion	Standard	Exception	Definition of terms
1. Cognitive behaviour therapy (CBT) in bulimia nervosa in adults			
In patients with bulimia nervosa, CBT specially adapted for the disorder should be offered to adult patients assessed as needing treatment in secondary care services.	CBT should be offered to all individuals with bulimia nervosa assessed as needing treatment in secondary care services.	Individuals who decline such an offer of treatment, who choose an alternative psychological intervention (such as interpersonal psychotherapy) and those with severe comorbidity of a type that will interfere with the patient benefiting from CBT (for example, severe depression, marked substance abuse).	The notes should indicate that the health care professional responsible has discussed the process and potential benefits of the intervention.
The course of treatment should normally be 16 to 20 individual sessions provided by a trained health care professional over four to five months.	The course of treatment should normally be 16 to 20 individual sessions provided by a trained health care professional over four to five months.		The notes should record if the patient completes a full course of treatment.

The course of the treatment should also be described in the notes and it should have followed the specific strategies and procedures employed in CBT–BN for bulimia nervosa (Fairburn et al., 1993). |

Criterion	Standard	Exception	Definition of terms
2. Cognitive behaviour therapy (CBT) in bulimia nervosa in adolescents			
Adolescents with bulimia nervosa may be treated with CBT-BN adapted as needed to suit their age, circumstances and level of development, including the family as appropriate.	CBT should be offered to the majority of adolescents with bulimia nervosa assessed as needing treatment in secondary care services.	Individuals with severe comorbidity or developmental problems of a type that will interfere with the patient benefiting from CBT.	The notes should indicate that the health care professional responsible has discussed the process and potential benefits of the intervention.
The course of treatment should normally be 16 to 20 individual sessions over four to five months.	The course of treatment should normally be 16 to 20 individual sessions provided by a trained health care professional over four to five months.		The notes should record if the patient completes a full course of treatment.
			The course of the treatment should also be described in the notes and it should have followed the specific strategies and procedures employed in CBT–BN for bulimia nervosa.

Criterion	Standard	Exception	Definition of terms
3. Psychological treatment in anorexia nervosa Adults with anorexia nervosa should be managed on an outpatient basis with psychological treatment provided by a health care professional competent in the psychological treatment of eating disorders. The course of treatment should normally last for at least six months.	Psychological treatment should be offered to all individuals with anorexia nervosa assessed as needing outpatient treatment in secondary care services. The course of treatment should normally be for at least six months.	Individuals who decline such an offer of treatment and those with severe comorbidity of a type that will interfere with the patient benefiting from psychological treatment (for example, severe depression, marked substance abuse).	The notes should indicate that the health care professional responsible has discussed the process and potential benefits of the intervention. The notes should record if the patient completes a full course of treatment. The course of the treatment should also be described in the notes and it should have followed the specific strategies set out for the chosen intervention.

Criterion	Standard	Exception	Definition of terms
4. Family interventions in anorexia nervosa Family interventions that directly address the eating disorder should be offered to children and adolescents with anorexia nervosa.	Family interventions that directly address the eating disorder should be offered to all families with a child or adolescent with anorexia nervosa.	Families who decline such an offer of treatment, and possibly where the child or adolescent is engaged in individual psychological treatment.	The notes should indicate that the health care professional responsible has discussed the process and potential benefits of the intervention. If the offer of intervention was not taken up, the notes should record whether the parent, child or both declined the offer and the number already in individual psychological treatment. The notes should record the form of family intervention (separate or conjoint) and if the family completed a full course of treatment. The course of the treatment should also be described in the notes and it should have followed the specific strategies and procedures employed in family interventions for anorexia nervosa.

Criterion	Standard	Exception	Definition of terms
5. Physical health review in anorexia nervosa All patients with enduring anorexia nervosa not under the care of secondary care services should be offered an annual health review by their GP.	Physical and mental health review offered by GP to 100 per cent of patients with enduring anorexia nervosa who are not in contact with secondary care services.	None.	The notes should indicate that the offer of a review was made to the patient and whether or not the patient attended for review.
6. Inpatient care of anorexia nervosa Patients with anorexia nervosa who require admission to a psychiatric unit should be admitted to a unit experienced in the treatment of eating disorders.	All patients requiring inpatient care should be admitted to a psychiatric unit experienced in the treatment of eating disorders.	Individuals who are admitted as psychiatric emergencies to general psychiatric wards.	An annual review of all admissions for anorexia in each PCT should be conducted for all services that have provided inpatient services for anorexia nervosa.

Criterion	Standard	Exception	Definition of terms
7. Patient satisfaction			
All patients treated in secondary care for an eating disorder should be asked to complete a satisfaction questionnaire at the end of treatment.	All patients should be asked to complete a satisfaction questionnaire at the end of treatment. The expected completion rate for the questionnaire is 50 per cent.	Individuals who decline to complete the questionnaire.	The report should specify the percentage of questionnaires returned and the characteristics of those who did and did not complete the questionnaire.
8. Atypical eating disorders			
In the absence of evidence to guide the management of atypical eating disorders (eating disorders not otherwise specified) other than as binge eating disorder, it is recommended that the clinician considers following the guidance on treatment of the eating problem that most closely resembles the individual's eating disorder.	Patients with atypical eating disorders are expected to comprise at least 40 per cent of patients assessed and taken on for treatment for eating disorders.	None.	The record system should record the diagnosis of all patients assessed and taken on for treatment in a service.

11 Appendices

Appendix 1:
Scope for the development of a clinical guideline on the management of anorexia nervosa, bulima nervosa and binge eating disorders

1. Objective

1.1. The National Institute for Clinical Excellence has commissioned a clinical guideline for patients and clinicians on the management of anorexia nervosa, bulimia nervosa and binge eating disorders. The guideline will provide advice on effective care using the best possible research evidence.

1.2. The commission received from the Department of Health and the National Assembly for Wales is in Figure 1.

1.3. The Institute's clinical guidelines will support the implementation of National Service Frameworks (NSF) in those aspects of care where a framework has been published. The statements in each NSF reflect the evidence, which was used at the time the framework was prepared. The clinical guidelines and technology appraisals published by the Institute after a NSF has been issued will have the effect of updating the framework.

Figure 1:
Remit from the Department of Health and the National Assembly for Wales

- We would wish the guideline to cover both primary and secondary care and to consider children as well as adults.

- We would like the guideline to give clear guidance to primary care on the situations under which someone should be referred urgently on to specialist services.

- We would like NICE to guide both primary care and general (non-specialised) psychiatric services in their treatment and referral choices (e.g whether drug treatments may be tried, whether to refer to clinical psychology, whether/when to refer to tertiary care).

---

2. Clinical need and practice

2.1.   Information on the incidence and prevalence of eating disorders is scarce. The prevalence of anorexia is estimated to be between 0.5 per cent and 1.0 per cent. Ninety per cent of people diagnosed as anorexic are women. The prevalence of bulimia is estimated to be between 1.0 per cent and 3.0 per cent. Ninety per cent of people diagnosed as bulimic are women. Because eating disorders are less common in males, they can go undetected.

2.2.   Severe eating disorders can result in long-term ill health or death.

2.3.   The World Health Organisation, The American Psychiatric Association, and the Eating Disorders Association have developed guidance in this area. The Faculty of Dental Surgery have developed guidance on the Management and Prevention of Dental Erosion.

3. Population

3.1.   The guideline will cover all people aged eight years and over with anorexia nervosa, bulimia nervosa or other binge eating disorders.

3.2.   Although the guideline will be of relevance to all patients with anorexia or bulimia, the guideline will not explicitly address the diagnosis or treatment of people with eating disorders in the context of a separate physical or other primary mental disorder of which a disorder of eating is a symptom.

3.3.   The guideline will provide advice on the involvement of family members and carers in the treatment and care of people with eating disorders.

3.4.   The guidance will be presented to ensure that patients and carers have the information they need and the opportunities to discuss with their clinicians the advantages, disadvantages and potential side effects of treatment so that they can make informed choices about their treatment options.

3.5.   The guideline will need to recognise best practice on confidentiality and consent of people under 18.

4. Health care setting

4.1.   The guideline will cover the care received from primary, secondary and tertiary health care professionals who have direct contact with and make decisions concerning the care of patients with these conditions.

4.2.   The guideline will also be relevant to the work but will not specifically cover the practice of other professionals such as A&E staff and those who work in education sectors.

4.3.   The guideline will offer guidance for the management of these conditions in:

    4.3.1.   Primary care

    4.3.2.   Decondary care including general (non-psychiatric) and non-specialised psychiatric services

    4.3.3.   Outpatient and day treatment services

    4.3.4.   Tertiary care and specialist services.

4.4.   The guideline will offer guidance on referral from primary care or non-specialist services to specialist care including urgent referrals.

4.5.   The guideline will address the interface between services and care shared between primary and secondary settings.

5.   Interventions and treatment

The guideline will include:

5.1.   Best practice advice on recognition, assessment and diagnosis

5.2.   Appropriate use of psychological interventions

    5.2.1.   Family interventions

    5.2.2.   Cognitive behavioural treatments

    5.2.3.   Other psychological therapies

5.3.   Appropriate management of dietary regimes

    5.3.1.   Type

    5.3.2.   Frequency

    5.3.3.   Duration

    5.3.4.   Nutritional replacement and parenteral feeding

5.4.   Management of people with acute physical health problems arising from their eating disorder

    5.4.1.   Assessment

    5.4.2.   Types of intervention

    5.4.3.   Interface with physical health services

5.5. Appropriate use of pharmacological treatments

    5.5.1. Type

        5.5.1.1. Antidepressants

        5.5.1.2. Antipsychotic

        5.5.1.3. Anxioloytics

        5.5.1.4. Appetite stimulants

    5.5.2. Dose

    5.5.3. Duration

    5.5.4. Discontinuation

    5.5.5. Changing drug regimes and sequencing in non-response

    5.5.6. The guideline assumes that prescribers will use the Summary of Product Characteristics to inform their prescribing decisions for individual patients.

5.6. Where appropriate, the guideline will provide advice on the recognition and management of strategies, which those suffering from an eating disorder may adopt including, for example, excessive exercise, use of benzodiazepines, laxative abuse.

5.7. Where the evidence is available to enable robust advice to be formulated, the guideline will address self-help approaches.

5.8. Advice on treatment options will be based on the best evidence available to the development group. When referring to pharmacological treatments, the guideline will normally recommend within the licence indications. Exceptionally, and only where the evidence clearly supports it, the guideline may recommend use outside the licence indications.

6. Presentation

The guideline will be available in three forms:

6.1. The full guideline containing the evidence base used by the developers.

6.2. A short form version, using a standard template, which will form the Institute's guidance to the NHS including a clinical practice algorithm.

6.3. The guideline will be accompanied by a version prepared specifically for patients and their carers. This patient/carer version will interpret the recommendations made in the Institute's short form version and will be designed to help patients to make informed choices about their care.

7. Status

7.1. This scoping statement is the subject of a four-week period of consultation with stakeholders. The scope was then re-drafted, submitted to the Guidelines Advisory Committee and subsequently the Institute's Guidance Executive, for approval. Once approved, it will be posted on the Institute's website, together with details of the Commissioning Brief and the name of the Collaborating Centre through which the guideline is being commissioned. The development of the guideline will begin in the autumn of 2001.

7.2. Information on the guidelines development process, stakeholder involvement and the progress of this guideline is available on the website http://www.nice.org.uk/.

Appendix 2:
Special advisors to the Guideline Development Group

Professor Marinos Elia
Professor of Clinical Nutrition and Metabolism, Fetal Origins of Adult Nutrition Division
University of Southampton, Southampton.

Dr Ian Forgacs
Department of Gastroenterology, King's College Hospital, London.

Dr Eric Johnson-Sabine
Eating Disorders Service, The Phoenix Wing, St Ann's Hospital, London.

Professor J Hubert Lacey
Department of Psychiatry, St George's Hospital Medical School, London.

Professor Tak Lee
Department of Respiratory Medicine & Allergy, King's College London, London.

Ms Fiona McKeown
Eating Disorders Service, The Phoenix Wing, St Ann's Hospital, London.

Dr Godama Prelevic
Department of Endocrinology, Middlesex Hospital, London.

Dr Paul Robinson
Royal Free Eating Disorders Service, London.

Mr Sam Clark-Stone
Clinical Coordinator, Gloucestershire Eating Disorders Project.

Ms Kate Trotter
Chief Dietician, The South London and Maudsley NHS Trust.

Dr Jeremy Shaw
Consultant in Restorative Dentistry, Birmingham Dental Hospital, Birmingham.

Dr Russell Viner
Consultant and Director of Adolescent Medicine, University College London Hospitals
and Great Ormond Street Hospital, London.

Appendix 3: Stakeholders who responded to early requests for evidence

All Wales Senior Nurses Advisory Group (Mental Health)

British Association for Counselling and Psychotherapy

British Medical Association

Eli Lilly and Company Limited

Health Technology Board of Scotland

National Collaborating Centre for Primary Care

Pain Society

Prodigy

Rethink Severe Mental Illness

Roche Products Limited

Royal College of General Practitioners

Royal College of Psychiatrists

Royal College of Speech and Language Therapists

Royal College of Surgery, Faculty of Dental Surgery

University of Leeds Innovations Limited

Appendix 4: Stakeholders and experts who responded to the first consultation draft of the Guideline

Stakeholders

Action for Sick Children

Association of the British Pharmaceuticals Industry (ABPI)

British Association for Counselling and Psychotherapy

British Association for Parenteral & Enteral Nutrition (BAPEN)

British Association of Behavioural & Cognitive Psychotherapy (BABCP)

British Dietetic Association

Chartered Society of Physiotherapy

College of Occupational Therapists

The Inner Cities Mental Health Group

National Centre for Eating Disorders

National Public Health Service for Wales

NHS Quality Improvement Scotland

Roche Products Limited

Royal College of Nursing (RCN)

Royal College of Paediatrics and Child Health

Royal College of Psychiatrists

The Survivors Trust

UK Council for Psychotherapy

Experts

Mr Sam Clark-Stone

Professor Marinos Elia

Professor Hubert Lacey

Professor Tak Lee

Roger Paxton

Dr Jeremy Shaw

Ms Kate Trotter

Professor Glenn Waller

Professor Timothy Walsh

Professor G.T. Wilson

Appendix 5: Researchers contacted to request information about unpublished or soon-to-be published studies

Dr Stewart Agras

Dr Leslie Arnold

Professor P.J.V. Beumont

Dr Cynthia M. Bulik

Dr Jacqueline C. Carter

Dr Scott J. Crow

Dr Martina de Zwaan

Dr Michael J. Devlin

Dr Ivan Eisler

Professor Manfred M. Fichter

Dr Chris Freeman

Dr Josie Geller

Dr Riccardo Dalle Grave

Dr Rosalyn Griffiths

Professor Katherine A. Halmi

Dr Phillipa Hay

Dr James Hudson

Professor Anita Jansen

Dr David Jimerson

Dr William Johnson

Dr Allan Kaplan

Dr Walter Kaye

Dr Jean L. Kristeller

Dr Daniel le Grange

Dr James Lock

Professor Susan McElroy

Dr Marsha D. Marcus

Dr James E. Mitchell

Dr Susan Paxton

Dr Kathleen Pike

Dr Howard Steiger

Dr Eric Stice

Dr Stephen Touyz

Professor Glenn C. Waller

Dr Timothy B. Walsh

Dr Denise Wilfley

Dr Terrence G. Wilson

Dr Blake Woodside

Appendix 6: Clinical questions

For all questions (unless otherwise stated) it is assumed that analysis of the questions should be by diagnostic grouping (AN, BN and BED) and age groups.

A. Psychological TG

1. **Does any psychological intervention produce benefits/harms on the specified outcomes in people with BN/BED compared to wait-list control?**
- Cognitive behavioural therapy for bulimia nervosa (CBT-BN) vs. wait-list control
- Exposure with response prevention (ERP) vs. wait-list control
- Supportive psychotherapy vs. wait-list control
- Dialectical behaviour therapy (DBT) vs. wait-list control
- Simple non-specialist treatments vs. wait-list control
- Interpersonal psychotherapy for bulimia nervosa vs. wait-list control
- Psychodynamic psychotherapy vs. wait-list control
- Behavioural self-management vs. wait-list control
- Psychological treatments vs. wait-list control

2. **Does CBT produce benefits/harms on the specified outcomes in people with BN compared to another psychological intervention?**
- CBT vs. treatments not focused on specific ED psychopathology
- CBT vs. behaviour therapy (BT)
- CBT vs. exposure with response prevention (ERP)
- CBT vs. interpersonal psychotherapy (IPT)
- CBT vs. psychodynamic psychotherapy
- CBT vs. supportive psychotherapy
- CBT vs. nutritional counselling (NC)
- CBT vs. simple non-specialist treatments

3. **Does another psychological intervention (other than CBT) produce benefits/harms on the specified outcomes in people with BN compared to another psychological intervention?**
- Exposure with response prevention (ERP) vs. supportive psychotherapy
- Exposure with response prevention (ERP) vs. nutritional counselling (NC)
- Behaviour therapy (BT) vs. interpersonal psychotherapy (IPT)
- Behaviour therapy (BT) vs. supportive psychotherapy
- Family therapy vs. any other psychological intervention

4. **Psychological interventions compared to drug treatment:**
Do psychological interventions alone produce benefits/harms on the specified outcomes in people with BN compared to antidepressants alone?

5. **Combination therapy:**

a. Does a combination of a psychological intervention and an antidepressant drug produce benefits/harms on the specified outcomes in people with BN compared to an antidepressant alone?

b. Does a combination of a psychological intervention and an antidepressant produce benefits/harms on the specified outcomes in people with BN compared to a psychological intervention alone?

6. **Predictors of response**

7. **Follow-up**

B. Service TG

1. Are screening tools effective in primary care (general medical settings) in identifying people with eating disorders?

2. Is there any evidence to support the specific sequencing or stepped provision of treatment? Can this be developed into referral guidance?

3. Type of Service:

a. Does specialist care produce benefits/harms in terms of the specified outcomes in people with BN/BED/AN compared to generalist care?

b. Does in-patient care produce benefits/harms in terms of the specified outcomes in people with BN/BED/AN compared to out-patient care?

c. Does in-patient care produce benefits/harms in terms of the specified outcomes in people with BN/BED/AN compared to day care?

d. Does out-patient care produce benefits/harms in terms of the specified outcomes in people with BN/BED/AN compared to day care?

4. Is the specified service setting/configuration associated with different levels of satisfaction/adherence to treatment in people with BN/BED/AN or their carers compared to the comparator service setting?

5. Does the identified service setting/configuration lead to lower risk of self-harm, suicide or death in people with BN/BED/AN compared to the comparator service setting?

6. Is treatment in the context of compulsory admission in people with BN/BED/AN associated with any benefits/harms or risks?

7. Does feeding in the context of active resistance in people with AN have any benefits/harms or risk?

C. Physical TG

1. How we identify eating disorders:
a. What are the physical signs?
b. What is the differential diagnosis?
c. What assessments should be done?
d. What are the diagnostic issues?

2. Risk Assessment/Management:
a. What service users are at risk of dying/or having poor outcome?
b. What factors indicate an increased need for monitoring?
c. What are the issues about sharing medical risk with carers/issues of confidentiality and capacity/refusal of treatment?

3. What is the best practice in the management of:
a. Osteoporosis
b. Osteopenia
c. Pubertal delay
d. Oestrogen deficiency
e. Growth stunting
f. Infertility
g. Polycystic ovarian syndrome (PCOS)
h. Brain loss/brain damage/neuropsychology/ventricular dilation
i. Bone marrow suppression/anaemia/leucopenia/thrombocytopenia
j. Renal/renal failure
k. Dental problems.

4. Drug treatment:
a. Do antipsychotics produce benefits/harms in the specified outcomes in people with BN/BED/AN compared to placebo?
b. Do antidepressants produce benefits/harms in the specified outcomes in people with BN/BED/AN compared to placebo?
c. Do appetite suppressants produce benefits/harms in the specified outcomes in people with BN/BED compared to placebo?
d. Do appetite stimulants produce benefits/harms in the specified outcomes in people with AN compared to placebo?
e. Do anticonvulsants produce benefits/harms in the specified outcomes in people with BN/BED/AN compared to placebo?
f. Do antiemetics produce benefits/harms in the specified outcomes in people with BN/BED/AN compared to placebo?
g. Do cannabinoids produce benefits/harms in the specified outcomes in people with BN/BED/AN compared to placebo?
h. Do anxiolytics produce benefits/harms in the specified outcomes in people with BN/BED/AN compared to placebo?
i. Does St. Johns Wort produce benefits/harms in the specified outcomes in people with BN/BED/AN compared to placebo?
j. Do antihistamines produce benefits/harms in the specified outcomes in people with BN/BED/AN compared to placebo?
k. Do antiepileptics produce benefits/harms in the specified outcomes in people with BN/BED/AN compared to placebo?

5. **Other physical interventions:**

a. Does nutritional/vitamin supplementation produce benefits/harms in the specified outcomes in people with BN/BED?

b. Does exercise/massage produce benefits/harms in the specified outcomes in people with BN/BED/AN?

c. Do alternative therapies (reflexology)/herbal medicine/mandometry/complementary medicine produce benefits/harms in the specified outcomes in people with BN/BED/AN?

d. Does nutritional or dietary management produce benefits/harms in the specified outcomes in people with BN/BED/AN?

e. Does nutritional or vitamin supplementation/nasogastric feeding/gastrotomy (PEG)/total parenteral nutrition (TPN)/enteral feeding improve weight gain/target weight in people with AN?

f. Does heat improve weight gain/target weight in people with AN?

g. Does forced feeding improve weight gain/target weight in people with AN?

h. Does jejunostomy improve weight gain/target weight in people with AN?

i. Does physiotherapy improve weight gain/target weight in people with AN?

6. **What are the effective methods for managing:**

a. Laxative abuse

b. Vomiting

c. Over-activity

d. Amphetamines

e. Stimulant abuse.

Appendix 7:
Physical Risk Assessment

Physical risk guidance
(Priority should be given to the overall physical examination of the patient)

System	Examination	Moderate risk	High risk
Nutrition	BMI	<15	<13
	BMI centiles	<3	<2
	Weight loss/wk	>0.5 kg	>1.0 kg
	Purpuric rash		+
Circulation	Systolic BP	<90 mm Hg	<80 mm Hg
	Diastolic BP	<60 mm Hg	<50 mm Hg
	Postural drop	>10 mm Hg	>20 mm Hg
	Pulse rate	<50 BPM	<40 BPM
	Extremities		Dark blue/cold
Musculo – skeletal (Squat Test*)	Unable to get up without using arms for balance	+	
	Unable to get up without using arms as leverage		+
	Unable to sit up without using arms as leverage	+	
	Unable to sit up at all		+
Temperature		<35°C	<34.5°C
Investigations	FBC, urea, electrolytes (including PO4), LFT, Albumin, Creatinine kinase, Glucose	Concern if outside normal limits	K <2.5 Na <130 Po4<0.5
	ECG	Rate <50	Rate <40 Prolonged QT interval

*The *squat test* gives a clinical indication of muscle power and may be used to monitor progress. The patient lies flat on a firm surface such as the floor and has to sit up without, if possible, using her hands. This is more sensitive to myopathic weakness.

Scoring:
- Grade 0: Completely unable to rise
- Grade 1: Able to rise only with use of hands
- Grade 2: Able to rise with noticeable difficulty
- Grade 3: Able to rise without difficulty.

PHYSICAL RISK ASSESSMENT

- In the management of these patients good practice involves discussion of issues of confidentiality and involvement of other parties

EXAMINATION

- BMI/BMI centile
- Height centile (for shunting)
- Tanner Staging if premenarchal
- BP lie and stand
- Pulse Rate
- Temperature
- Sit up and squat test
- Look for signs of peripheral shutdown, check feet
- Skin breakdown

INVESTIGATIONS

- Hb, WCC, platelets (FBC)
- U&E, renal function, LFT (if abn. check PI/INR)
- Glucose
- Mg, Ca, Phosph,
- ECG

MODERATE RISK

- SEE TABLE (for guidance). Priority should be given to physical examination
- Weekly monitoring
- Consider need for admission if weight continues to fall
- Good practice to actively encourage involvement of carers

HIGH RISK

- SEE TABLE (for guidance). Priority should be given to physical examination
- CONSIDER URGENT MEDICAL ADMISSION
- Consult specialist

IF VOLUNTARY ADMISSION REFUSED: ASSESS CAPACITY

- Understand the nature of the health risk
- To assess the risks and benefits of treatment/no treatment
- Able to weigh up the information rationally
- Make a fully informed choice with full capacity
- Consider use of Mental Health Act 1983/Children Act 1989

THE MANAGEMENT OF PHYSICAL RISK

MANAGING RISK DURING REFEEDING

- Start multivitamin and mineral supplements before feeding begins
- Feeding – small and often
- Rest
- Warm
- Fluids
- Avoid medication
- Monitor cardiac status
- Monitor bowel sounds
- Monitor electrolytes – U&E & PO4

DEHYDRATION

- Push fluids
- Monitor U&E
- Monitor intake/output
- Monitor cardiac function

HIGH CVS/RHYTHM RISK

- Avoid drugs
- CK – cardiac
- Check electrolytes
- Monitor ECG

LOW POTASSIUM

- Check magnesium
- Oral replacement
- Consider protein pump inhibitor

HYPOGLYCAEMIA RISK

- If glucose <2.0
- Meals 2–3 hours
- Check glucose 2am if abnormal during the day

LOW PHOSPHATE

- Refeed with milk products
- Oral replacement

ALWAYS CONSULT PHYSICIAN/PAEDIATRICIAN COLLEAGUES IF CONCERNED. CONSIDER WHETHER PATIENT IS BEST MANAGED ON MEDICAL WARD OR EATING DISORDERS UNIT

Appendix 8:
Search strategies for the identification of clinical studies

1. General search filters

a. MEDLINE, EMBASE, PsycINFO, CINAHL – OVID interface

1.   eating disorder/ or eating disorders/
2.   (eating adj2 disorder$).mp. [mp=ti, sh, ab, it, tn, ot, dm, mf, dv, rw, hw, ty, id]
3.   appetite disorder/
4.   anorexia nervosa/
5.   (anorexia adj1 nervosa).mp. [mp=ti, sh, ab, it, tn, ot, dm, mf, dv, rw, hw, ty, id]
6.   bulimia/or bulimi$.mp.
7.   binge eating disorder/
8.   (bing$ or overeat$ or (compulsive adj2 (eat$ or vomit$)) or (food$ adj2 bing$) or (self?induc$ adj2 vomit$) or (restrict$ adj2 eat$)).mp.
9.   or/1–8
10. 'Appetite Disorder'/si [Side Effect]
11. 'Eating Disorders'/si [Side Effect]
12. 'Eating Disorders'/ci [Chemically Induced]
13. or/10–12
14. 9 not 13

b. Cochrane Database of Systematic Reviews – Cochrane library

((EATING-DISORDERS*:ME or ANOREXIA-NERVOSA*:ME or BULIMIA*:ME or eating disorder or appetite disorder or anorexia nervosa or bulimia or binge* or overeat*) or (compulsive and (eat* or vomit*)) or (food* and bing*) or (self-induc* and vomit*))

c. Cochrane Controlled Trials Register – Cochrane Library

((EATING-DISORDERS*:ME or ANOREXIA-NERVOSA*:ME or BULIMIA*:ME or eating disorder or appetite disorder or anorexia nervosa or bulimia or binge* or overeat*) or (compulsive and (eat* or vomit*)) or (food* and bing*) or (self-induc* and vomit*))

d. Database of Reviews of Effectiveness – Cochrane Library

((EATING-DISORDERS*:ME or ANOREXIA-NERVOSA*:ME or BULIMIA*:ME or eating disorder or appetite disorder or anorexia nervosa or bulimia or binge* or overeat*) or (compulsive and (eat* or vomit*)) or (food* and bing*) or (self-induc* and vomit*))

e. Evidence-Based Mental Health – Website

1. 'eating disorder' or 'appetite disorder' or 'anorexia nervosa' or bulimia
2. binge or overeat* or (compulsive and (eat* or vomit*)) or (food* and bing*)
3. (self-induc* and vomit*) or (restrict* and eat*)
4. or/1–3

f. NHS R&D Health Technology Assessment Programme – Website

('eating disorder' or 'appetite disorder' or 'anorexia nervosa' or bulimia or binge or overeat* or (compulsive and (eat* or vomit*)) or (food* and bing*) or (self-induc* and vomit*) or (restrict* and eat*))

g. National Research Register – Website

((EATING-DISORDERS*:ME or ANOREXIA-NERVOSA*:ME or BULIMIA*:ME or eating disorder or appetite disorder or anorexia nervosa or bulimia or binge* or overeat*) or (compulsive and (eat* or vomit*)) or (food* and bing*) or (self-induc* and vomit*))

2. Systematic review search filters

a. MEDLINE, EMBASE, PsycINFO, CINAHL – OVID interface

(((meta analysis or literature review or research review).fc. and ((medline or medlars or embase or scisearch or psychinfo or psycinfo or psychlit or psyclit or cinahl or cochrane).ti,ab,sh. or (hand search$ or manual search$ or electronic database$ or bibliographic database$ or POOLING or POOLED ANALYSIS or PETO or DER SIMONIAN or DERSIMONIAN or FIXED EFFECT or RANDOM EFFECT or (MANTEL adj2 HAENZEL)).tw.)) or (exp meta analysis/ or (meta-analy$ or metaanaly$ or meta analy$ or (systematic$ adj25 review$) or (systematic$ adj25 overview) or (QUANTITATIVE$ adj25 REVIEW) or (QUANTITATIVE$ adj25 OVERVIEW) or (METHODOLOGIC$ adj25 REVIEW) or (METHODOLOGIC$ adj25 OVERVIEW) or INTEGRATIVE RESEARCH REVIEW$ or RESEARCH INTEGRATION or QUANTITATIVE$ SYNTHESIS).mp. or DATA SYNTHESIS.tw.) or ((review or review, tutorial or review, academic).pt. and ((medline or medlars or embase or scisearch or psychinfo or psycinfo or psychlit or psyclit or cinahl or cochrane).ti,ab,sh. or (hand search$ or manual search$ or electronic database$ or bibliographic database$ or pooling or pooled analys$ or fixed effect or random effect or (mantel adj2 haenzel) or peto or der?simonian).tw.)) or (meta-analysis.pt,sh. or (meta-analy$ or metaanaly$ or meta analy$ or (systematic$ adj25 review$) or (systematic$ adj25 overview) or (quantitative$ adj25 review) or (quantitative$ adj25 overview) or (methodologic$ adj25 review) or (methodologic$ adj25 overview) or integrative research review$ or research integration or quantitative$ synthesis or data synthesis).tw.))

not (letter/ or comment/)

Animal$/ not (animal$/ and human$/)

3. Randomised Controlled Trials search filter

b. MEDLINE, EMBASE, PsycINFO, CINAHL – OVID interface

1.   exp clinical trials/ or (clinical adj2 trial$).mp.
2.   Double-Blind Method/ or Double-Blind Procedure/ or Double-Blind Studies/
3.   Single-Blind Method/ or Single-Blind Procedure/
4.   exp Crossover Design/ or Cross-Over Studies/ or Crossover Procedure/
5.   cross?over.mp.
6.   random$.mp. or (random$.pt. or exp random assignment/)
7.   (single?blind$ or single blind$).mp.
8.   (double?blind$ or double blind$).mp.
9.   (treble?blind$ or treble blind$).mp.
10. (triple?blind$ or triple blind$).mp.
11. or/1–10
12. (animal not (human and animal)).sh.
13. Animal$/ not (animal$/ and human$/)
14. meta-analysis/ or meta-analysis.pt. or systematic review/
15. 11 not (12 or 13 or 14)

4. Antidepressant drug search filter

(Antidepressant$ or tricyclic$ or imipramine or amitriptyline or clomipramine or nortriptyline or *desipramine* or fluoxetine or sertraline or paroxetine or citalopram or fluvoxamine or bupropion or trazodone or nefazodone or phenelzine or isocarboxazid$ or moclobemide or *brofaromine* or *tranylcypromine* or mianserin or mirtazapine)

(Drugs in italics are not currently used in the UK)

5. Cognitive behavioural therapy search filter

((COGNITIV$ and BEHAVIO$ and THERAP$) or (COGNITI$ and (TECHNIQUE$ or THERAP$ or RESTRUCTUR$ or CHALLENG$)) or (ATTRIBUTION$ or (SELF and (INSTRUCT$ or MANAGEMENT$ or ATTRIBUTION$)) or (RET or (RATIONAL and EMOTIV$))))

Appendix 9:
Clinical study data extraction form

Information about each study was entered into an Access database using specially designed forms (see below for an example).

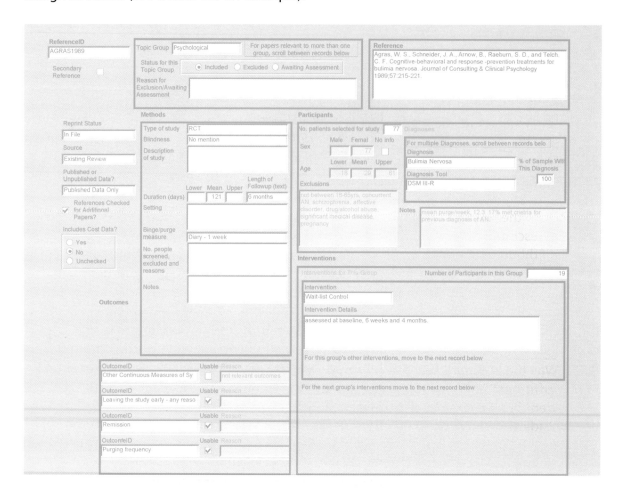

Appendix 10: Clinical study quality checklists

Table 1. Quality checklist for a systematic review
(notes for reviewer are presented in italics)

Checklist completed by:	Report reference ID:
SECTION 1: VALIDITY	
Evaluation criteria	**Comments**
1.1 Does the review address an appropriate and clearly focused question?	*Unless a clear and well-defined question is specified, it will be difficult to assess how well the study has met its objectives or how relevant it is to the question you are trying to answer on the basis of its conclusions.*
1.2 Does the review include a description of the methodology used?	*A systematic review should include a detailed description of the methods used to identify and evaluate individual studies. If this description is not present, it is not possible to make a thorough evaluation of the quality of the review, and it should be rejected as a source of Level 1 evidence. (Though it may be useable as Level 4 evidence, if no better evidence can be found.)*
1.3 Was the literature search sufficiently rigorous to identify all relevant studies?	*Consider whether the review used an electronic search of at least one bibliographic database (searching for studies dating at least 10 years before publication of the review). Any indication that hand searching of key journals, or follow up of reference lists of included studies were carried out in addition to electronic database searches can normally be taken as evidence of a well conducted review.*
1.4 Was study quality assessed and taken into account?	*A well conducted systematic review should have used clear criteria to assess whether individual studies had been well conducted before deciding whether to include or exclude them. At a minimum, the authors should have checked that there was adequate concealment of allocation, that the rate of drop out was minimised, and that the results were analysed on an 'intention to treat' basis1. If there is no indication of such an assessment, the review should be rejected as a source of Level 1 evidence. If details of the assessment are poor, or the methods considered to be inadequate, the quality of the review should be downgraded.*

SECTION 2: OVERALL ASSESSMENT			
		Comments	Code
2.1	Low risk of bias	All or most criteria met.	A
	Moderate risk of bias	Most criteria partly met	B
	High risk of bias	Few or no critria met.	C

Table 2. Quality checklist for a randomised controlled trial
(notes for reviewer are presented in italics)

Checklist completed by:		Report reference ID:	
SECTION 1: INTERNAL VALIDITY			
Evaluation criteria		**Comments**	
1.1	Was the assignment of subjects to treatment groups randomised?	*If there is no indication of randomisation, the study should be rejected. If the description of randomisation is poor, or the process used is not truly random (e.g. allocation by date, alternating between one group and another) or can otherwise be seen as flawed, the study should be given a lower quality rating.*	
1.2	Was an adequate concealment method used?	*Centralised allocation, computerised allocation systems, or the use of coded identical containers would all be regarded as adequate methods of concealment, and may be taken as indicators of a well conducted study. If the method of concealment used in regarded as poor, or relatively easy to subvert, the study must be given a lower quality rating, and can be rejected if the concealment method is seen as inadequate.*	
SECTION 2: OVERALL ASSESSMENT			
		Comments	Code
2.1	Low risk of bias	All or most criteria met.	A
	Moderate risk of bias	Most criteria partly met	B
	High risk of bias	Few or no critria met.	C

Appendix 11: Predicting the outcome of treatment and recovery review

Anorexia Nervosa

Pre-treatment predictors of outcome

Predictor	Studies finding a positive result	Studies finding a negative result
Low BMI at presentation or admission or minimum BMI*	Kachele *et al.*, 2001 Lowe *et al.*, 2001 (low during course) Tanaka *et al.*, 2001 Zipfel *et al.*, 2000 Howard *et al.*, 1999 (day tx) Nielsen *et al.*, 1998 (on SMR) Herzog *et al.*, 1997b Hebebrand *et al.*, 1996, 1997 (<13) Casper & Jabine, 1996 Gowers *et al.*, 1994 *Steinhausen & Siedel, 1993* *(trend)* Santonastaso *et al.*, 1987 Burns & Crisp, 1984 Steinhausen & Glanville, 1983 Goldberg *et al.*, 1980 Hsu *et al.*, 1979	Ben-Tovim *et al.*, 2001 Herzog *et al.*, 1997a Strober *et al.*, 1997 Bryant Waugh *et al.*, 1988 Remschmidt *et al.*, 1988 Morgan *et al.*, 1983 Lee *et al.*, 2003
Medical emergency pre-admission/ lab findings/ somatic complaints	Saccomani *et al.*, 1998 Herzog *et al.*, 1997a & b Deter & Herxog 1994 Goldberg *et al.*, 1980 *Suematsu et al., 1985 (trend)*	
Bulimic sub-type*	Bulik *et al.*, 2000 (BN EDI scale) Fichter & Quadflieg, 1999 (B) Ostuzzi *et al.*, 1999 (ANB) Saccomani *et al.*, 1998 (B) Herzog *et al.*, 1997a (P) Gowers *et al.*, 1994 (V) Deter & Herzog, 1994 (P) *Santonastaso et al., 1991 (trend)* Santonastaso *et al.*, 1987 (VorL) Nussbaum *et al.*, 1985 (V) Hsu *et al.*, 1979 (ANB or V) Stonehill & Crisp, 1977 (V) Willi & Hagemann, 1976 (L)	Eddy *et al.*, 2002 Strober *et al.*, 1997 Steinhausen & Seidel, 1993 Toner *et al.*, 1986 Morgan *et al.*, 1983 Casper & Jabine, 1996 *Continued*

Predictor	Studies finding a positive result	Studies finding a negative result
Bulimic subtype* *Continued*	Theander, 1970 (V) Ward et al., 2003 Suematsu et al., 1985	
Premorbid associality/ personality difficulties/ interpersonal problems or distrust	Bizeul et al., 2001 (distrust) Herzog et al., 1997a (in comb with purging) Strober et al., 1997 (poor social relating) Morgan et al., 1983 Hsu et al., 1979 Morgan & Russell, 1975 Suematsu et al., 1985	
Previous treatment*	Bryant Waugh et al., 1988 Burns & Crisp, 1984 Steinhausen & Glanville, 1983 Eckert, 1979 Halmi et al., 1979 Morgan & Russell 1975 Santanastaso et al., 1997	Strober et al., 1997
Family disturbance	Strober et al., 1997 (hostility towards family lengthens time to recovery) Ratnasuriya et al., 1991 Burns & Crisp, 1984 Morgan et al., 1983 Hsu et al., 1979 Morgan & Russell, 1975 Suematsu et al., 1985 Lee et al., 2003	Theander, 1970
Body image disturbance/ dissatisfaction, low desired weight during treatment or at follow-up	Ben-Tovim et al., 2001 Strober et al., 1999 (atypical do better) Goldberg et al., 1980 Crisp et al., 1979 (size estimation) Suematsu et al., 1985	
Older age at presentation (those above 20 have worse outcome)	Lee et al., 2003 Kachele, 2001 (older poorer outcome) (with treatment length) Nielsen et al., 1998 (20–29 highest risk of death) Deter & Herzog, 1994 Deter et al., 1989 (older age poorer) Hsu et al., 1979	Ben-Tovim et al., 2001 Gowers et al., 1994

Post-treatment predictors of outcome

Predictor	Studies finding a positive result	Studies finding a negative result
Inadequate weight gain*	Lowe *et al.*, 2001 (low BMI during course of disorder) Zipfel *et al.*, 2000 Fichter & Quadflieg, 1999 Russell & Gross, 2000 (<BMI 19) Howard *et al.*, 1999 (<BMI 19)	Richards *et al.*, 2003
General psychopathology	Ivarsson *et al.*, 2000 (mood disorder) Eckert *et al.*, 1995 (affective or anxiety disorder) Rastam *et al.*, 1995 (PD)/2003 (GAF) Herpetz-Dahlmann *et al.*, 2001 (psychiatric disorders inc PD) Lowe *et al.*, 2001 (mood & substance disorder) Saccomani *et al.*, 1998 (PD or mood disorder) Schork *et al.*, 1994	Bulik *et al.*, 2000 (depression) Saccomani *et al.*, 1998 (anxiety disorder)
Low desired weight/drive for thinness/dieting	Richards *et al.*, 2003 Kachele *et al.*, 2001 Bulik *et al.*, 2000 Eckert *et al.*, 1995	
Poor social adjustment	Herpetz-Dahlmann *et al.*, 2001 (social contacts & sexuality) Lowe *et al.*, 2001 (living alone, no children) Stonehill & Crisp, 1977 Willi & Hagemann, 1976 (those who marry do better)	Eckert *et al.*, 1995 (less sensitive measure)

Findings may be confounded by severity, duration of disorder or chronicity.

Bulimia Nervosa
Pre-treatment predictors of outcome

Predictor	Studies finding a positive result	Studies finding a negative result
BPD features	Steiger et al., 1994b (those with stably high BSI scores had high DFT) Garner et al., 1990 (BSI trend) Johnson et al., 1990	
Concurrent substance misuse	Flament et al., 1996 Fichter et al., 1994a Garner et al., 1990 (higher MCMI scores though non-clinical)	
Motivation for/ stage of change	Richards et al., 2003 Wolk & Devlin, 2001 (IPT only) Treasure et al., 1999	
History of obesity	Fairburn et al., 2003 Bulik et al., 1998 Fairburn et al., 1995 Maddocks & Kaplan, 1991	Garner, 1990
Higher levels of binge eating and/or purging	Thiels et al., 2000 (B) (in abbreviated tx) Mussell et al., 2000(V) Bulik et al., (1999) (B) Wilson et al., 1999 (B&V) Bulik et al., 1998 (EDI BN) Esplen et al., 1998 (P) Turnbull et al., 1997 (B) (in abbreviated tx) Olmsted et al., 1994 Fahy & Russell, 1993 Keller et al., 1992 Olmsted et al., 1991 (V) (in abbreviated tx) Garner et al., 1990 (B) Mitchell et al., 1989 (B&V)	Agras et al., 2000 Keel et al., 1999 Esplen et al., 1998 (B) Cooper et al., 1996 (P) Fairburn et al., 1995 (by 3–11 years follow-up) Fairburn, Peveler et al., 1993 Rossiter et al., 1993 (P) Maddocks & Kaplan, 1991 Walsh et al., 1991 (B&L) Garner et al., 1990 (V) Mitchell et al., 1986

Post-treatment predictors of outcome

Predictor	Studies finding a positive result	Studies finding a negative result
Social maladjustment/ lack of a satisfactory stable relationship/ interpersonal distrust	Fairburn *et al.*, 2003 Agras *et al.*, 2000 Reas *et al.*, 2000 (marital status) Reiss & Johnson-Sabine, 1995 Collings & King, 1994 Olmsted *et al.*, 1994 (interpersonal distrust) Johnson-Sabine *et al.*, 1992 Maddocks *et al.*, 1992 (ID) Fallon *et al.*, 1991 Garner *et al.*, 1990 (composite)	
Post-treatment depressive features	Agras *et al.*, 2000 Bulik *et al.*, 1998 (univariate anal only) Collings & King 1994 Maddocks *et al.*, 1992 Fallon *et al.*, 1991 (major dep) Garner *et al.*, 1990 (dysthymia) (composite) Hsu & Sobkiewicz 1989 Wilson *et al.*, 1986 Swift *et al.*, 1985	
Higher ED cognitions/body dissatisfaction or body image disturbance/ drive for thinness	Fairburn *et al.*, 2003 (DR mediator) Keel *et al.*, 1999 (BSQ) Bulik *et al.*, 1998 (univariate anal only) Fairburn *et al.*, 1993 Maddocks *et al.*, 1992 Johnson-Sabine *et al.*, 1992 Garner *et al.*, 1990 (DFT) Mitchell *et al.*, 1989 (BD) Swift *et al.*, 1985	
Abstinence during/ by end of treatment binge eating/ binge eating frequency (good outcome)	Fairburn *et al.*, 2003 (pred comp behaviours) Richards *et al.*, 2003 Mussell *et al.*, 2000 Bulik *et al.*, 1998 Maddocks *et al.*, 1992 Swift *et al.*, 1985	*Continued*

Post-treatment predictors of outcome (continued)

Predictor	Studies finding a positive result	Studies finding a negative result
Lower social class/income	Reas *et al.*, 2000 (income) Reiss & Johnson-Sabine, 1995 Johnson-Sabine *et al.*, 1992 Collings & King, 1994	
Post-treatment purging frequency	Olmsted *et al.*, 1994 Garner *et al.*, 1990 Mitchell *et al.*, 1989 Swift *et al.*, 1985	
Comorbidity/ general psychiatric symptoms	Bulik *et al.*, 1998 Collings & King, 1994 Rossiter *et al.*, 1993 (trend cluster B features) Fallon *et al.*, 1991 (GAF)	Fairburn *et al.*, 2003

Appendix 12: Search strategies for the identification of health economic evidence

12.1

Databases searched: MEDLINE, PreMEDLINE, EMBASE (Excerpta Medica Database, CINAHL (Cumultive Index to Nursing and Allied Health Literature), PsycINFO, Cochrane Database of Systematic Reviews (CDSR), Cochrane Controlled Trials Register (CCTR), Database of Abstracts of Reviews of Effectiveness (DARE).

Interface used: OVID.

Date of search: August 2002.

Combined search strategy used:

1. (burden adj2 illness).mp.
2. (burden adj2 disease).mp.
3. (cost$ adj2 evaluat$).mp.
4. (cost$ adj2 benefit$).mp.
5. (cost$ adj2 utilit$).mp.
6. (cost$ adj2 minimi$).mp.
7. (cost$ adj2 illness).mp.
8. (cost$ adj2 disease).mp.
9. (cost$ adj2 analys$).mp.
10. (cost$ adj2 assess$).mp.
11. (cost$ adj2 study).mp.
12. (cost$ adj2 studies).mp.
13. (cost$ adj2 allocation).mp.
14. (cost$ adj2 outcome$).mp.
15. (cost$ adj2 consequence$).mp.
16. (cost$ adj2 effect$).mp.
17. (cost$ adj2 treatment$).mp.
18. (economic adj2 evaluat$).mp.
19. (economic adj2 analysis$).mp.
20. (economic adj2 study).mp.
21. (economic adj2 studies).mp.
22. (economic adj2 assess$).mp.
23. (economic adj2 consequence$).mp.
24. (economic adj2 outcome$).mp.
25. (resource$ adj2 allocation$).mp.
26. (resource$ adj2 utili$).mp.
27. expenditure$.mp.
28. exp economics/
29. exp 'costs and cost analysis'/
30. exp 'health economics'/
31. or/1–30
AND

1. eating disorder/ or eating disorders/
2. (eating adj2 disorder$).mp. [mp=ti, sh, ab, it, tn, ot, dm, mf, dv, rw, hw, ty, id]
3. appetite disorder/
4. anorexia nervosa/
5. (anorexia adj1 nervosa).mp. [mp=ti, sh, ab, it, tn, ot, dm, mf, dv, rw, hw, ty, id]
6. bulimia/ or bulimi$.mp.
7. binge eating disorder/
8. (bing$ or overeat$ or (compulsive adj2 (eat$ or vomit$)) or (food$ adj2 bing$) or (self?induc$ adj2 vomit$) or (restrict$ adj2 eat$)).mp.
9. or/1-8.

12.2

Databases searched: HTA (Health Technology Assessment), NHS EED (NHS Economic Evaluation Database), OHE HEED (Office of Health Economics Health Economic Evaluations Database).

Interfaces used: NHS Centre for Reviews and Dissemination website and OHE HEED CD-ROM.

Date of search: August 2002.

Abbreviated search strategy used:

EATING-DISORDERS*:ME or (eating NEXT disorder*) OR (appetite NEXT disorder*) OR (anorexia NEXT nervosa) OR (bulimia) OR (bing* OR overeat*) OR (compulsive NEXT eat*) OR (vomit*).

Appendix 13: Quality checklists for economic studies

13.1 Full economic evaluations

Author: **Date:**

Title:

	Yes	No	NA
Study design			
1. The research question is stated	☐	☐	
2. The viewpoint(s) of the analysis are clearly stated		☐	☐
3. The alternatives being compared are relevant	☐	☐	
4. The rationale for choosing the alternative programmes or interventions compared is stated	☐	☐	
5. The alternatives being compared are clearly described	☐	☐	
6. The form of economic evaluation used is justified in relation to the question addressed	☐	☐	
Data collection			
1. The source of effectiveness data used is stated	☐	☐	
2. Details of the design and results of effectiveness study are given	☐	☐	☐
3. The primary outcome measure(s) for the economic evaluation are clearly stated	☐	☐	
4. Methods to value health states and other benefits are stated	☐	☐	
5. Details of the subjects from whom valuations were obtained are given	☐	☐	
6. Indirect costs (if included) are reported separately	☐	☐	☐
7. Quantities of resources are reported separately from their unit costs	☐	☐	☐
8. Methods for the estimation of quantities and unit costs are described	☐	☐	
9. Currency and price data are recorded	☐	☐	
10. Details of currency of price adjustments for inflation or currency conversion are given	☐	☐	☐
11. Details of any model used are given	☐	☐	☐
12. The choice of model used and the key parameters on which it is based are justified	☐	☐	☐
Analysis and interpretation of results			
1. Time horizon of costs and benefits is stated	☐	☐	
2. The discount rate(s) is stated	☐	☐	☐
3. The choice of rate(s) is justified	☐	☐	☐
4. An explanation is given if costs or benefits are not discounted	☐	☐	☐

	Yes	No	NA
5. Details of statistical tests and confidence intervals are given for stochastic data	☐	☐	☐
6. The approach to sensitivity analysis is given	☐	☐	
7. The choice of variables for sensitivity analysis is given	☐	☐	
8. The ranges over which the variables are varied are stated	☐	☐	
9. Relevant alternatives are compared	☐	☐	
10. Incremental analysis is reported	☐	☐	☐
11. Major outcomes are presented in a disaggregated as well as aggregated form	☐	☐	
12. The answer to the study question is given	☐	☐	
13. Conclusions follow from the data reported	☐	☐	
14. Conclusions are accompanied by the appropriate caveats	☐	☐	

13.2 Partial economic evaluations

Author: **Date:**

Title:

	Yes	No	NA
Study design			
1. The research question is stated	☐	☐	
2. The viewpoint(s) of the analysis are clearly stated and justified	☐	☐	
Data collection			
1. Details of the subjects from whom valuations were obtained are given	☐	☐	
2. Indirect costs (if included) are reported separately	☐	☐	☐
3. Quantities of resources are reported separately from their unit costs	☐	☐	
4. Methods for the estimation of quantities and unit costs are described	☐	☐	
5. Currency and price data are recorded	☐	☐	
6. Details of currency of price adjustments for inflation or currency conversion are given	☐	☐	☐
7. Details of any model used are given	☐	☐	☐
8. The choice of model used and the key parameters on which it is based are justified	☐	☐	☐
Analysis and interpretation of results			
1. Time horizon of costs is stated		☐	☐
2. The discount rate(s) is stated	☐	☐	☐
3. Details of statistical tests and confidence intervals are given for stochastic data	☐	☐	☐
4. The choice of variables for sensitivity analysis is given	☐	☐	
5. Appropriate sensitivity analysis is performed	☐	☐	
6. The answer to the study question is given	☐	☐	
7. Conclusions follow from the data reported	☐	☐	
8. Conclusions are accompanied by the appropriate caveats	☐	☐	

Appendix 14:
Data extraction form for economic studies

Reviewer: **Date of Review:**

Authors:

Publication Date:

Title:

Country:

Language:

Economic study design:

☐ CEA   ☐ CCA
☐ CBA   ☐ CA
☐ CUA
☐ CMA

Modelling:

☐ No   ☐ Yes

Source of data for effect size measure(s):

                                        ☐ Meta-analysis
☐ RCT   ☐ RCT
☐ Quasi experimental study   ☐ Quasi experimental study
☐ Cohort study   ☐ Cohort study
☐ Mirror image (before-after) study   ☐ Mirror image (before-after) study
                                        ☐ Expert opinion

Comments:..

Primary outcome measure(s) (please list):

....

Interventions compared (please describe):

Treatment:...

Comparator:...

Setting (please describe):

....

....

Patient population characteristics (please describe):

....

....

Perspective of analysis:

☐ Societal   ☐ Other: ....
☐ Patient and family
☐ Health care system
☐ Health care provider
☐ Third party payer

Time frame of analysis:..

Cost data:

☐ Primary   ☐ Secondary

If secondary please specify:...

Costs included:

Direct medical	*Direct non-medical*	*Lost productivity*
☐ direct treatment	☐ social care	☐ income forgone due to illness
☐ inpatient	☐ social benefits	☐ income forgone due to death
☐ outpatient	☐ travel costs	☐ income forgone by caregiver
☐ day care	☐ caregiver out-of-pocket	
☐ community health care	☐ criminal justice	
☐ medication	☐ training of staff	
or		
☐ staff		
☐ medication		
☐ consumables		
☐ overhead		
☐ capital equipment		
☐ real estate	Others:	

Currency: .... **Year of costing:**..

Was discounting used? ☐ Yes, for benefits and costs ☐ Yes, but only for costs ☐ No

Discount rate used for costs: ....

Discount rate used for benefits: ....

Result(s): ....

....

....

Comments, limitations of the study:

....

....

....

Quality checklist score (Yes/NA/All): ..../........../..........

Appendix 15:
Model structure

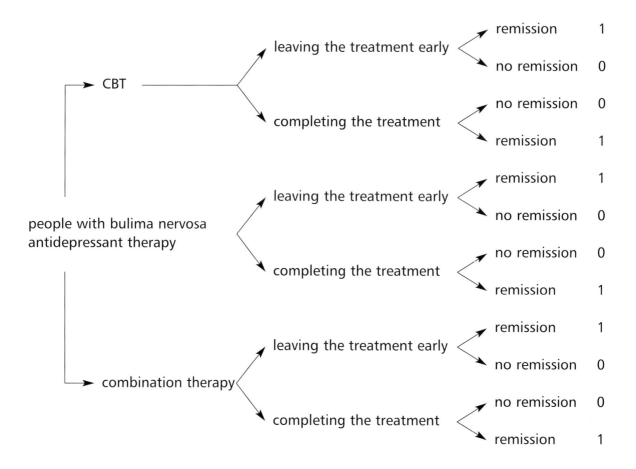

Appendix 16: Model parameters

Parameter	Base case	Minimum value	Maximum value	Source
Staff unit costs				
Clinical psychologist per hour of client contact	£65.00	–	–	Netten et al. (2002)
General practitioner per hour of patient contact	£91.00	–	–	Netten et al. (2002)
Specialist per hour of patient contact	£27.00	– –	£207.00	Netten et al. (2002)
Length of CBT sessions	50 minutes	40 minutes	60 minutes	Fairburn (1991), personal communication
Length of GP visits	9.36 minutes	4 minutes	15 minutes	Netten et al. (2002), personal communication
Length of specialist outpatient visits	15 minutes	10 minutes	20 minutes	Agras (1992), personal communication
Number of CBT sessions	20	–	–	Treatment manual, personal communication
Average drop out time CBT	11.5 weeks	–	–	Agras (1992, 1994)
Number of AD visits	4	3	8	Agras (1992), personal communication
Length of AD	16 weeks	–	24 weeks	Personal communication, clinical evidence review
Average drop out time AD	7.42 weeks	–	9.5 weeks	Agras (1992, 1994)

Parameter	Base case	Minimum value	Maximum value	Source
Drug unit costs				
Fluoxetine (20mg, 30cap/pack)	£7.61	–	–	BNF 45
Prozac (60mg, 30cap/pack)	£47.61	–	–	BNF 45
Total treatment costs				
Cost per patient leaving CBT early	£650.00	Dependent on the component parameter values	Dependent on the component parameter values	Calculated
Cost per patient completing CBT	£1083.3	Dependent on the component parameter values	Dependent on the component parameter values	Calculated
Cost per patient leaving AD early	£74.05	Dependent on the component parameter values	Dependent on the component parameter values	Calculated
Cost per patient completing AD	£148.10	Dependent on the component parameter values	Dependent on the component parameter values	Calculated

Parameter	Base case	Minimum value	Maximum value	Source
Clinical efficacy				
Relative risk of no remission AD vs. CBT	1.28	1.09	1.50	Clinical evidence review (Paragraph 7.4)
Absolute risk of no remission AD	0.807	0.667	0.913	Clinical evidence review (Paragraph 7.4)
Absolute risk of no remission CBT	0.630	Dependent on the component parameter values	Dependent on the component parameter values	Calculated
Probability of no remission when leaving the treatment early	1.00	–	–	Clinical evidence review (intention-to-treat analysis)
Drop out				
Relative risk of leaving the treatment early AD vs. CBT	1.49	–	–	Clinical evidence review (Paragraph 7.4)
Absolute risk of leaving the treatment early AD	0.40	–	–	Clinical evidence review (Paragraph 7.4)
Absolute risk of leaving the treatment early CBT	0.268	–	–	Calculated

AD: antidepressant therapy
CBT: cognitive behaviour therapy

Appendix 17: Diagnostic criteria for eating disorders

Eating disorder	DSM-IV-TR	ICD-10
Anorexia nervosa	*307.1*	*F50.0*
Criteria	a. Refusal to maintain body weight at or above a minimally normal weight for age and height (e.g. weight loss leading to maintenance of body weight less than 85% of that expected; or failure to make expected weight gain during period of growth, leading to body weight less than 85% of that expected).	a. Body weight is maintained at least 15% below that expected (either lost or never achieved), or Quetelet's body-mass index is 17.5 or less. Prepubertal patients may show failure to make the expected weight gain during the period of growth.
	b. Intense fear of gaining weight or becoming fat, even though underweight.	b. The weight loss is self-induced by avoidance of 'fattening foods'. One or more of the following may also be present: self-induced vomiting; self-induced purging; excessive exercise; use of appetite suppressants and/or diuretics.
	c. Disturbance in the way in which one's body weight or shape is experienced, undue influence of body weight or shape on self-evaluation, or denial of the seriousness of the current low body weight.	c. There is body-image distortion in the form of a specific psychopathology whereby a dread of fatness persists as an intrusive, overvalued idea and the patient imposes a low weight threshold on himself or herself.
	d. In postmenarcheal females, amenorrhoea, i.e. the absence of at least three consecutive menstrual cycles. (A woman is considered to have amenorrhoea if her periods occur only following hormone, e.g. oestrogen, administration.)	d. A widespread endocrine disorder involving the hypothalamic – pituitary – gonadal axis is manifest in women as amenorrhoea and in men as a loss of sexual interest and potency. (An apparent exception is the persistence of vaginal bleeds in anorexic women who are receiving replacement hormonal therapy, most commonly taken as a contraceptive pill.) There may also be elevated levels of growth hormone, raised levels of cortisol, changes in the peripheral metabolism of the thyroid hormone, and abnormalities of insulin secretion.
		e. If onset is prepubertal, the sequence of pubertal events is delayed or even arrested (growth ceases; in girls the breasts do not develop and there is a primary amenorrhoea; in boys the genitals remain juvenile). With recovery, puberty is often completed normally, but the menarche is late.
Subtypes	**Restricting type:** During current episode of Anorexia Nervosa, the person has not regularly engaged in binge-eating or purging behaviour. **Binge-eating/purging type:** During the current episode of Anorexia Nervosa the person has regularly engaged in binge-eating or purging behaviour.	

Eating disorder	DSM-IV-TR	ICD-10
Bulimia nervosa	*307.51*	*F50.2*
Criteria	a. Recurrent episodes of binge eating. An episode of binge eating is characterised by both of the following: (1) eating, in a discrete period of time (e.g. within any 2-hour period), an amount of food that is definitely larger than most people would eat during a similar period of time and under similar circumstances; (2) a sense of lack of control over eating during the episode (e.g. a feeling that one cannot stop eating or control what or how much one is eating).	a. There is a persistent preoccupation with eating, and an irresistible craving for food; the patient succumbs to episodes of overeating in which large amounts of food are consumed in short periods of time.
	b. Recurrent inappropriate compensatory behaviour in order to prevent weight gain, such as self-induced vomiting; misuse of laxatives, diuretics, enemas, or other medications; fasting or excessive exercise.	b. The patient attempts to counteract the 'fattening' effects of food by one or more of the following: self-induced vomiting; purgative abuse, alternating periods of starvation; use of drugs such as appetite suppressants, thyroid preparations or diuretics. When bulimia occurs in diabetic patients they may choose to neglect their insulin treatment.
	c. The binge eating and inappropriate compensatory behaviours both occur, on average, at least twice a week for 3 months.	c. The psychopathology consists of a morbid dread of fatness and the patient sets herself or himself a sharply defined weight threshold, well below the premorbid weight that constitutes the optimum or healthy weight in the opinion of the physician. There is often, but not always, a history of an earlier episode of anorexia nervosa, the interval between the two disorders ranging from a few months to several years. This earlier episode may have been fully expressed, or may have assumed a minor cryptic form with a moderate loss of weight and/or a transient phase of amenorrhoea.
	d. Self-evaluation is unduly influenced by body shape and weight.	
	e. The disturbance does not occur exclusively during episodes of Anorexia Nervosa.	
Subtypes	**Purging type:** During the current episode, the person has regularly engaged in self-induced vomiting or the misuse of laxatives. **Non-purging type:** During the current episode of Bulimia Nervosa, the person has used other inappropriate compensatory behaviors, such as fasting or excessive exercise, but has not regularly engaged in self-induced vomiting or the misuse of laxatives, diuretics, or enemas.	

Appendix 18: Studies included/ excluded in the comparisons covered by the Clinical Evidence Table

Please refer to the data CD attached to the inside back cover.

(The CD should start automatically when inserted; if it fails to do so, double-click on eating_disorders.html, and then click on 'Clinical evidence tables' when the page opens. Macintosh users: double-click on eating_disordersMAC.html.)

12 References

Agras, W.S., Dorian, B., Kirkley, B.G., Arnow, B. & Backman, J. (1987). Imipramine in the treatment of bulimia: A double-blind controlled study. *International Journal of Eating Disorders, 6,* 29–38.

Agras, W.S., Schneider, J.A., Arnow, B., Raeburn, S.D. & Telch, C.F. (1989). Cognitive-behavioral and response-prevention treatments for bulimia nervosa. *Journal of Consulting & Clinical Psychology, 57,* 215–221.

Agras, W.S., Rossiter, E.M., Arnow, B., Schneider, J.A., Telch, C.F., Raeburn, S.D., Bruce, B., Perl, M. & Koran, L.M. (1992). Pharmacologic and cognitive-behavioral treatment for bulimia nervosa: A controlled comparison. *American Journal of Psychiatry, 149,* 82–87.

Agras, W.S., Rossiter, E.M., Arnow, B., Telch, C.F., Raeburn, S.D., Bruce, B. & Koran, L.M. (1994). One-year follow-up of psychosocial and pharmacologic treatment for bulimia nervosa. *Journal of Clinical Psychiatry, 55,* 179–183.

Agras, W.S., Telch, C.F., Arnow, B., Eldredge, K.L., Detzer, M.J., Henderson, J. & Marnell, M. (1995). Does interpersonal therapy help patients with binge eating disorder who fail to respond to cognitive-behavioral therapy? *Journal of Consulting & Clinical Psychology, 63,* 356–360.

Agras, W.S., Walsh, B.T., Fairburn, C.G., Wilson, C.T. & Kramer, H.C. (2000a). A multi-centre comparison of Cognitive-Behavioral Therapy and Interpersonal Psychotherapy for bulimia nervosa. *Archives of General Psychiatry, 54,* 459–465.

Agras, W.S., Crow, S.J., Halmi, K.A., Mitchell, J.E., Wilson, G.T. & Kraemer, H.C. (2000). Outcome predictors for the cognitive behavior treatment of bulimia nervosa: Data from a multisite study. *American Journal of Psychiatry, 157*(8), 1302–1308.

Agras, W.S. (2001). The consequences and costs of the eating disorders. *24*(2), 371–379.

APA (1994). American Psychiatric Association Work Group on Eating Disorders. Practice guideline for the treatment of patients with eating disorders (revision 2000). *American Journal of Psychiatry, 157*, 1–39.

Anstine, D. & Grinenko, D. (2000). Rapid screening for disordered eating in college-aged females in the primary care setting. *Journal of Adolescent Health, 26*(5), 338–342.

Arii, I., Yamashita, T., Kinoshita, M., Shimizu, H., Nakamura, M. & Nakajima, T. (1996). Treatment for inpatients with anorexia nervosa: Comparison of liquid formula with regular meals for improvement from emaciation. *Psychiatry & Clinical Neurosciences, 50,* 55–59.

Arnold, L.M., McElroy, S., Hudson, J.I., Welge, J.A., Bennett, A.J. & Keck, P.E. (2002). A placebo-controlled, randomised trial of fluoxetine in the treatment of binge-eating disorder. *Journal of Clinical Psychiatry, 63,* 1028–1033.

Attia, E., Haiman, C., Walsh, B.T. & Flater, S.R. (1998). Does Fluoxetine augment the inpatient treatment of anorexia nervosa? *American Journal of Psychiatry, 155,* 548–551.

Babyak, M. *et al.* (2000). Exercise treatment for major depression: Maintenance of therapeutic benefit at 10 months. *Psychosomatic Medicine, 62,* 633–638.

Bachar, E., Latzer, Y., Kreitler, S. & Berry, E.M. (1999). Empirical comparison of two psychological therapies. *Journal of Psychotherapy Practise and Research, 8,* 115–128.

Bachrach, L.K., Guido, D., Katzman, D., Litt, I.F. & Marcus, R. (1990). Decreased bone density in adolescent girls with anorexia nervosa. *Pediatrics, 86,* 440–447.

Bailer, U., de Zwaan, M., Leisch, F., Strnad, A., Lennkh-Wolfsberg, C., El-Giamal, N., Hornik, K. & Kasper, S. (2002). Guided self-help versus cognitive behavioural group therapy in the treatment of bulimia nervosa. *British Journal of Psychiatry* (in press).

Beglin, S.J. & Fairburn, C.G. (1992). What is meant by the term 'binge'? *American Journal of Psychiatry, 149*(1), 123–124.

Ben-Tovim, D.I., Walker, K., Gilchrist, .P, Freeman, R., Kalucy, R. & Esterman, A. (2001). Outcome in patients with eating disorders: A five-year study. *The Lancet, 357*(9264), 1254–1257.

Bergh, C., Brodin, U., Lindberg, G. & Sodersten, P. (2002). Randomised controlled trial of a treatment for anorexia and bulimia nervosa. *Proceedings of the National Academy of Sciences of the United States of America, 99,* 9486–9491.

Berlin, J.A. (1997). Does blinding of readers affect the results of meta-analyses? University of Pennsylvania Meta-analysis Blinding Study Group. *Lancet, 350 (9072),* 185–186.

Beumont, P.J., Abraham, S.F, Argall, W.J., George, C.W. & Glaun, D.E. (1978). The onset of anorexia nervosa. *Australian & New Zealand Journal of Psychiatry, 12,* 145–149.

Beumont, P.J., Russell, J.D., Touyz, S.W., Buckley, C., Lowinger, K., Talbot, P. & Johnson, G.F.S. (1997). Intensive nutritional counselling in bulimia nervosa: A role for supplementation with fluoxetine? *Australian & New Zealand Journal of Psychiatry, 31,* 514–524.

Bianchi, A.S., Toy, E.C. & Baker, I.B. (1998). The evaluation of involuntary weight loss. *Primary Care Update for Ob/Gyns, 5*(6), 263–267.

Biederman, J., Herzog, D., Rivinus, T.M., Harper, G.P., Ferber, R.A., Rosenbaum, J.F., Harmatz, J.S., Tondorf, R., Orsulak, P.J. & Schildkraut, J.J. (1985). Amitriptyline in the treatment of anorexia nervosa: A double-blind, placebo-controlled study. *Journal of Clinical Psychopharmacology, 5,* 10–16.

Biller, B.M., Saxe, V., Herzog, D.B., Rosenthal, D.I., Holzman, S. & Klibanski, A. (1989). Mechanisms of osteoporosis in adult and adolescent women with anorexia nervosa. *Journal of Clinical Endocrinology and Metabolism, 68,* 548–554.

Birchall, H., Palmer, R.L., Waine, J., Gadsby, K. & Gatward, N. (2002). Intensive day programme treatment for severe anorexia nervosa – the Leicester experience. *Psychiatric Bulletin, 26,* 334–336.

Birmingham, C.L., Goldner, E.M. & Bakan, R. (1994). Controlled trial of zinc supplementation in anorexia nervosa. *International Journal of Eating Disorders, 15,* 251–255.

Bizeul, C., Sadowsky, N. & Rigaud, D. (2001). The prognostic value of initial EDI scores in anorexia nervosa patients: A prospective follow-up study of 5–10 years. Eating Disorder Inventory. *European Psychiatry, 16*(4), 232–238.

Braun, D.L., Sunday, S.R. & Halmi, K.A. (1994). Psychiatric comorbidity in patients with eating disorders. *Psychological Medicine, 24,* 859–867.

Briggs, A.H., Goeree, R., Blackhouse, G. & O'Brien, B.J. (2002). Probabilistic analysis of cost-effectiveness models: Choosing between treatment strategies for gastroesophageal reflux disease. *Medical Decision Making,* July–August, 290–308.

Briggs, A.H. & Gray, A.M. (1999). Handling uncertainty when performing economic evaluation of health care interventions. *NICE Health Technology Assessment, 3*(2).

Brinch, M., Isager, T. & Tolstrup, K. (1988). Anorexia nervosa and motherhood: Reproduction pattern and mothering behaviour of 50 women. *Acta Psychiatrica Scandinavica, 77,* 611–617.

Brinch, M., Isager, T. & Tolstrup, K. (1988). Patients' evaluation of their former treatment for anorexia nervosa (AN). Nordisk psykiatrisk tidsskrift. *Nordic Journal of Psychiatry, 42,* 445–448.

British Medical Association and the Royal Pharmaceutical Society of Great Britain (2003). *British National Formulary (BNF), 45.*

Brown, A. (1997). Eating disorders – the developing mixed economy. *Mental Health Research Review, 4,* 32–35.

Bryant-Waugh, R., Knibbs, J., Fosson, A., Kaminski, Z. & Lask, B. (1988). Long-term follow-up of patients with early onset anorexia nervosa. *Archives of Disease in Childhood, 63*(1), 5–9.

Bryant-Waugh, R. (2000). Overview of eating disorders. In B. Lask & R. Bryant-Waugh (Eds.), *Anorexia nervosa and related eating disorders in childhood and adolescence* (pp.27-40). Hove: Psychology Press.

Bryant-Waugh, R.J. & Lask, B.D. (1995). Eating disorders in children. *Journal of Child Psychoogy & Psychiatry, 36*(2), 191–202.

Bryant-Waugh, R.J., Lask, B.D., Shafran, R.L. & Fosson, A.R. (1992). Do doctors recognise eating disorders in children? *Archives of Disease in Childhood, 67*(1), 103–105.

Bulik, C.M., Sullivan, P.F., Carter, F.A., McIntosh, V.V. & Joyce, P.R. (1998). The role of exposure with response prevention in the cognitive-behavioural therapy for bulimia nervosa. *Psychol. Med., 28*(3), 611–623.

Bulik, C.M., Sullivan, P.F., Fear, J.L., Pickering, A., Dawn, A. & McCullin, M. (1999). Fertility and reproduction in women with anorexia nervosa: A controlled study. *Journal of Clinical Psychiatry, 60,* 130–135.

Bulik, C.M., Sullivan, P.F., Wade, T. & Kendler, K.S. (2000). Twin studies of eating disorders: A review. *International Journal of Eating Disorders, 27,* 1–20.

Bulik, C.M., Sullivan, P.F., Fear, J.L. & Pickering, A. (2002). Outcome of anorexia nervosa: Eating attitudes, personality and parental bonding. *International Journal of Eating Disorders, 28*(2), 139–147.

Burns, T. & Crisp, A.H. (1984). Outcome of anorexia nervosa in males. *British Journal of Psychiatry, 145,* 319–325.

Buston, K. (2002). Adolescents with mental health problems: What do they say about health services? *Journal of Adolescence, 25,* 231–242.

Carney, C.P. & Andersen, A.E. (1996). Eating disorders. Guide to medical evaluation and complications. *Psychiatric Clinics of North America, 19*(4), 657–679.

Carruba, M.O., Cuzzolaro, M., Riva, L., Bosello, O., Liberti, S., Castra, R., Dalle, Grave R., Santonastaso, P., Garosi, V. & Nisoli, E. (2001). Efficacy and tolerability of moclobemide in bulimia nervosa: A placebo-controlled trial. *International Clinical Psychopharmacology, 16,* 27–32.

Carter, J. & Moss (1984). Screening for anorexia and bulimia nervosa in a college population: Problems and limitations. *Addictive Behaviour, 9*(4), 417–419.

Carter, J. & Fairburn, C.C. (1998). Cognitive behavioral self-help for binge eating disorder: A controlled effectiveness study. *Journal of Consulting & Clinical Psychology, 66,* 616–623.

Carter, J., Olmsted, M., Kaplan, A.S., McCabe, R.E., Mills, J.S. & Aime, A. (2003). Self-help for bulimia nervosa: A randomised controlled trial. *American Journal of Psychiatry, 160,* 973–978.

Casper, R.C. (1996). Introduction to special issue. *Journal of Youth and Adolescence, 25, 413–418.*

Casper, Regina, C. & Jabine, L.N. (1996). An eight-year follow-up: Outcome from adolescent compared to adult onset anorexia nervosa. *Journal of Youth & Adolescence, 25*(4), 499–517.

Castro, J., Lazaro, L., Pons, .F, Halperin, I. & Toro, J. (2001). Adolescent anorexia nervosa: The catch-up effect in bone mineral density after recovery. *Journal of the American Academy of Child and Adolescent Psychiatry, 40,* 1215–1221.

Channon, S., de Silva, P., Hemsley, D. & Perkins, R. (1989). A controlled trial of cognitive-behavioural and behavioural treatment of anorexia nervosa. *Behavioural Research and Therapy, 27,* 529–535.

Chen, E., Touyz, S.W., Beumont, P.J., Fairburn, C.G., Griffiths, R., Butow, P., Russell, J., Schotte, D. E., Gertler, R. & Basten, C. (2003). Comparison of group and individual cognitive-behavioural therapy for patients with bulimia nervosa. *International Journal of Eating Disorders, 33,* 241–254.

Cochrane Collaboration. (2003). Review Manager (RevMan) [Computer program]. Version 4.2 for Windows. Oxford, England: The Cochrane Collaboration.

Cole *et al.* (1995). Body mass index reference curves for the UK, 1990. *Arch Dis Child, 73*(1), 25–29.

Cole, T.J., Bellizzi, M.C., Flegal, K.M., *et al.* (2000). Establishing a standard definition for child overweight and obesity worldwide: International survey. *British Medical Journal, 320,* 1240–1243.

Cooper, Z. & Fairburn, C. (1987). The Eating Disorder Examination: A semi-structured interview for the assessment of the specific psychopathology of eating disorders. *International Journal of Eating Disorders, 6,* 1–8.

Cooper, P.J. & Steere, J.A. (1995). Comparison of two psychological treatments for bulimia nervosa: Implications for models of maintenance. *Behaviour Research and Therapy, 33*, 875–885.

Cooper, P.J., Coker, S. & Fleming, C. (1996). An evaluation of the efficacy of supervised cognitive behavioral self-help bulimia nervosa. *J. Psychosom Res., 40*(3), 281–287.

Cooper, P.J., Watkins, B., Bryant-Waugh, R. & Lask, B. (2002). The nosological status of early onset anorexia nervosa. *Psychol Med., 32*(5), 873–880.

Cotton, M.A., Ball, C. & Robinson, P. (2003). Four simple questions can help screen for eating disorders. *Journal of General Internal Medicine.*

Crisp, A.H., Callender, J.S., Halek, C. & Hsu, L.K.G. (1992). Long-term mortality in anorexia nervosa: A 20-year follow-up of the St George's and Aberdeen Cohorts. *British Journal of Psychiatry, 161,* 80–87.

Crisp, A.H., Hsu, L.K. & Stonehill, E. (1979). Personality, body weight and ultimate outcome in anorexia nervosa. *Journal of Clinical Psychiatry, 40*(8), 332–325.

Crisp, A.H., Norton, K., Gowers, S., Halek, C., Bowyer, C., Yeldham, D., Levett, G. & Bhat, A. (1991). A controlled study of the effect of therapies aimed at adolescent and family psychopathology in anorexia nervosa *British Journal of Psychiatry, 59,* 325–333.

Crisp, A.H. (1995). The dyslipophobias: A view of the psychopathologies involved and the hazards of construing anorexia nervosa and bulimia nervosa as 'eating disorders'. *Proc Nutr Soc., 54*(3), 701–709.

Crisp, A.H. (2000). Stigmatisation of people with mental illnesses. *British Journal of Psychiatry, 177,* 4–7.

Crow, S., Praus, B. & Thuras, P. (1999). Mortality from eating disorders – A 5–10-year record linkage study. *International Journal of Eating Disorders, 26,* 97–101.

Crow, S.J. & Peterson, C.B. (2003). The economic and social burden of eating disorders: A review. In M. Maj *et al.* (Eds), *Eating Disorders*. John Wiley & Sons Ltd.

Dally, P.J. (1969). *Anorexia Nervosa*. London: Heinemann Medical Books.

Danziger, Y., Mukamel, M., Zeharia, A., Dinari, G. & Mimouni, M. (1994). Stunting of Growth in Anorexia nervosa during the prepubertal and pubertal period. *Israeli Journal of Medical Science, 30,* 581–584.

Dare, C. & Crowther, C. (1995). Living dangerously: Psychoanalytic psychotherapy of anorexia nervosa. In G. Szmukler, C. Dare & J. Treasure (Eds.), *Eating disorders: Handbook of theory, treatment and research.* Chichester: John Wiley & Sons.

Dare, C., Eisler, I., Russell, G., Treasure, J. & Dodge, L. (2001). Psychological therapies for adults with anorexia nervosa: Randomised controlled trial of out-patient treatments. *British Journal of Psychiatry, 178,* 216–221.

Deeks, J.J. (2002). Issues in the selection of a summary statistic for meta-analysis of clinical trials with binary outcomes. *Statistics in Medicine, 21*(11), 1575–1600.

Deering, S. (2000). Eating disorders: Recognition, evaluation and implications for obstetrician/gynecologists. *Primary Care Update for Ob/Gyns, 8*(1), 31–35.

Department of Health (2003). A commitment to carers; Help for relatives, partners and friends of people with a mental health problem. http://www.rethink.org/carers/.

DerSimonian, R. & Laird, N. (1986).Meta-analysis in Clinical Trials. *Controlled Clinical Trials, 7,* 177–188.

Deter, H.C., Herzog, W. & Petzold, E. (1992). The Heidelberg-Mannheim study: long-term follow-up of anorexia nervosa patients at the university medical center – background and preliminary results. In W. Herzog *et al.* (Eds.), *The course of eating disorders: Long-term follow-up studies of anorexia and bulimia nervosa* (pp.71–84). Berlin: Springer.

Deter, H.C. & Herzog, W. (1994). Anorexia nervosa in a long-term perspective: Results of the Heidelberg-Mannheim Study. *Psychosomatic Medicine, 56*(1), 20–27.

Deter, H.C., Kopp, W., Zipfel, S. & Herzog, W. (1998). Male anorexia nervosa patients in long-term follow-up. *Nervenarzt, 69*(5), 419–426.

Dolan, R.J., Mitchell, J. & Wakeling, A.: (1988). Structural brain changes in patients with anorexia nervosa. *Psychological Medicine, 18,* 349–353.

Eating disorders: A guide for the primary care physician (2002). *Primary Care; Clinics in Office Practice, 29*(1), 81–98.

Eccles, M. & Mason, J. (2001). How to develop cost-conscious guidelines. *Health Technology Assessment, 5*(16*),* 1–69.

Eccles, M., Freemantle, N. & Mason, J. (1998). North of England evidence-based guideline development project: Methods of developing guidelines for efficient drug use in primary care. *British Medical Journal, 316,* 1232–1235.

Eckert, E.D., Halmi, K.A., Marchi, P., Grove, W. & Crosby, R. (1995). Ten-year follow-up of anorexia nervosa: Clinical course and outcome. *Psychological Medicine, 25,* 143–156.

Eckert, E.D., Goldberg, S.C., Halmi, K.A., Casper, R.C. & Davis, J.M. (1979). Behaviour therapy in anorexia nervosa. *British Journal of Psychiatry, 134,* 55–59.

Eddy, K.T., Keel, P.K., Dorer, D.J., Delinsky, S.S., Franko, D.L. & Herzog, D.B. (2002). Longitudinal comparison of anorexia nervosa subtypes. *International Journal of Eating Disorders, 31*(2), 191–201.

Eiro, M., Katoh, T. & Watanabe, T. (2002). Use of a proton-pump inhibitor for metabolic disturbances associated with anorexia nervosa. *New England Journal of Medicine, 346*(2), 140.

Eisler, I., Dare, C., Hodes, M., Russell, G., Dodge, E. & Le Grange, D. (2000). Family therapy for adolescent anorexia nervosa: The results of a controlled comparison of two family interventions. *Journal of Child Psychology & Psychiatry & Allied Disciplines, 41,* 727–736.

Eldredge, K.L., Agras, W.S., Arnow, B., Telch, C.F., Bell, S., Castonguay, L. & Marnell, M. (1997). The effects of extending cognitive-behavioural therapy for binge eating disorder among initial treatment non-responders. *International Journal of Eating Disorders, 21,* 347–352.

Fairburn, C.G. (1981). A cognitive behavioural approach to the treatment of bulimia. *Psychol Med., 11*(4), 707–711.

Fairburn, C.G., Marcus, M.D. & Wilson, G.T. (1993). Cognitive-behavioral therapy for binge eating and bulimia nervosa: A comprehensive treatment manual. In C.G. Fairburn & G.T. Wilson (Eds.), *Binge eating: Nature, assessment and treatment* (pp.361–404). New York: Guilford Press.

Fairburn, C.G. (1995). *Overcoming binge eating disorders.* New York: Guilford Press.

Fairburn C.G., Cooper Z., Doll H.A., Norman P. & O'Connor M. (2000). The natural course of bulimia nervosa and binge eating disorder in young women. *Archives of General Psychiatry, 57,* 659–665.

Fairburn, C.G. & Harrison, P.J. (2003). Eating disorders. *The Lancet, 361,* 407–416.

Fairburn C.G. & Peveler (1990). Bulimia nervosa and a stepped care approach to management. *Gut., 31*(11), 1220–1222.

Fairburn, C.G. & Cooper, Z. (1984). Binge-eating, self-induced vomiting and laxative abuse: A community study. *Psychol Med., 14*(2), 401–410.

Fairburn, C.G. & Cooper, P.J. (1982). Self-induced vomiting and bulimia nervosa: An undetected problem. *Br Med J (Clin Res Ed), 17,* 284(6323), 1153–1155.

Fairburn, C.G., Welch, S.L., Norman, P.A., O'Connor, M.E. & Doll, H.A. (1996). Bias and bulimia nervosa: How typical are clinic cases? *Am J Psychiatry, 153*(3), 386–391.

Fairburn, C.G. & Beglin (1990). Studies of the epidemiology of bulimia nervosa. *Am J Psychiatry, 147*(4), 401–408.

Fairburn, C.G., Jones, R., Peveler, R. & Hope, R.A. (1993). Psychotherapy and bulimia nervosa. Longer-term effects of interpersonal psychotherapy, behaviour therapy and cognitive behavior therapy. *Archives of General Psychiatry, 50,* 419–428.

Fairburn, C.G., Jones, R., Peveler, R., Carr, S.J., Solomon, R.A., O'Conner, M., Burton, J. & Hope, R.A. (1991). Three psychological treatments for bulimia nervosa: A comparative trial. *Archives of General Psychiatry, 48,* 463–469.

Fairburn, C.G., Jones, R., Peveler, R., Hope, T. & O'Connor, M. (1993). Predictors of 12 month outcome in bulimia nervosa and the influence of attitudes to shape and weight. *Journal of Consulting & Clinical Psychology, 61,* 696–698.

Fairburn, C.G., Kirk, J., O'Conner, M. & Cooper, P.J. (1986). A comparison of two psychological treatments for bulimia nervosa. *Behaviour Research and Therapy, 24,* 629–643.

Fairburn, C.G., Norman, P.A., Welch, S.L., O'Connor, M., Doll, H.A. & Peveler, R. (1995). A prospective study of outcome in bulimia nervosa and the long-term effects of three psychological treatments. *Archives of General Psychiatry, 52,* 304–312.

Fairburn, C.G., Cowen, P.J. & Harrison, P.J. (1999) .Twin studies and the aetiology of eating disorders. *International Journal of Eating Disorders, 26,* 349–358.

Fairburn, C.G., Cooper Z., Doll H., Norman P. & O'Connor M. (2000). The natural course of bulimia nervosa and binge eating disorder in young women. *Archives of General Psychiatry, 57,* 659–665.

Fairburn, C.G. & Harrison, P.J. (2003). Eating disorders. *The Lancet, 361*(9355), 407–416.

Faris, P.L., Meller, W.H., Goodale, R.L., Oakman, S.A., Hofbauer, R.D., Marshall, A.M., Daughters, R.S., Banerjee-Stevens, D., Eckert, E.D.& Hartman, B.K. (2000). 5-HT3 antagonist therapy of bulimia nervosa: A peripherally active agent for a central nervous system eating disorder? *Gastroenterology, 119,* 271–272.

Faris, P.L., Won Kim, S., Meller, W.H., Goodale, R.L., Oakman, S.A., Hofbauer, R.D., Marshall, A.M., Daughters, R.S., Banerjee-Stevens, D., Eckert, E.D. & Hartman, B.K. (2000). Effect of decreasing afferent vagal activity with ondansetron on symptoms of bulimia nervosa: a randomised, double-blind trial. *The Lancet, 355,* 792–797.

Fassino, S., Leombruni, P., Daga, G., Brustolin, A., Migliaretti, G., Cavallo, F. & Rovera, G. (2002). Efficacy of citalopram in anorexia nervosa: A pilot study. *European Neuropsychopharmacology, 12*(5), 453–459.

Fichter, M.M. & Quadflieg, N. (1999). Six-year course and outcome of anorexia nervosa. *International Journal of Eating Disorders, 26*(4), 359–385.

Fichter, M.M., Leible, K., Rief, W., Brunner, E., Schmidt-Auberger, S. & Engel, R.R. (1991). Fluoxetine versus placebo: A double-blind study with bulimic inpatients undergoing intensive psychotherapy. *Pharmacopsychiatry, 24,* 1–247.

Fichter, M., Kruger, R., Rief, W., Holland, R. & Dohne, J. (1996). Fluvoxamine in prevention of relapse in bulimia nervosa: Effects on eating-specific psychopathology. *Journal of Clinical Psychopharmacology, 16,* 9–18.

Field, T., Schanberg, S., Kuhn, C., Field, T., Fierro, K., Henteleff, T., Mueller, C., Yando, R., Shaw, S. & Burman, I. (1998). Bulimic adolescents benefit from massage therapy. *Adolescence, 33,* 555–563.

Fluoxentine for anorexia nervosa (2001). *Nurses Drug Alert, 25,* 47–48.

Fluoxetine Bulimia Nervosa Collaborative Study Group (1992). Fluoxetine in the treatment of bulimia nervosa. A multicenter, placebo-controlled, double-blind trial. *Archives of General Psychiatry, 49,* 139–147.

Franko, D.L., Blais, M.A., Becker, A.E., Delinsky, S.S., Greenwood, D.N., Flores, A.T., Eddy, K.T. & Herzog, D.B. (2001). Pregnancy complications and neonatal outcomes in women with eating disorders. *American Journal of Psychiatry, 158,* 1461–1466.

Freeman, C., Barry, F., Dunkeld-Turnbull, J. & Henderson (1988). Controlled trial of psychotherapy for bulimia nervosa. *British Medical Journal, 296,* 521–525.

Freeman, C., Sinclair, F., Turnball, J. & Annandale, A. (1985). Psychotherapy for bulimia: A controlled study. *Journal of Psychiatric Research, 19,* 473–478.

Freund, K.M., Graham, S.M., Lesky, L.G. & Moskovitz, M.A. (1993). Detection of bulimia nervosa in a primary care setting. *Journal of General Internal Medicine, 8*(5), 236–242.

Garner & Garfinkel (1979). The Eating Attitudes Test: An index of the symptoms of anorexia nervosa. *Psychol Med., 9*(2), 273–279.

Garner, D.M., Olmsted, M.P. & Polivy, J. (1983). Development and validation of a multidimensional eating disorders inventory for anorexia nervosa and bulimia. *Int J Eat Dis, 2,* 15–34.

Garner, D.M., Rockert, W., Davis, R., Garner, M.V., Olmsted, M. & Eagle, M. (1993). Comparison of cognitive-behavioural and supportive-expressive therapy for bulimia nervosa. *American Journal of Psychiatry, 150,* 37–46.

Garvin, V. & Striegel-Moore, R.H. (2001). Health services research for eating disorders in the United States: A status report and a call to action. In R.H. Striegel-Moore *et al.* (Eds.), *Eating disorders: Innovative directions in research and practice.* Washington D.C.: APA.

Geist, R., Heinmaa, M., Stephens, D., Davis, R. & Katzman, D.K. (2000). Comparison of family therapy and family group psychoeducation in adolescents with anorexia nervosa. *Canadian Journal of Psychiatry – Revue Canadienne de Psychiatrie, 45,* 173–178.

Goldberg, S.C., Eckert, E.D., Casper, R.C., Halmi, K.A., Davis, J.M. & Roper, M.T. (1980). Factors influencing hospital differences in weight gain in anorexia nervosa. *Journal of Nervous and Mental Disease, 168*(3), 181–183.

Goldberg, S.C., Casper, R.C. & Eckert, E.D. (1980). Effects of cyproheptadine in anorexia nervosa. *Psychopharmacology Bulletin, 16,* 29–30.

Goldberg, S.C., Halmi, K.A., Eckert, E D., Casper, R.C. & Davis, J.M. (1979). Cyproheptadine in anorexia nervosa. *British Journal of Psychiatry, 134,* 67–70.

Goldbloom, D.S., Olmsted, M.P., Davies, R. & Shaw, B. (1997). A randomised control trial of fluoxetine and cognitive behavioural therapy for bulimia nervosa: Short-term outcome. *Behavioural Research and Therapy, 35,* 803–811.

Goldbloom, D.S. & Kennedy, S.H. (1995). Medical complications of anorexia nervosa. In K.D. Brownell & C.G. Fairburn (Eds.), *Eating disorders and obesity: A comprehensive handbook.* New York: Guilford.

Golden, N.H., Ashtari, M., Kohn, M.R., Patel, M., Jacobson, M.S., Fletcher, A. & Shenker, I.R. (1996). Reversibility of cerebral ventricular enlargement in anorexia nervosa, demonstrated by quantitative magnetic resonance imaging. *Journal of Pediatrics, 128,* 296–301.

Golden, N.H. (1992). Osteopenia in adolescents with anorexia nervosa. *Children's Hospital Quaterly, 4,* 143–148.

Goldfarb, L.A., Fuhr, R., Tsujimoto, R.N. & Fischman, S.E. (1987). Systematic desensitisation and relaxation as adjuncts in the treatment of anorexia nervosa: A preliminary study. *Psychological Reports, 60,* 511–518.

Goldstein, D.J., Wilson, M.G., Thomson, V.L., Potvin, J.H. & Rampey, A.H. (1995). Long-term fluoxetine treatment of bulimia nervosa. *British Journal of Psychiatry, 166,* 660–666.

Gordon, C.M., Grace, E., Emans, S.J., Feldman, H.A., Goodman, E., Becker, K.A., Rosen, C.J., Gundberg, C.M. & LeBoff, M.S. (2002). Effects of oral dehydroepiandrosterone on bone density in young women with anorexia nervosa: A randomised trial. *Journal of Clinical Endocrinology and Metabolism, 87,* 4935–4941.

Gordon, C.M., Grace, E., Emans, J., Goodman, E., Crawford, M.H. & Leboff, M.S. (1999). Changes in bone turnover markers and menstrual function after short-term oral DHEA in young women with anorexia nervosa. *Journal of Bone and Mineral Research, 14,* 136–145.

Gorin, A.A. (2001). A controlled trial of cognitive-behavioural therapy with and without spousal involvement for binge eating disorder. *Dissertation Abstracts International: Section B: the Sciences & Engineering, 61.*

Gowers, S., Norton, K., Halek, C. & Crisp, A.H. (1994). Outcome of out-patient psychotherapy in a random allocation treatment study of anorexia nervosa. *International Journal of Eating Disorders, 15,* 165–177.

Gowers, S.G. & Shore, A. (1999). The stigma of eating disorders. *Int J Clin Pract, 53*(5), 386–388.

Gowers, S.G. & Shore, A. (2001). Development of weight and shape concerns in the aetiology of eating disorders. *Br J Psychiatry, 179,* 236–242.

Griffiths, R.A. & Channon-Little, L. (1993). The hypnotisability of patients with bulimia nervosa and partial syndromes participating in a controlled treatment outcome study. *Contemporary Hypnosis, 10,* 81–87.

Griffiths, R.A., Hadzi-Pavlovic, D. & Channon-Little, L. (1994). A controlled evaluation of hypnobehavioural treatment for bulimia nervosa: Immediate pre-post treatment effects. *European Eating Disorders Review, 2,* 202–220.

Griffiths, R.A., Hadzi-Pavlovic, D. & Channon-Little, L. (1996). The short-term follow-up effect of hypnobehavioural and cognitive behavioural treatment for bulimia nervosa. *European Eating Disorders Review, 4,* 12–31.

Griffiths, R.A., Hazi-Pavlovic, D. & Channon-Little, L. (1997). Are there differences in response to psychological treatment for recruited and nonrecruited bulimic patients? *European Eating Disorders Review, 5,* 131–140.

Grinspoon, S., Thomas, E., Pitts, S., Gross, E., Mickley, D., Miller, K., Herzog, D. & Klibanski, A. (2000). Prevalence and predictive factors for regional osteopenia in women with anorexia nervosa. *Annals of Internal Medicine, 133,* 790–794.

Grinspoon, S., Baum, H., Lee, K., Anderson, E., Herzog, D. & Klibanski, A. (1996). Effects of short-term recombinant human insulin-like growth factor I administration on bone turnover in osteopenic women with anorexia nervosa. *Journal of Clinical Endocrinology & Metabolism, 81,* 3864–3870.

Grinspoon, S., Herzog, D. & Klibanski, A. (1997). Mechanisms and treatment options for bone loss in anorexia nervosa. *Psychopharmacol Bull, 33*(3), 399–404.

Grinspoon, S., Thomas, L., Miller, K., Herzog, D. & Klibanski, A. (2002). Effects of recombinant human IGF-I and oral contraceptive administration on bone density in anorexia nervosa. *Journal of Clinical Endocrinology & Metabolism, 87,* 2883–2891.

Gross, H., Ebert, M.H. & Faden, V.B. (1983). A double-blind trial of Delta9-tetrahydrocannabinol in primary anorexia nervosa. *Journal of Clinical Psychopharmacology, 3,* 165–171.

Halbreich, U. & Kahn, L.S. (2000). Selective oestrogen receptor modulators – current and future brain and behaviour applications. *Expert Opinion in Pharmacotherapy, 1,* 1385–1398.

Hall, A. & Crisp, A.H. (1987). Brief psychotherapy in the treatment of anorexia nervosa. Outcome at one year. *British Journal of Psychiatry, 151,* 185–191.

Hall, A. & Hay, P.J. (1991). Eating disorder patient referrals from a population region 1977–1986. *Psychol Med, 21*(3), 697–701.

Halmi, K.A., Goldberg, S.C., Casper, R.C., Eckert, E.D. & Davis, J.M. (1979). Pre-treatment predictors of outcome in anorexia nervosa. *British Journal of Psychiatry, 134,* 71–78.

Halmi, K.A. & Goldberg, S.C. (1978). Cyproheptadine in anorexia nervosa. *Psychopharmacology Bulletin, 14,* 31–33.

Halmi, K.A., Eckert, E. & Falk, J.R. (1983). Cyproheptadine, an antidepressant and weight-inducing drug for anorexia nervosa. *Psychopharmacology Bulletin, 19,* 103–105.

Halmi, K.A., Eckert, E., LaDue, T.J. & Cohen, J. (1986). Anorexia nervosa. Treatment efficacy of cyproheptadine and amitriptyline. *Archives of General Psychiatry, 43,* 177–181.

Hart, S., Field, T., Hernandez-Reif, M., Nearing, G., Shaw, S., Schanberg, S. & Kuhn, C. (2001). Anorexia nervosa symptoms are reduced by massage therapy. *Eating Disorders, 9,* 289–299.

Harwood, M.P. & Newton, T. (1995). Dental aspects of bulimia nervosa: Implications for the health care team. *European Eating Disorders Review, 3*(2), 93–102.

Hay, P.J. (1998). Eating disorders: Anorexia nervosa, bulimia nervosa and related syndromes – An overview of assessment and management. *Australian Prescriber, 21*(4), 100–103.

Hay, P.J., Marley, J. & Lemar, S. (1998). Covert eating disorders: The prevalence, characteristics and help-seeking of those with bulimic eating disorders in general practice. *Primary Care Psychiatry, 4*(2), 95–99.

Hay, P.J. & Bacaltchuk, J. (2003). Psychotherapy for bulimia nervosa and binging. *Cochrane Database Syst Rev., (1)*, CD000562.

Hebebrand, J., Himmelmann, G.W., Herzog, W., Herpertz-Dahlmann, B.M., Steinhausen, H.C., Amstein, M., Seidel, R., Deter, H.C., Remschmidt, H. & Schafer, H. (1997). Prediction of low body weight at long-term follow-up in acute anorexia nervosa by low body weight at referral. *American Journal of Psychiatry, 154*(4), 566–569.

Hebebrand, J., Himmelmann, G.W., Wewetzer, C., Gutenbrunner, C., Heseker, H., Schafer, H. & Remschmidt, H. (1996). Body weight in acute anorexia nervosa and at follow-up assessed with percentiles for the body mass index: Implications of a low body weight at referral. *International Journal of Eating Disorders, 19*(4), 347-357.

Hebebrand, J., Wehmeier, P.M. & Remschmidt, H. (2000). Letter to the editor: Weight criteria for diagnosis of anorexia nervosa. *American Journal of Psychiatry, 157,* 1024.

Hebebrand, J., Himmelmann, G.W., Heseker, H. *et al*. (1996). Use of percentiles for the body mass index in anorexia nervosa: diagnostic, epidemiological, and therapeutic considerations. *International Journal of Eating Disorders, 19,* 359–369.

Herpertz-Dahlmann, B., Muller, B., Herpertz, S., Heussen, N., Hebebrand, J. & Remschmidt, H. (2001). Prospective 10-year follow-up in adolescent anorexia nervosa – course, outcome, psychiatric comorbidity and psychosocial adaptation. *Journal of Child Psychology and Psychiatry, 42*(5), 603–612.

Herzog, D.B., Keller, M.B., Sacks, N.R., Yeh, C.J. & Lavori, P.W. (1992). Psychiatric comorbidity in treatment-seeking anorexics and bulimics. *J Am Acad Child Adolesc Psychiatry, 31*(5),810–818.

Herzog, D.B., Nussbaum, K.M. & Marmor, A.K. (1996). Comorbidity and outcome in eating disorders. *Psychiatric Clinics of North America, 19*(4), 843–859.

Herzog, W., Deter, H.C., Fiehn, W. & Petzold, E. (1997). Medical findings and predictors of long-term physical outcome in anorexia nervosa: A prospective, 12-year follow-up study. *Psychological Medicine, 27*(2), 269–279.

Herzog, W., Greenwood, D.N, Dorer, D.J. *et al.* (2000). Mortality in eating disorders: A descriptive study. *International Journal of Eating Disorders, 28,* 20–26.

Herzog, W., Schellberg, D. & Deter, H.C. (1997). First recovery in anorexia nervosa patients in the long-term course: A discrete-time survival analysis. *Journal of Consulting and Clinical Psychology, 65*(1), 169–177.

Herzog, T., Hartmann, A. & Falk, C. (1996). The short-term effects of psychodynamic in-patient treatment of anorexia nervosa with and without an explicit focus on eating pathology – A controlled study. *Psychotherapie Psychosomatik Medizinische Psychologie, 46,* 11–22.

Herzog, W., Deter, H.C., Fiehn, W. & Petzold, E. (2003). Medical findings and predictors of long-term physical outcome in anorexia nervosa – A prospective, 12-year follow-up study. *Psychological Medicine, 27,* 269–279.

Higgins, J.P.T. & Thompson, S.G. (2002). Quantifying heterogeneity in a meta-analysis. *Statistics in Medicine, 21*(11), 1539–1558.

Hodes, M., Timimi, S. & Robinson, P. (1997). Children of mothers with eating disorders. A preliminary study. *European Eating Disorders Review, 5,* 1–24.

Hoek, H.W. (1991). The incidence and prevalence of anorexia nervosa in primary care. *Psychological Medicine, 21,* 455–460.

Hoek, H.W. (2003). Distribution of eating disorders. In M. Maj *et al.* (Eds.), *Eating disorders.* John Wiley & Sons Ltd.

Hoek, H.W. (1991). The incidence and prevalence of anorexia nervosa in primary care. *Psychological Medicine, 21,* 455–460.

Holderness, C.C., Brooks-Gunn, J. & Warren, M.P. (1994). Co-morbidity of eating disorders and substance abuse review of the literature. *International Journal of Eating Disorders, 16*(1), 1–34.

Horne, R.L., Ferguson, J.M., Pope, H.G., Hudson, J.I., Lineberry, C.G., Ascher, J. & Cato, A. (1988). Treatment of bulimia with bupropion: A multicenter controlled trial. *Journal of Clinical Psychiatry, 49,* 262–266.

Howard, W.T., Evans, K.K., Quintero-Howard, C.V., Bowers, W.A. & Andersen, A.E. (1999). Predictors of success or failure of transition to day hospital treatment for inpatients with anorexia nervosa. *American Journal of Psychiatry, 156*(11), 1697–1702.

Howlett, M, McClelland, L. & Crisp, A.H. (1995). The cost of illness that defies. *Postgraduate Medical Journal, 71,* 36–39.

Hsu, L.K., Crisp, A.H. & Callender, J.S. (1992). Psychiatric diagnoses in recovered and unrecovered anorectics 22 years after onset of illness: A pilot study. *Compr Psychiatry, 33*(2), 123–127.

Hsu, L.K. (1995). Outcome of bulimia nervosa. In K.D. Brownell & C.G. Fairburn (Eds.), *Eating disorders and obesity* (pp.238–246).

Hsu, L.K., Rand, W., Sullivan, S., Liu, D.W., Mulliken, B., McDonagh, B. & Kaye, W.H. (2001). Cognitive therapy, nutritional therapy and their combination in the treatment of bulimia nervosa. *Psychological Medicine, 31,* 871–879.

Hsu, L.K., Crisp, A.H. & Harding, B. (1979) Outcome of anorexia nervosa. *The Lancet,* 61–65.

Hudson, J.I., McElroy, S., Raymond, N.C., Crow, S., Keck, P.E., Carter, M.D., Mitchell, J.E., Strakowski, M.D., Pope, H.G., Coleman, B.S. & Jonas, J.M. (1998). Fluvoxamine in the treatment of binge-eating disorder: A multicenter placebo-controlled, double-blind trial. *American Journal of Psychiatry, 155,* 1756–1762.

Huseman, C.A., Pearson, P.H., Madison, J.& Leuschen, M.P. (1990). Bulimia as a form of self-addiction: Treatment with naltrexone hydrochloride (Trexan(TM)) – a pilot study. *Clinical Trials Journal, 27,* 77–83.

Iketani, T., Kiriike, N., Nakanishi, S. & Nakasuji, T. (1995). Effects of weight gain and resumption of menses on reduced bone density in patients with anorexia nervosa. *Biological Psychiatry, 37,* 521–527.

Irwin, M. (1984). Early onset anorexia nervosa. *Southern Medical Journal, 77,* 611–614.

Isner, J.M., Roberts, W.C., Heymsfield, S.B. & Yageer, J. (1985). Anorexia nervosa and sudden death. *Annals of Internal Medicine, 102,* 49–52.

Ivarsson, T., Rastam, M., Wentz, E., Gillberg, I.C. & Gillberg, C. (2000). Depressive disorders in teenage-onset anorexia nervosa: A controlled longitudinal, partly community-based study. *Comprehensive Psychiatry, 42*(5), 398–403

Jacobi, C., Dahme, D. & Dittmann, R. (2002). Cogntive-behavioural, fluoxetine and combined treatment for bulimia nervosa: Short-and long-term results. *European Eating Disorders Review, 10,* 179–198.

Jadad, A.R., Moore, R.A., Carroll, D., Jenkinson, C., Reynolds, D.J., Gavaghan, D.J. & McQuay, H.J. (1996). Assessing the quality of reports of randomised clinical trials: Is blinding necessary? *Controlled Clinical Trials, 17*(1), 1–12.

Jansen, A., Elgersma, H., Nederkoorn, C. & Smeets, T. (2002). What makes treatment of bulimia nervosa successful? Paper presented at the European Association for Cognitive and Behaviour Therapies Congress, 18–21 September, Maastricht.

Jansen, A., Van den Hout, M.A., De Loof, C., Zandbergen, J. & Griez, E. (1989). A case of bulimia successfully treated by cue exposure. *J Behav Ther Exp Psychiatry, 20*(4), 327–332.

Johnson, W.G., Jarrel,l M.P., Chupurdia, K.M. & Williamson, D.A. (1994). Repeated binge/purge cycles in bulimia nervosa: Role of glucose and insulin. *Int J Eat Disord, 15*(4), 331–341.

Johnson, J.G., Spitzer, R.L. & Williams, J.B. (2001). Health problems, impairment and illnesses associated with bulimia nervosa and binge eating disorder among primary care and obstetric gynaecology patients. *Psychological Medicine, 31,* 1455–1466.

Jones, R., Peveler, R., Hope, R.A. & Fairburn, C.G. (1993). Changes during treatment for bulimia nervosa: A comparison of three psychological treatments. *Behaviour Research and Therapy,* 4797786975485.

Kachele, H., Kordy, H. & Mattias, R. (2001). Research Group Treat. Therapy amount and outcome of in-patient psychodynamic treatment of eating disorders in Germany: Data from a multi-center study. *Psychotherapy Research, 11*(3), 239–257.

Kachele, H. (1999). Eine multizentrishe Studie zu Aufwand und Erfolg bei psychodynamischer Therapie von Essstorungen. *Psychotherapy, Psychosomatik, Midizinische Psychologie, 49,* 100–108.

Kanerva, R., Rissanen, A. & Sarna, S. (1994). Fluoxetine in the treatment of anxiety, depressive symptoms and eating-related symptoms in bulimia nervosa. *Journal of Psychiatry, 49,* 237–242.

Kaplan, A.S. (2002). Psychological treatments for anorexia nervosa: A review of published studies and promising new directions. *Canadian Journal of Psychiatry, 47,* 235–242.

Kaplan, D.W., Blythe, M., Diaz, A., Feinstein, R.A., Fisher, M.M., Klein, J.D. *et al.* (2003). Identifying and treating eating disorders. *Pediatrics, 111*(1), 204–211.

Katz, R.L., Keen, C.L., Litt, I.F., Hurley, L.S., Kellams-Harrison, K.M. & Glader, L.J. (1987). Zinc deficiency in anorexia nervosa. *Journal of Adolescent Health Care, 8,* 400–406.

Katzman, D.K., Lambe, E.K., Mikulis, D.J., Ridgley, J.N., Goldbloom, D.S. & Zipursky, R.B. (1996). Cerebral gray matter and white matter volume deficits in adolescent girls with anorexia nervosa. *Journal of Pediatrics, 129,* 794–803.

Kaye, W.H., Nagata, T., Weltzin, T.E., Hsu, L.K., Sokol, M.S., McConaha, C., Plotnicov, K.H., Weise, J. & Deep, D. (2001). Double-blind placebo-controlled administration of fluoxetine in restricting- and restricting-purging-type anorexia nervosa. Biological Psychiatry, 49, 644–652.

Keel, P.K., Dorer, D.J., Eddy, K.T. *et al.* (2003). Predictors of mortality in eating disorders. *Archives of General Psychiatry, 60,* 179–183.

Keel, P.K. & Mitchell, J.E. (1997). Outcome in bulimia nervosa. *American Journal of Psychiatry, 154,* 313.

Keel, P.K., Mitchell, J.E., Miller, K.B., Davis, T.L. & Crow, S.J. (1999). Long-term outcome of bulimia nervosa. *Archives of General Psychiatry, 56*(1), 63–69.

Keel, P.K., Mitchell, J.E., Davis, T.L. & Crow, S.J. (2002). Long-term impact of treatment in women diagnosed with bulimia nervosa. International Journal of Eating Disorders, 31, 151–158.

Keilen, M., Treasure, T., Schmidt, U. & Treasure, J. (1994). Quality of life measurements in eating disorders, angina and transplant candidates: Are they comparable? *Journal of the Royal Society of Medicine, 87*(8), 441–444.

Kendall, T.J.G., Pilling, S., Barnes, T.R.E. *et.al.* (2003). *Schizophrenia: Full national clinical guideline on core interventions in primary and secondary care.* London: Gaskell.

King, M.B. (1989). Eating disorders in a general practice population. Prevalence, characteristics and follow-up at 12 to 18 months. *Psychological Medicine Monograph Supplement, 14,* 1–34.

Kingston, K., Szmukler, G., Andrewes, D., Tress, B. & Desmond, P. (1996). Neuropsychological and structural brain changes in anorexia nervosa before and after refeeding. *Psychological Medicine, 26,* 15–28.

Kirkley, B.G., Schneider, J.A., Agras, W.S. & Bachman, J.A. (1985). Comparison of two group treatments for bulimia. *Journal of Consulting & Clinical Psychology, 53,* 43–48.

Klibanski, A., Biller, B.M.K., Schoenfeld, D.A., Herzog, D.B. & Saxe, V.C. (1995). The effects of estrogen administration on trabecular bone loss in young women with anorexia nervosa. *Journal of Clinical Endocrinology & Metabolism, 80,* 898–904.

Kohn, M.R., Ashtari, M., Golden, N.H., Schebendach, J., Patel, M., Jacobson, M.S. & Shenker, I.R. (1997). Structural brain changes and malnutrition in anorexia nervosa. *Annals of the New York Academy of Science, 817,* 398–399.

Koran, L.M., Agras, W.S., Rossiter, E.M. *et al.* (1995). Comparing the cost-effectiveness of psychiatric treatments: Bulimia nervosa. *Psychiatry Research, 58,* 13–21.

Krauth, C., Buser, K. & Vogel, H. (2002). How high are the costs of eating disorders – anorexia nervosa and bulimia nervosa – for German society? *European Journal of Health Economics, 3,* 244–250.

Kreipe, R.E. & Birndorf, S.A. (2000). Eating disorders in adolescents and young adults. *Medical Clinics of North America, 84*(4), 1027–1049.

Krieg, J.C., Pirke, K.M., Lauer, C. & Backmund, H. (1988). Endocrine, metabolic and cranial computed tomographic findings in anorexia nervosa. *Biological Psychiatry, 23,* 377–387.

Kumetz, N.C. (1983). Bulimia: A descriptive and treatment study. PhD Thesis The University of Texas Health Science Center at Dallas.

Lacey, J.H. (1983). Bulimia nervosa, binge eating and psychogenic vomiting: A controlled treatment study and long-term outcome. *Br Med J (Clin Res Ed), 286*(6378), 1609–1613.

Lacey, J.H. & Crisp, A.H. (1980). Hunger, food intake and weight: The impact of clomipramine on a refeeding anorexia nervosa population. *Postgraduate Medical Journal, 56,* 79–85.

Lacey, J.H. & Smith, G. (1987). Bulimia nervosa. The impact of pregnancy on mother and baby. *British Journal of Psychiatry, 150,* 777–781.

Laederach-Hofmann, K., Graf, C., Horber, F., Lippuner, K., Lederer, S., Michel, R. & Schneider, M. (1999). Imipramine and diet counseling with psychological support in the treatment of obese binge eaters: A randomised, placebo-controlled double-blind study. *International Journal of Eating Disorders, 26,* 231–244.

Laessle, R.G., Beumont, P.J.V., Butow, P., Lennerts, W., O'Conner, M., Pirke, K.M., Touyz, S.W. & Waadt, S. (1991). A comparison of nutritional management with stress management in the treatment of bulimia nervosa. *British Journal of Psychiatry, 159,* 250-261.

Laessle, R.G., Waadt, S. & Pirke, K.M. (1987). A structured behaviourally-orientated group treatment for bulimia nervosa. *Psychotherapy & Psychosomatics, 48,* 141-145.

Lambe, E.K., Katzman, D.K., Mikulis, D.J., Kennedy, S.H. & Zipursky, R.B. (1997). Cerebral gray matter volume deficits after weight recovery from anorexia nervosa. *Archives of General Psychiatry, 54,* 537-542.

Lask, B., Fosson, A., Rolfe, U. & Thomas, S. (1993). Zinc deficiency and childhood-onset anorexia nervosa. *Journal of Clinical Psychiatry, 54,* 63–66.

Le Grange, D., Eisler, I., Dare, C. & Russell, G. (1992). Evaluation of family treatments in adolescent anorexia nervosa: A pilot study. *International Journal of Eating Disorders, 12,* 347–357.

Le Grange, D. & Gelman, T. (1998). Patients' perspective of treatment in eating disorders: A preliminary study. *South African Journal of Psychology, 28*(3).

Lee, N.F. & Rush, A.J. (1986). Cognitive-behavioural group therapy for bulimia. *International Journal of Eating Disorders, 5,* 599–615.

Leibowitz, S.F. & Alexander, J.T.(1998). Hypothalamic serotonin in control of eating behaviour, meal size and body weight. *Biological Psychiatry, 44,* 851–864.

Leitenberg, H., Rosen, J.C., Gross, J., Nudelman, S. & Vara, L.S. (1988). Exposure plus response-prevention treatment of bulimia nervosa. *Journal of Consulting & Clinical Psychology, 56,* 535–541.

Leitenberg, H., Rosen, J.C., Wolf, J., Vara, L.S., Detzer, M.J. & Srebnik, D. (1994). Comparison of cognitive-behaviour therapy and desipramine in the treatment of bulimia nervosa. *Behavioural Research and Therapy, 32,* 37–45.

Lemouchoux, C., Millar, H. & Naji, S. (2001). Eating disorders in Scotland: Starved of resources? *Psychiatric Bulletin, 21*(7), 256–260.

Lock, J. & Le Grange, D. (2001). Can family-based treatment of anorexia be manualised? *Journal of Psychotherapy Practice Research, 10*(4), 253–261.

Loeb, K.L., Wilson, G.T., Gilbert, J.S. & Labouvie, E. (2000). Guided and unguided self-help for binge eating. *Behaviour Research and Therapy, 38,* 259–272.

Lowe, B., Zipfel, S., Buchholz, C., Dupont, Y., Reas, D.L. & Herzog, W. (2001). Long-term outcome of anorexia nervosa in a prospective 21-year follow-up study. *Psychological Medicine, 31*(5), 881–890.

Lucas, A.R., Melton, L.J. III, Crowson, C.S. & O'Fallon, W.M. (1999). Long-term fracture risk among women with anorexia nervosa: A population-based cohort study. *Mayo Clin. Proc, 74,* 972–977.

Luck, A.J., Morgan, J.F., Reid, F., O'Brien, A., Brunton, J., Price, C., Perry, L. & Lacey, J.H. (2002). The SCOFF questionnaire and clinical interview for eating disorders in general practice: Comparative study. *British Medical Journal, 325*(7367), 755–756.

Mann, T. (1996). Clinical guidelines: Using clinical guidelines to improve patient care within the NHS. Department of Heath NHS Executive.

Maugars, Y.M., Berthelot, J.M., Forestier, R., Mammar, N., Lalande, S., Venisse, J.L. & Prost, A.M. (1996). Follow-up of bone mineral density in 27 cases of anorexia nervosa. *European Journal of Endocrinology, 135,* 591–597.

MacDonald, C. (2002). Treatment resistance in anorexia nervosa and the pervasiveness of ethics in clinical decision-making. *Canadian Journal of Psychiatry, 47,* 267–270.

McCann, U.D. & Agras, W.S. (1990). Successful treatment of non-purging bulimia nervosa with desipramine: A double-blind, placebo-controlled study. *American Journal of Psychiatry, 147,* 1509–1513.

McClain, C.J., Stuart, M.A., Vivian, B., McClain, M., Talwalker, R., Snelling, L. & Humphries, L. (1992). Zinc status before and after zinc supplementation of eating disorder patients. *Journal of the American College of Nutrition, 11,* 694–700.

McElroy, S.L., Casuto, L.S., Nelson, E.B., Lake, K.A., Soutullo, C.A., Keck, P.E. Jr. & Hudson, J.I. (2000). Placebo-controlled trial of sertraline in the treatment of binge eating disorder. *American Journal of Psychiatry, 157,* 1004–1006.

McElroy, S., Arnold, L.M., Shapira, N.A., Keck, P.E., Rosenthal, N.R., Karim, R., Kamin, M. & Hudson, J.I. Topiramate in the treatment of binge eating disorder associated with obesity: A randomised, placebo-controlled trial. American Journal of Psychiatry (in press).

McIntosh, V.V., Jordan, J., Carter, F.A., Luty, S.E., McKenzie, J.M., Bulik, C.M., Frampton, C.M.A. & Joyce, P.R. Three psychotherapies for anorexia nervosa: A randomised controlled trial. Submitted for publication.

Meads, C., Gold, L. & Burls, A. (2001). How effective is out-patient care compared to in-patient care for the treatment of anorexia nervosa? A systematic review. *European Eating Disorders Review, 9,* 229–241.

Mehler, P.S. (2001). Diagnosis and care of patients with anorexia nervosa in primary care settings. *Annals of Internal Medicine,* 1048–1059.

Mehler, P.S. & Linas, S. (2002). Use of a proton-pump inhibitor for metabolic disturbances associated with anorexia nervosa. *New England Journal of Medicine, 347,* 373–374.

Mitchell, J.E. & Groat, R.A. (1984). Placebo-controlled, double-blind trial of amitriptyline in bulimia. *Journal of Clinical Psychopharmacology, 4*(4), 186–193.

Mitchell, J.E., Hatsukami, D., Eckert, E.D. & Pyle, R.L. (1985). Characteristics of 275 patients with bulimia. *American Journal of Psychiatry, 142*(4), 482–485.

Mitchell, J.E., Pomeroy, C., Seppala, M. & Huber, M. (1988). Diuretic use as a marker for eating problems and affective disorders among women. *Journal of Clinical Psychiatry, 49*(7), 267–270.

Mitchell, J.E., Christenson, G., Jennings, J., Huber, M., Thomas, B., Pomeroy, C. & Morley, J.A (1989). Placebo-controlled, double-blind crossover study of naltrexone hydrochloride in outpatients with normal weight bulimia. *Journal of Clinical Psychopharmacology, 9,* 94–97.

Mitchell, J.E., Fletcher, L., Hanson, K., Mussell, M.P., Seim, H., Crosby, R. & Al Banna, M. (2001). The relative efficacy of fluoxetine and manual-based self-help in the treatment of outpatients with bulimia nervosa. *Journal of Clinical Psychopharmacology, 21,* 298–304.

Mitchell, J.E., Pyle, R.L., Eckert, E.D., Hatsukami, D., Pomeroy, C. & Zimmerman, R. (1990). A comparison study of antidepressants and structured intensive group psychotherapy in the treatment of bulimia nervosa. *Archives of General Psychiatry, 47,* 149–157.

Mitchell, J.E., Pomeroy, C. & Adson, D. (1997). Managing medical complications. In D. Garner & P. Garfinkel (Eds.), *Handbook of treatment for eating disorders* (2nd ed.) (pp.383–393). New York: Guilford Press.

Mitchell, J.E., Peterson, C.B. & Agras, S. (1999). Cost-effectiveness of psychotherapy for eating disorders. In N.E. Miller (Ed.), *Cost-effectiveness of psychotherapy.* Oxford: Oxford University Press.

Mitchell, J.E., Halmi, K., Wilson, G.T., Agras, W.S., Kraemer, H. & Crow, S. (2002). A randomised secondary treatment study of women with bulimia nervosa who fail to respond to CBT. *International Journal of Eating Disorders, 32*(3), 271–281.

Morgan, H.G., Purgold, J. & Welbourne, J. (1983). Management and outcome in anorexia nervosa. A standardised prognostic study. *British Journal of Psychiatry, 143,* 282–287.

Morgan, H.G. & Russell, G.F. (1975). Value of family background and clinical features as predictors of long-term outcome in anorexia nervosa: Four-year follow-up study of 41 patients. *Psychological Medicine, 5*(4), 355–371.

Morgan, J.F., Lacey, J.H. & Sedgwick, P.M. (1999). Impact of pregnancy on bulimia nervosa. *British Journal of Psychiatry, 174,* 135–140.

Morgan, J.F., Reid, F. & Lacey, J.H. (1999). The SCOFF questionnaire: Assessment of a new screening tool for eating disorders. *British Medical Journal, 319,* 1467–1468.

Mumford, D.B. & Whitehouse, A.M. (1998). Increased prevalence of bulimia nervosa among Asian schoolgirls. *British Medical Journal, 297,* 718–719.

National Institute for Clinical Excellence (NICE) (2002). *The guideline development process – information for National Collaborating Centres and Guideline Development Groups.* London: National Institute for Clinical Excellence.

Nauta, H., Hospers, H., Kok, G. & Jansen, A. (2000). A comparison between a cognitive and a behavioural treatment for obese binge eaters and obese non-binge eaters. *Behaviour Therapy, 31,* 441–461.

Netten, A., Rees, T. & Harrison, G. (2002). Unit costs of health and social care. Personal Social Services Research Unit, Canterbury.

Neumärker, K.J. (1997). Mortality and sudden death in anorexia nervosa. *International Journal of Eating Disorders, 21,* 205–212.

Neumärker, K.J. (2000). Mortality rates and causes of death. *European Eating Disorders Review, 8,* 181–187.

Neumärker, K.J., Dudeck, U., Meyer, U., Neumarker, U., Schulz, E. & Schonheit, B. (1997). Anorexia nervosa and sudden death in childhood: Clinical data and results obtained from quantitative neurohistological investigations of cortical neurons. *Eur.Arch.Psychiatry Clin.Neurosci., 247,* 16–22.

Nicholls, D. & Stanhope, R. (2000). Medical complications of anorexia nervosa in children and young adolescents. *European Eating Disorders Review, 8,* 170–178.

Nielsen, S., Emborg, C. & Molbak, A.G. (2002). Mortality in concurrent type 1 diabetes and anorexia nervosa. *Diabetes Care, 25,* 309–312.

Nielsen, S., Moller-Madsen, S., Isager, T., Jorgensen, J., Pagsberg, K. & Theander, S. (1998). Standardised mortality in eating disorders – a quantitative summary of previously published and new evidence. *Journal of Psychosomatic Research, 44,* 413–434

Nielsen, S. (2002). Eating disorders in females with type 1 diabetes: An update of a meta-analysis. *European Eating Disorders Review, 10,* 241–254.

Nielsen, S. (2001). Epidemiology and mortality of eating disorders. *Eating Disorders, 24,* 201–214.

Noordenbos, G. (1988). Eating disorders in primary care: Early identification and intervention by general practitioners. In W. Vandereycken & G. Nordenbos (Eds.), *The prevention of eating disorders* (pp.214–229). London: Athlone Press.

Nussbaum, M., Baird, D., Sonnenblick, M., Cowan, K. & Shenker, I.R. (1985). Short stature in anorexia nervosa patients. *Journal of Adolescent Health Care, 6*(6), 453–455.

Office of Health Economics (1994). *Eating disorders.* London: OHE.

Ogg, E.C., Millar, H.R., Pusztai, E.E. & Thom, A.S. (1997). General practice consultation patterns preceding diagnosis of eating disorders. *International Journal of Eating Disorders, 22*(1), 89–93.

O'Herlihy, A., Worrall, A., Banerjee, S. et al. (2001). *National Inpatient Child and Adolescent Psychiatry Study (NICAPS): Final report to the Department of Health.* London. Royal College of Psychiatrists' Research Unit.

Ostuzzi, R., Didonna, F. & Micciolo, R. (1999). One-year weight follow-up in anorexia nervosa after inpatient psycho-nutritional rehabilitative treatment. *Eat Weight Disord, 4*(4), 194–197.

Patton, G.C. (1988). Mortality in eating disorders. *Psychological Medicine, 18*(4), 947–951.

Perry, L., Morgan, J., Reid, F., Brunton, J., O'Brien, A., Luck, A. & Lacey, H. (2002). Screening for symptoms of eating disorders: Reliability of the SCOFF screening tool with written compared to oral delivery. *International Journal of Eating Disorders, 32*(4), 466–472.

Pertschuk, M.J., Forster, J., Buzby, G. & Mullen, J.L. (1981). The treatment of anorexia nervosa with total parenteral nutrition. *Biological Psychiatry, 16,* 539–550.

Pike, K.M., Walsh, B.T., Vitousek, K., Wilson, G.T. & Bauer, J. (2003). Cognitive behavioral therapy in the post-hospital treatment of anorexia nervosa. *American Journal of Psychiatry* (in press).

Pillay, M. & Crisp, A.H. (1981). The impact of social skills training within an established inpatient treatment programme for anorexia nervosa. *British Journal of Psychiatry, 139,* 533–539.

Pope, H.G. Jr & Hudson, J.I. (1982). Treatment of bulimia nervosa with antidepressants. *Psychopharmacology, 78,* 176–179.

Pope, H.G. Jr, Keck, P.E., McElroy, S. & Hudson, J.I. (1989). A placebo-controlled study of trazodone in bulimia nervosa. *Journal of Clinical Psychopharmacology, 9,* 254–259.

Pope, H.G., Hudson, J.I., Jonas, J.M. & Yurgelum-Todd, D. (1985). Antidepressant treatment of bulimia: A two-year follow-up study. *Journal of Clinical Psychopharmacology, 5,* 320–327.

Pope, H.G., Hudson, J.I., Jonas, J.M. & Yurgelum-Todd, D. (1983). Bulimia treated with imipramine: A placebo-controlled, double-blind study. *American Journal of Psychiatry, 140,* 554–558.

Pyle, R.L., Mitchell, J.E., Eckert, E.D., Hatsukami, D., Pomeroy, C. & Zimmerman, R. (1990). Maintenance treatment and six-month outcome for bulimic patients who respond to initial treatment. *American Journal of Psychiatry, 147,* 871–875.

Ratnasuriya, R.H., Eisler, I., Szmukler, G.I. & Russell, G.F. (1991). Anorexia nervosa: Outcome and prognostic factors after 20 years. *British Journal of Psychiatry, 158,* 495–502.

Reeves, R.S., McPherson, R.S., Nichaman, M.Z., Harrist, R.B., Foreyt, J.P. & Goodrick, G.K. (2001). Nutrient intake of obese female binge eaters. *Journal of the American Dietetic Association, 101,* 209–215.

Remschmidt, H., Wienand, F. & Wewetzer, C. (1988). Long-term prognosis in anorexia nervosa. *Monatsschr Kinderheilkd, 136*(11), 726–731.

Ricca, V., Mannucci, E., Mezzani, B. et al. (2001). Psychopathological and clinical features of outpatients with an eating disorder not otherwise specified. *Eat Weight Disord, 6,* 157–165.

Ricca, V., Mannucci, E., Moretti, S., Di Bernardo, M., Zucchi, T., Cabras, P.L. & Rotella, C.M. (2000). Screening for binge eating disorder in obese outpatients. *Comprehensive Psychiatry, 41,* 111–115.

Rigotti, N.A., Neer, R.M., Skates, S.J., Herzog, D.B. & Nussbaum, S.R. (1991). The clinical course of osteoporosis in anorexia nervosa. A longitudinal study of cortical bone mass. *Journal of the American Medical Association, 265,* 1133–1138.

Robb, A.S., Silber, T.J., Orrell-Valente, J.K., Valadez-Meltzer, A., Ellis, N., Dadson, M.J. & Chatoor, I. (2002). Supplemental nocturnal nasogastric refeeding for better short-term outcome in hospitalised adolescent girls with anorexia nervosa. *American Journal of Psychiatry, 159,* 1347–1353.

Robin, A.L., Siegel, P.T., Koepke, T., Moye, A.W. & Tice, S. (1994). Family therapy versus individual therapy for adolescent females with anorexia nervosa. *Journal of Developmental and Behavioural Pediatrics, 15,* 111–116.

Robin, A.L., Siegel, P.T., Moye, A.W., Gilroy, M., Dennis, A.B. & Sikand, A. (1999). A controlled comparison of family versus individual therapy for adolescents with anorexia nervosa. *American Academy of Child and Adolescent Psychiatry, 38,* 1482–1489.

Robinson, P. (2003). Day treatments. In J. Treaure, U. Schmidt & E. van Furth (Eds.), *Handbook of eating disorders* (2nd ed.). John Wiley & Sons.

Robinson, P.H. (2000). Review article: Recognition and treatment of eating disorders in primary and secondary care. *Alimentary Pharmacology & Therapeutics, 14*(4), 367–377.

Romano, S.J., Halmi, K.A., Sarkar, N.P., Koke, S.C. & Lee, J.S. (2002). A placebo-controlled study of fluoxetine in continued treatment of bulimia nervosa after successful acute fluoxetine treatment. *American Journal of Psychiatry, 159,* 96–102.

Rome, ES. (1996). Eating disorders in adolescents and young adults: What's a primary care clinician to do? *Clevland Clinic Journal of Medicine, 63*(7), 387–395.

Rosenvinge, J.H. & Klusmeier, A.K. (2000). Treatment for eating disorders from a patient satisfaction perspective: A Norwegian replication of a British study. *European Eating Disorders Review, 8,* 293–300.

Rosenvinge, J.H., Martinussen, M. & Ostensen, E. (2000). The comorbidity of eating disorders and personality disorders: A meta-analytic review of studies published between 1983 and 1998. *Eating Weight Disorders, 5*(2), 52–61.

Rosenvinge, J.H., Perry, J.A., Bjørgum, L., Bergersen, T.D., Silvera, D.H. & Holte, A. (2001). A new instrument measuring disturbed eating patterns in community populations: Development and initial validation of a 5-item scale (EDS-5). *European Eating Disorder Review, 9,* 123–132.

Ruggiero, G.M., Laini, V., Mauri, M.C., Ferrari, V.M., Clemente, A., Lugo, F., Mantero, M., Redaelli, G., Zappulli, D. & Cavagnini, F. (2001). A single-blind comparison of amisulpride, fluoxetine and clomipramine in the treatment of restricting anorectics. *Progress in Neuro-Psychopharmacology & Biological Psychiatry, 25,* 1049–1059.

Russell, G.F. (1985). Pre-menarchal anorexia nervosa and its sequelae. *Journal of Psychiatric Research, 19,* 363–369.

Russell, G.F., Szmukler, G.I., Dare, C. & Eisler, I. (1987). An evaluation of family therapy in anorexia nervosa and bulimia nervosa. *Archives of General Psychiatry, 44,* 1047–1056.

Russell, G.F., Treasure, J. & Eisler, I. (1998). Mothers with anorexia nervosa who underfeed their children: Their recognition and management. *Psychological Medicine, 28,* 93–108.

Russell, J. & Gross, G. (2000). Anorexia nervosa and body mass index. *American Journal of Psychiatry, 157*(12), 2060.

Russell, G.F. (2001). Involuntary treatment in anorexia nervosa. *Psychiatr Clin North Am, 24*(2), 337–349.

Sabine, E.J., Yonace, A., Farrington, A.J., Barrnat, K.H. & Wakeling, A. (1983). Bulimia nervosa: A placebo-controlled double-blind therapeutic trial of mianserin. *British Journal of Clinical Pharmacology, 15,* 1955–2025.

Saccomani, L., Savoini, M., Cirrincione, M., Vercellino, F. & Ravera, G. (1998). Long-term outcome of children and adolescents with anorexia nervosa: Study of comorbidity. *Journal of Psychosomatic Research, 44*(5), 565–571.

Safer, D.L., Telch, C.F. & Agras, W.S. (2001). Dialectical behaviour therapy for bulimia nervosa. *American Journal of Psychiatry, 158,* 632–634.

Santonastaso, P., Favaretto, G. & Canton, G. (1987). Anorexia nervosa in Italy: Clinical features and outcome in a long-term follow-up study. Psychopathology, 20(1), 8–17.

Santonastaso, P., Pantano, M., Panarotto, L. & Silvestri, A. (1991). A follow-up study on anorexia nervosa: Clinical features and diagnostic outcome. *European Psychiatry, 6,* 177–185.

Schork, E.J., Eckert, E.D. & Halmi, K.A. (1994). The relationship between psychopathology, eating disorder diagnosis and clinical outcome at 10-year follow-up in anorexia nervosa. *Comprehensive Psychiatry, 35*(2), 113–123.

Seeman, E., Szmukler, G.I., Formica, C., Tsalamandris, C. & Mestrovic, R. (1992). Osteoporosis in anorexia nervosa: The influence of peak bone density, bone loss, oral contraceptive use and exercise. *Journal of Bone Mineral Research, 7,* 1467–1474.

Serfaty, M.A., Turkington, D., Heap, M., Ledsham, L. & Jolley, E. (1999). Cognitive therapy versus dietary counselling in the outpatient treatment of anorexia nervosa: Effects of the treatment phase. *European Eating Disorders Review, 7,* 334–350.

Silber, T.J., D'Angelo & Lawrence, J. (1991). The role of the primary care physician in the diagnosis and management of anorexia nervosa. *Psychosomatics, 32*(2), 221–225.

Solanto, M.V., Jacobson, M.S., Hellers, L., Golden, N.H. & Hertz, S. (1994). Rate of weight gain of inpatients with anorexia nervosa under behavioural contracts. *Pediatrics, 93,* 989–991.

Soyka, L.A., Grinspoon, S., Levitsky, L.L., Herzog, D.B. & Klibanski, A. (1999). The effects of anorexia nervosa on bone metabolism in female adolescents. *Journal of Clinical Endocrinology and Metabolism, 84,* 4489–4496.

Sriegel-Moore, R., Silberstein, L.R. & Rodin, J. (1986). Toward an understanding of risk factors for bulimia. *American Psychologist, 41,* 246–263.

Stefanis, N., Mackintosh, C., Abraha, H.D., Treasure, J. & Moniz, C. (1998). Dissociation of bone turnover in anorexia nervosa. *Annals of Clinical Biochemistry, 35,* 709–716.

Steiner, H., Smith, C., Rosenkranz, R.T. & Litt, I. (1991). The early care and feeding of anorexics. *Child Psychiatry and Human Development, 21,* 163–167.

Steinhausen, H.C. (2002). The outcome of anorexia nervosa in the 20th century. *American Journal of Psychiatry, 159,* 1284–1293.

Steinhausen, H.C. & Glanville, K. (1983). A long-term follow-up of adolescent anorexia nervosa. *Acta Psychiatrica Scandinavica, 68(*1), 1–10.

Steinhausen, H.C. & Seidel, R. (1993). Outcome in adolescent eating disorders. *International Journal of Eating Disorders, 14*(4), 487–496.

Stice, E. (2002). Risk and maintenance factors for eating pathology: A meta-analytic review. *Psychological Bulletin, 128,* 825–848.

Stice, E. & Agras, W.S. (1998). Predicting onset and cessation of bulimic behaviors during adolescence: A longitudinal grouping analysis. *Behaviour Therapy, 29,* 257–276.

Stonehill, E. & Crisp, A.H. (1977). Psychoneurotic characteristics of patients with anorexia nervosa before and after treatment and at follow-up four to seven years later. *Journal of Psychosomatic Research, 21*(3), 189–193.

Striegel-Moore, R.H., Leslie, D., Petrill, S.A., Garvin, V. & Rosenheck, R.A. (2000). One-year use and cost of inpatient and outpatient services among female and male patients with an eating disorder: Evidence from a national database of health insurance claims. *International Journal of Eating Disorders, 23,* 161–167.

Striegel-Moore, R.H., Silberstein, L.R. & Rodin, J. (1986). Toward an understanding of risk factors for bulimia. *Am Psychol, 41*(3), 246–263.

Strober, M., Freeman, R. & Morrel, W. (1997). The long-term course of severe anorexia nervosa in adolescents: Survival analysis of recovery, relapse and outcome predictors over 10–15 years in a prospective study. *International Journal of Eating Disorders, 22,* 339.

Strober, M., Freeman, R. & Morrell, W. (1999). Atypical anorexia nervosa: Separation from typical cases in course and outcome in a long-term prospective study. *International Journal of Eating Disorders, 25*(2), 135–142.

Strober, M., Freeman, R. & Morrell, W. (1997). The long-term course of severe anorexia nervosa in adolescents: Survival analysis of recovery, relapse and outcome predictors over 10–15 years in a prospective study. *International Journal of Eating Disorders, 22*(4), 339–360.

Strober, M. (1984). Stressful life events associated with bulimia in anorexia nervosa: Empirical findings and theoretical speculations. *International Journal of Eating Disorders, 3,* 3–16.

Sullivan, P.F. (1995). Mortality in anorexia nervosa. *American Journal of Psychiatry, 152,* 1073–1074.

Sundgot-Borgen, J., Rosenvinge, J.H., Bahr, R. & Schneider, L.S. (2002). The effect of exercise, cognitive therapy and nutritional counseling in treating bulimia nervosa. *Medicine & Science in Sports & Exercise, 34,* 190–195.

Swayze, V.W., Andersen, A., Arndt, S., Rajarethinam, R., Fleming, F., Sato, Y. & Andreasen ,N.C. (1996). Reversibility of brain tissue loss in anorexia nervosa assessed with a computerised Talairach 3-D proportional grid. *Psychological Medicine, 26,* 381–390.

Tanaka, H., Kiriike, N., Nagata, T. & Riku, K. (2001). Outcome of severe anorexia nervosa patients receiving inpatient treatment in Japan: An eight-year follow-up study. *Psychiatry and Clinical Neurosciences, 55*(4), 389–396.

Tchanturia, K., Morris, R., Surguladze, S. & Treasure, J. (2003). Perceptual and cognitive set shifting tasks in acute anorexia nervosa and following recovery. *Eat. Weight. Disord* (in press).

Tchanturia, K., Serpell, L., Troop, N. & Treasure, J. (2001). Perceptual illusions in eating disorders: Rigid and fluctuating styles. *J Behav Ther Exp Psychiatry, 32,* 107–115.

Telch, C.F., Agras, W.S. & Linehan, M.M. (2001). Dialectical behaviour therapy for binge eating disorder. *Journal of Consulting & Clinical Psychology, 69,* 1061–1065.

Telch, C.R., Agras, W.S., Wilfley, D.E. & Kenardy, J. (1980). Group cognitive behavioural treatment for the non-purging bulimic: An initial evaluation. *Journal of Consulting & Clinical Psychology, 58,* 629–635.

Theander, S. (1970). Anorexia nervosa. A psychiatric investigation of 94 female patients. *Acta Psychiatrica Scandinavica Suppl., 214,* 1–194.

Thien, V., Thomas, A., Markin, D. & Birmingham, C.L. (2000). Pilot study of a graded exercise programme for the treatment of anorexia nervosa. *International Journal of Eating Disorders, 28,* 101–106.

Toner, B.B., Garfinkel, P.E. & Garner, D.M. (1986). Long-term follow-up of anorexia nervosa. *Psychosomatic Medicine, 48*(7), 520–529

Tozzi, F., Sullivan, P., Fear, J., McKenzie, J. & Bulik, C.M. (2003). Causes and recovery in anorexia nervosa: The patient's perspective. *International Journal of Eating Disorders, 33,* 143–154.

Treasure, J., Gavan, K., Todd, G. & Schmidt, U. (2003). Changing the environment in eating disorders: Working with carers/families to improve motivation and facilitate change. *European Eating Disorders Review, 11,* 25–37.

Treasure, J., Murphy, T., Szmukler, G., Todd, G., Gavan, K. & Joyce, J. (2001). The experience of caregiving for severe mental illness: A comparison between anorexia nervosa and psychosis. *Social Psychiatry and Psychiatric Epidemiology, 36,* 343–347.

Treasure, J.L., Russell, G.F., Fogelman, I. & Murby, B. (1987). Reversible bone loss in anorexia nervosa. *British Medical Journal (Clin.Res.Ed), 295,* 474–475.

Treasure, J.L. & Russell, G.F. (1988). Intrauterine growth and neonatal weight gain in babies of women with anorexia nervosa. *British Medical Journal (Clin.Res.Ed), 296,* 1038.

Treasure ,J.L. (1998). *Anorexia nervosa and bulimia* (1st ed.) (pp.858–902). Edited by Royal College Psychiatrists. London: Gaskell.

Treasure, J.L. & Schmidt, U. (2002). Anorexia nervosa. *Clin Evid, 8,* 903–913.

Treasure, J.L. & Schmidt, U. (2001). Needs assessment and eating disorders. In G. Thornicroft, C. R. Brewin & J. Wing (Eds.), *Measuring mental health needs* (2nd ed.). London: Gaskell (in press).

Treasure, J.L. & Ward, A. (1997). Cognitive analytical therapy (CAT) in eating disorders. *Clinical Psychology and Psychotherapy, 4,* 62–71.

Treasure, J.L, Katzman, M., Schmidt, U., Troop, N., Todd, G. & de Silva, P. (1999). Engagement and outcome in the treatment of bulimia nervosa: First phase of a sequential design comparing motivation enhancement therapy and cognitive behavioural therapy. *Behaviour Research and Therapy, 37,* 405–418.

Treasure, J.L., Schmidt, U., Troop, N., Tiller, J., Todd, G. & Turnbull, S. (1996). Sequential treatment for bulimia nervosa incorporating a self-care manual. *British Journal of Psychiatry, 168,* 84–98.

Treasure, J.L., Schmidt, U., Troop, N., Tiller, J., Todd, G., Keilen, M. & Dodge, E. (1994). First step in managing bulimia nervosa: Controlled trial of a therapeutic manual. *British Medical Journal, 308,* 686–689.

Treasure, J.L., Todd, G., Brolly, M., Tiller, J., Nehmed, A. & Denman, F. (1995). A pilot study of a randomised trial of cognitive analytical therapy vs educational behavioural therapy for adult anorexia nervosa. *Behavioural Research and Therapy, 33,* 363–367.

Troop, N., Schmidt, U., Tiller, J., Todd, G., Keilen, M. & Treasure, J.L. (1996). Compliance with a self-care manual for bulimia nervosa: Predictors and outcome. *British Journal of Clinical Psychology, 35,* 435–438.

Turnbull, S.J., Schmidt, U., Troop, N., Tiller, J., Todd, G. & Treasure, J.L. (1997). Predictors of outcome for two treatments for bulimia nervosa. *International Journal of Eating Disorders, 21,* 17–22.

Turnbull, S., Ward, A., Treasure, J.L., Jick, H. & Derby, L. (1996). The demand for eating disorder care. *British Journal of Psychiatry, 169,* 705–712.

Turnbull, W., Treasure, J.L. & Derby, L. (1996). The demand for eating disorders care. Epidemiological study using the General Practice Research Database. *British Journal of Psychiatry, 169,* 705–712.

Turner, H. & Bryant-Waugh, R. (2003). Eating disorder not otherwise specified (EDNOS) profiles of clients presenting at a community eating disorder service. *European Eating Disorders Review* (in press).

Valla, A., Groenning, I.L., Syversen, U. & Hoeiseth, A. (2000). Anorexia nervosa: Slow regain of bone mass. *Osteoporosis International, 11,* 141–145.

Vandereycken, W. & Pierloot, R. (1982). Pimozide combined with behaviour therapy in the short-term treatment of anorexia nervosa. A double-blind placebo-controlled cross-over study. *Acta Psychiatrica Scandinavica, 66,* 445–450.

Vandereycken, W. (1984). Neuroleptics in the short-term treatment of anorexia nervosa. A double-blind placebo-controlled study with sulpiride. *British Journal of Psychiatry, 144,* 288–292.

Vestergaard, P., Emborg, C., Stoving, R.K., Hagen, C., Mosekilde, L. & Brixen, K. (2002). Fractures in patients with anorexia nervosa, bulimia nervosa and other eating disorders – a nationwide register study. *International Journal Eating Disorders, 32,* 301–308.

Vogelantz-Holm, N., Wonderlich, S.A, Lewis, B. *et al.* (2000). Longitudinal predictors of binge eating, intense dieting and weight concerns in a national sample of women. *Behaviour Therapy, 31,* 221–235.

Vos, T. *et al.* (2001). The burden of mental disorders in Victoria. *Social Psychiatry Psychiatric Epidemiology, 36,* 53–62.

Wallin, U., Kronovall, P. & Majewski M.L. (2000). Body awareness therapy in teenage anorexia nervosa: Outcome after two years. *European Eating Disorders Review, 8,* 19–30.

Walsh, J.M., Wheat, M.E. & Freund, K. (2000). Detection, evaluation and treatment of eating disorders: The role of the primary care physician. *Journal of General Internal Medicine, 15*(8), 577–590.

Walsh, B.T. (1986). Medication in the treatment of bulimia. *Adolescent Psychiatry, 13,* 437–445.

Walsh, B.T., Fairburn, C.G., Mickley, D., Sysko, R., & Parides, M.K. (2003). Treatment of bulimia nervosa in a primary care setting. Submitted for publication.

Walsh, B.T., Gladis, M., Roose, S.P., Stewart, J.W. & Glassman, A.H. (1987). A controlled trial of phenelzine in bulimia. *Psychopharmacology Bulletin, 23,* 49–51.

Walsh, B.T., Gladis, M., Roose, S.P., Stewart, J.W. & Glassman, A.H. (1988). Phenelzine vs placebo in 50 patients with bulimia. *Archives of General Psychiatry, 45,* 471–475.

Walsh, B.T., Hadigan, C.M., Devlin, M.J., Gladis, M. & Roose, S.P. (1991). Long-term outcome of antidepressant treatment for bulimia nervosa. *Journal of Psychiatry, 148,* 1206–1212.

Walsh, B.T., Stewart, J.W., Roose, S.P., Gladis, M. & Glassman, A.H. (1984). Treatment of bulimia with phenelzine. A double-blind, placebo-controlled study. *Archives of General Psychiatry, 41,* 1105–1109.

Walsh, B.T., Stewart, J.W., Roose, S.P., Gladis, M. & Glassman, A.H. (1985). A double-blind trial of phenelzine in bulimia. *Journal of Psychiatric Research, 19,* 485–489.

Walsh, B.T., Wilson, G.T., Loeb, K.L., Devlin, M.J., Pike, K.M., Roose, S.P., Fleiss, J. & Waternaux, C. (1997). Medication and psychotherapy in the treatment of bulimia nervosa. *American Journal of Psychiatry, 154,* 523–531.

Walsh, B.T., Stewart, J.W., Wright, L., Harrison, W., Roose, S.P. & Glassman, A.H. (1982). Treatment of bulimia with monoamine oxidase inhibitors. *American Journal of Psychiatry, 139*(12), 1629–1630.

Ward, A., Brown, N. & Treasure, J.L. (1997). Persistent osteopenia after recovery from anorexia nervosa. *International Journal of Eating Disorders, 22,* 71–75.

Weizman, A., Tyano, S., Wijsenbeek, H. & Ben David, M. (1985). Behaviour therapy, pimozide treatment and prolactin secretion in anorexia nervosa. *Psychotherapy & Psychosomatics, 43,* 136–140.

Wezel-Meijler, G. & Wit, J.M. (1989). The offspring of mothers with anorexia nervosa: A high-risk group for undernutrition and stunting? *European Journal of Peadiatrics, 149,* 130–135.

Wilfley, D.E., Agras, W.S., Telch, C.F., Rossiter, E.M., Schneider, J.A., Cole, A.G., Sifford, L.A. & Raeburn, S.D. (1993). Group cognitive behavioural and group interpersonal psychotherapy for thenonpurging bulimic individual: A controlled comparison. *Journal of Consulting & Clinical Psychology, 61,* 296–305.

Wilfley, D., Welch, S.S., Stein, R.I., Spurrell, E.B., Cohen, L.R., Saelens, B.E., Dounchis, J.Z., Frank, M.A., Wiseman, C.V & Matt, G.E. (2002). A randomised comparison of group cognitive behavioural therapy and group interpersonal psychotherapy for the treatment of overweight individuals with binge-eating disorder. *Archives of General Psychiatry, 25,* 713–721.

Wilhelm, K. & Clarke, D. (1998). Eating disorders from a primary care perspective. *Medical Journal of Australia, 168,* 458–463.

Whitehouse, A.M., Cooper, P.J., Vize, C.V., Hill, C. & Vogel, L. (1992). Prevalence of eating disorders in three Cambridge general practices: Hidden and conspicuous morbidity. *British Journal of General Practice, 42*(355), 57–60.

Willi, J. & Hagemann, R. (1976). Long-term course of anorexia nervosa. *Schweiz Med Wochenschr, 106*(43), 1459–1465.

Williams, P., Hand, D. & Tarnopolsky, A. (1982). The problem of screening for uncommon disorders – a comment on the Eating Attitudes Test. *Psychol Med, 12*(2), 431–434.

Williamson, D.A., Thaw, J.M. & Varnado-Sullivan, P.J. (2001). Cost-effectiveness analysis of a hospital-based cognitive-behavioural treatment programme for eating disorders. *Behaviour Therapy, 32,* 459–477.

Wilson, G.T., Eldredge, K.L., Smith, D. & Niles, B. (1991). Cognitive behavioural treatment with and without response prevention for bulimia. *Behaviour Research and Therapy, 29,* 575–583.

Wilson, G.T., Fairburn, C.C., Agras, W.S., Walsh, B.T. & Kraemer, H. (2002). Cognitive-behavioural therapy for bulimia nervosa: Time course and mechanisms of change. *Journal of Consulting & Clinical Psychology, 70,* 267–274.

Wilson, G.T., Loeb, K.L., Walsh, B.T., Labouvie, E., Petkova, E., Liu, X. & Waternaux, C. (1999). Psychological versus pharmacological treatments of bulimia nervosa: Predictors and processes of change. *Journal of Consulting & Clinical Psychology, 67,* 451–459.

Wilson *et al.* (1986). Treatment of bulimia nervosa: When CBT fails. *Behav Res Ther.*

Wolf, E.M. & Crowther, J.H. (1992). An evaluation of behavioural and cognitive-behavioural group interventions for the treatment of bulimia nervosa in women. *International Journal of Eating Disorders, 11,* 3–15.

Wolk, S.L. & Devlin, M.J. (2001). Stage of change as a predictor of response to psychotherapy for bulimia nervosa. *International Journal of Eating Disorders, 30,* 96–100.

Zipfel, S., Löwe, B., Reas, D.L. *et al.* (2000). Long-term prognosis in anorexia nervosa: Lessons from a 21-year follow-up study. *The Lancet, 355,* 712–722.

Zipfel, S., Seibel, M.J., Lowe, B., Beumont, P.J., Kasperk, C. & Herzog, W. (2001). Osteoporosis in eating disorders: A follow-up study of patients with anorexia and bulimia. *Journal of Clinical Endocrinology and Metabolism, 86,* 5227–5233.

13 Abbreviations

A&E	Accident and emergency
AGREE	Appraisal of Guidelines Research and Evaluation
APA	American Psychiatric Association
BED	Binge eating disorder
BMI	Body mass index
BPS	British Psychological Society
CAMHS	Child and adolescent mental health services
CAT	Cognitive analytic therapy
CBT	Cognitive behaviour therapy
CEBMH	Centre for Evidence Based Mental Health
CEFAHP	Clinical Effectiveness Forum for the Allied Health Professions
CEMH	Centre for Economics in Mental Health
CHAI	Commission for Health Care, Audit and Improvement
CI	Confidence interval
CMR	Crude mortality rate
CORE	British Psychological Society Centre for Outcomes Research and Effectiveness
COT	College of Occupational Therapists
CRU	Royal College of Psychiatrists College Research Unit
DHEA	Dehyroepiandosterone
DSM-IV	Diagnostic and Statistical Manual of Mental Disorders, Fourth edition
EAT	Eating attitudes test
EDE	Eating disorders examination
EDI	Eating disorders inventory
EDNOS	Eating disorders not otherwise specified
EDSIG	Eating disorders special interest group
EEG	Electroencephalography
ERP	Exposure with response prevention
GDG	Guideline development group
GSH	Guided self-help
ICD10	International Classification of Diseases, 10th Edition
IoP	Institute of Psychiatry
IPT	Interpersonal Psychotherapy
MANOVA	Multivariate analysis of variance
MAOI	Monoamine-oxidase inhibitors

N	Number of studies
n	Number of participants
NCCMH	National Collaborating Centre for Mental Health
NG	Nasogastric
NICAPS	National Inpatient Child and Adolescent Psychiatry Study
NHS	National Health Service
NICE	National Institute for Clinical Excellence
NNT	Number needed to treat
OCD	Obsessive-compulsive disorder
OR	Odds ratio
PEG	Percutaneous endoscopic gastrostomy
PSH	Pure self-help
RCGP	Royal College of General Practitioners
RCN	Royal College of Nursing
RCT	Randomised controlled trials
RCPsych	Royal College of Psychiatrists
RPS	Royal Pharmaceutical Society
RR	Relative risk, risk ratio
SCIE	Social Care Institute of Excellence
SMR	Standardised Mortality Rate
SSRI	Selective serotonin reuptake inhibitors
TPN	Total parenteral nutrition
WHO	World Health Organisation

14 Glossary

Adherence: The behaviour of taking medicine according to treatment dosage and schedule as intended by the prescriber. In this guideline, the term 'adherence' is used in preference to 'compliance', but is not synonymous with 'concordance', which has a number of meanings.

Affective disorder: A syndrome in which an individual experiences a significant alteration in affect or mood. Whether depressed or elated, this change of mood is accompanied by alteration in the individual's activity levels.

Anorexia nervosa: A syndrome in which the individual maintains a low weight as a result of a preoccupation with body weight, construed either as a fear of fatness or pursuit of thinness. Weight is maintained at least 15 per cent below that expected or body mass index (calculated as weight in kilograms divided by height in metres squared) is below 17.5. Weight loss is self-induced by exercise, vomiting or purgation, and avoidance of fattening foods. A widespread endocrine disorder involving the hypothalamo-pituitary-gonadal axis is present. In females this is manifest as amenorrhoea and in males by loss of sexual interest and impotence. Other psychosocial features such as mood disorder, obsessive-compulsive symptoms and social withdrawal are common.

Atypical eating disorder: This term is used to denote eating disorders of clinical severity that do not meet the diagnostic criteria for anorexia nervosa or bulimia nervosa. The equivalent American term is 'eating disorder not otherwise specified'.

Behavioural weight control (BWC): Behavioural treatments that have weight loss as their goal.

Behaviour therapy (BT): Behavioural treatments that include many features of cognitive behaviour therapy for bulimia nervosa (CBT-BN) but have little or no emphasis on the direct modification of ways of thinking.

Binge eating disorder (BED): A syndrome in which an individual experiences repeated uncontrolled episodes of overeating but does not use extreme compensatory weight-control behaviours. It is a provisional new eating disorder diagnosis in DSM-IV.

Bulimia nervosa: A syndrome characterised by recurrent episodes of binge eating and by compensatory behaviour (vomiting, purging, fasting or exercising) in order to prevent weight gain. Binge eating is accompanied by a subjective feeling of loss of control over eating. This is a normal weight syndrome in which the body mass index (BMI) is maintained above 17.5 kg/m^2.

Cognitive analytic therapy (CAT): A specific time-limited, problem-focused psychotherapy developed by Ryle (Ryle & Kerr, 2002). It integrates cognitive, behavioural and psychodynamic principles.

Cognitive behaviour therapy (CBT): A psychological intervention that is designed to enable people to establish links between their thoughts, feelings or actions and their current or past symptoms and to re-evaluate their perceptions, beliefs or reasoning about the target symptoms. The intervention should involve at least one of the following: (1) monitoring thoughts, feelings or behaviour with respect to the symptom; (2) being helped to use alternative ways of coping with the target symptom; (3) reducing stress.

Cognitive behaviour therapy for binge eating disorder (CBT-BED): A specific form of CBT derived from CBT-BN, and adapted to suit patients with BED.

Cognitive behaviour therapy for bulimia nervosa (CBT-BN): A specific form of CBT devised for patients with bulimia nervosa. It typically involves 16 to 20 hour-long one-to-one treatment sessions over four to five months. Its focus is not only on helping patients change their eating habits but also on addressing the ways of thinking (most especially the over-evaluation of shape and weight) that maintain them. It has been described in several treatment manuals, the one used in most of the more recent treatment trials being that by Fairburn and colleagues (Fairburn *et al.*, 1993).

Cognitive behaviour therapy plus exposure with response prevention (CBT+ERP): A treatment that combines elements of CBT-BN with repeated sessions of exposure to situations that would normally trigger either binge eating or purging.

Confidence interval: The range within which the 'true' values (e.g. size of effect of an intervention) are expected to lie with a given degree of certainty (e.g. 95 per cent or 99 per cent). Confidence intervals represent the probability of random errors, but not systematic errors – or bias.

Controlled trial: An experiment in which investigators allocate eligible people into groups to receive or not to receive one or more interventions that are being compared.

Costing study: This is the simplest economic study, measuring only the costs of given interventions. It does not provide answers to efficiency questions.

Cost-benefit analysis: A type of full economic evaluation that compares alternatives in which the costs and consequences vary. Both costs and benefits are measured in monetary units. If benefits exceed costs, the evaluation would be a basis for recommending the treatment. It can address the question of whether a treatment or policy is socially worthwhile in the broadest sense.

Cost-consequence analysis: An analysis in which both outcomes and costs of alternative treatments or policy options are described. However, multiple outcomes are measured and there is no attempt to reduce everything to a single ratio.

Cost-effectiveness analysis: A type of full economic evaluation that compares competing alternatives of which the costs and consequences vary. The outcomes are measured in the same non-monetary (natural) unit. It expresses the result in the form of an incremental (or average or marginal) cost-effectiveness ratio.

Cost-minimisation analysis: A type of full economic evaluation where the costs of equally effective alternative treatments are compared. The aim is to find the least costly alternative.

Cost-of-illness/economic burden studies: An economic analysis of the total costs incurred by a society due to a specific disease.

Costs (direct): The costs of all the goods, services and other resources that are consumed in the provision of a health intervention. They can be medical or non-medical.

Costs (indirect): The lost productivity suffered by the national economy as a result of an employee's absence from the workplace through illness, decreased efficiency or premature death.

Cost-utility analysis: A type of full economic evaluation that compares competing alternatives of which the costs and consequences vary. It measures and values the impact of a treatment or policy alternative in utility units (see QALY). The result is expressed in the form of a cost-utility ratio.

Decision analysis: An explicit, quantitative, systematic approach to decision making under conditions of uncertainty, in which the probability of each possible event, along with the consequences of those events, is explicitly stated.

Dialectical behaviour therapy (DBT): A multifaceted and intensive psychological treatment designed for patients with borderline personality disorder (Linehan, 1993a, 1993b). A simplified and abbreviated form of the treatment has been developed for patients with bulimia nervosa or binge eating disorder (Telch *et al.*, 2000, 2001). It primarily focuses on enhancing patients' emotion regulation skills. It involves 20 two-hour group sessions once a week. Details are provided by Wiser and Telch (1999).

Dietary counselling: Also termed 'nutritional counselling'. A form of treatment in which the primary goal is the modification of what the patient eats as well as relevant eating habits and attitudes. It is not a well-defined intervention and is practised in a variety of ways. It is usually implemented by dietitians.

Drop out: A term no longer used to indicate leaving a study before its completion (the term 'leaving the study early' is now preferred).

Economic evaluation: Technique developed to assess both costs and consequences of alternative health strategies and to provide a decision making framework.

Eating disorder focused family therapy: A specific form of family therapy that focuses on directly addressing the eating disorder in addition to addressing family and individual issues. The best-tested version (sometimes called the 'Maudsley method') has been manualised by Lock *et al.* (2001).

Eating disorders not otherwise specified (EDNOS): Eating disorders that closely resemble anorexia nervosa and bulimia nervosa, but are considered atypical as they do not meet the precise diagnostic criteria for these conditions.

Effectiveness: The extent to which a specific intervention, when used under ordinary circumstances, does what it is intended to do. Clinical trials that assess effectiveness are sometimes called management trials.

Efficacy: The extent to which an intervention produces a beneficial result under ideal conditions. Clinical trials that assess efficacy are sometimes called explanatory trials and are restricted to participants who fully co-operate. The randomised controlled trial is the accepted 'gold standard' for evaluating the efficacy of an intervention.

Exposure with response prevention (ERP): This form of treatment was originally based on an 'anxiety reduction' model of bulimia nervosa according to which self-induced vomiting negatively reinforces binge eating by removing fears of secondary weight gain (Rosen & Leitenberg, 1982). The model on which it is based has evolved over the years (Carter & Bulik, 1994) and various versions of the treatment have been tested (e.g. Rosen & Leitenberg, 1982; Jansen *et al.*, 1989; Schmidt & Marks, 1989). Each involves repeated exposure to cues that precede binge eating or purging with the response (binge eating or purging) being prevented. The treatment is typically combined with elements of cognitive behaviour therapy. Treatment sessions that involve in vivo exposure may last up to three hours. ERP has been describes as 'time-intensive, expensive and logistically complicated' (Bulik *et al.*, 1998, p.620).

Family interventions: Family sessions with a treatment function based on systemic, cognitive behavioural or psychoanalytic principles, which may include psychoeducational, problem-solving and crisis management work and specific interventions with the identified patient. With eating disorders, the focus is on the eating disorder and how this impacts family relationships, emphasising in the early stages of treatment the necessity for parents to take a central role in supporting their child's efforts to eat.

Family therapy: See Family interventions.

Feeding against the will of the patient: Using any method of feeding that requires that the individual be restrained to allow the feeding to take place.

Focal supportive psychotherapy: A collective term used in this Guideline for the various types of supportive psychological treatment that have been evaluated in the treatment of patients with eating disorders. These are varied in nature but they have in common their focus on supporting patients in their attempts to address difficulties in their life. Some have included limited emphasis on changing eating habits. These treatments should not be confused with more general forms of supportive psychotherapy or with counselling.

Forest plot: A graphical display of results from individual studies on a common scale, allowing visual comparison of trial results and examination of the degree of heterogeneity between studies.

Guided self-help (GSH): A self-help programme for bulimia nervosa in which a clinical professional provides support and encouragement.

Guideline recommendation: A systematically developed statement that is derived from the best available research evidence, using predetermined and systematic methods to identify and evaluate evidence relating to the specific condition in question.

Insulin purging: The omission or intentional under-dosing with insulin, sometimes done by patients with bulimia nervosa and diabetes.

Interpersonal psychotherapy (IPT): A specific form of focal psychotherapy that is designed to help patients identify and address current interpersonal problems. It was originally developed for the treatment of depression (Klerman *et al.*, 1984) but has been adapted for the treatment of bulimia nervosa (IPT-BN; Fairburn, 1997).

Interpersonal psychotherapy for binge eating disorder (IPT-BED): A specific form of IPT derived from IPT-BN and adapted to suit patients with BED.

Interpersonal psychotherapy for bulimia nervosa (IPT-BN): A specific form of IPT adapted for the treatment of bulimia nervosa (IPT-BN; Fairburn, 1997). In IPT–BN there is no emphasis on directly modifying eating habits; rather, it is expected that they will change as interpersonal functioning improves. IPT-BN involves the same number and pattern of treatment sessions as CBT-BN.

Meta-analysis: The use of statistical techniques in a systematic review to integrate the results of the included studies. Also used to refer to systematic reviews that use meta-analysis.

Number of people leaving the study early: For the purposes of the guideline, the number of people leaving the study early due to any reason is taken as a proxy for treatment acceptability, whereas the number of people leaving the study early due to adverse events is taken as a proxy for treatment tolerability. An exception to this is when the comparison group is a wait-list control, in which case this assumption is not made.

Number needed to harm: The number of people (calculated statistically) who need to be treated to cause one bad outcome. The lower the number needed to harm, the higher the likelihood of harm.

Number needed to treat: The number of people who need to be treated to prevent one bad outcome (i.e. a good outcome). It is the inverse of the risk difference.

Nutritional counselling: See Dietary counselling.

Odds ratio: A measure of the relative benefit of the experimental treatment that can be obtained by dividing the experimental odds by the control odds.

Patient: The terms 'patient' or 'person with eating disorder, anorexia nervosa, bulimia nervosa or binge eating disorder, etc.', are used in this guideline to identify the person presently or formerly with the condition and/or receiving services in the present or past.

Psychodynamic psychotherapy: Regular individual therapy sessions with a trained psychotherapist, or a therapist under supervision, based on a psychodynamic or psychoanalytic model, which use a variety of strategies, including exploratory insight-oriented, supportive or directive activity, applied flexibly, working with transference, but with the therapists using a less strict technique than that used in psychoanalysis.

Psychological treatment not otherwise specified: A residual category that is used for psychological treatments other than those individually specified.

Pure self-help (PSH): A self-help programme for bulimia nervosa which patients follow on their own without the support of a professional.

Quality-adjusted life years (QALY): A form of utility measure, calculated by estimating the total life-years gained from a treatment and weighting each year with a quality-of-life score in that year.

Randomisation: A method used to generate a random allocation sequence, such as using tables of random numbers or computer-generated random sequences. The method of randomisation should be distinguished from concealment of allocation, because if the latter is inadequate selection bias may occur despite the use of randomisation. For instance, a list of random numbers may be used to randomise participants, but if the list were open to the individuals responsible for recruiting and allocating participants, those individuals could influence the allocation process, either knowingly or unknowingly.

Randomised controlled trial (RCT): Also termed 'randomised clinical trial'. An RCT is an experiment in which investigators randomly allocate eligible people into groups to receive or not to receive one or more interventions that are being compared. The results are assessed by comparing outcomes in the different groups. Through randomisation, the groups should be similar in all aspects apart from the treatment they receive during the study.

Refeeding: Increasing nutritional intake and restoring weight to within a normal range in the treatment of anorexia nervosa

Relative risk: Also known as risk ratio; the ratio of risk in the intervention group to the risk in the control group. The risk (proportion, probability or rate) is the ratio of people with an event in a group to the total in the group. A relative risk (RR) of 1 indicates no difference between comparison groups. For undesirable outcomes, an RR that is less than 1 indicates that the intervention was effective in reducing the risk of that outcome.

Relaxation therapy: A psychological treatment that focuses on enhancing patients' ability to relax physically and psychologically.

Selective serotonin reuptake inhibitors (SSRIs): Medicines that inhibit the reuptake of serotonin into the presynaptic neurone thus increasing neurotransmission. Although they 'selectively' inhibit serotonin reuptake, they are not serotonin specific. Some of the drugs in this class also inhibit the reuptake of noradrenaline and/or dopamine. As a class, these drugs are associated with less anticholinergic side effects and are less likely to cause postural hypotension or sedation.

Self-help: This involves following a self-help programme for bulimia nervosa, either with support and encouragement from a clinical professional (guided self-help) or on one's own (pure self-help). The self-help programmes studied to date have taken the form of self-help books (Cooper, 1995; Fairburn, 1995; Schmidt & Treasure, 1995).

Sensitivity analysis: Sensitivity analysis is a technique used in economic analysis or decision making to allow for uncertainty by testing whether plausible changes in the values of the main variables affect the results of the analysis.

Simplified dialectical behaviour therapy (simplified DBT): A simplified and abbreviated version of DBT.

Social skills training: A psychological treatment that focuses on enhancing patients' social skills.

Standard dosage: The recommended dosage range listed in the *British National Formulary*; this normally reflects the information contained in the manufacturers' Summary of Product Characteristics as well as advice from an external panel of experts.

Stepped-care model: A sequence of treatment options to offer simpler and less expensive interventions first and more complex and expensive interventions if the patient has not benefited, based on locally agreed protocols.

Supportive therapy: A non-specific form of supportive psychotherapy.

Weighted mean difference: A method of meta-analysis used to combine measures on continuous scales (such as weight), where the mean, standard deviation and sample size in each group are known. The weight given to each study (e.g. how much influence each study has on the overall results of the meta-analysis) is determined by the precision of its estimate of effect and, in the statistical software used by the NCCMH, is equal to the inverse of the variance. This method assumes that all of the trials have measured the outcome on the same scale.